Dualistic Equilibrium in Neurotransmission and Beyond: Unraveling the Pathophysiology and Unlocking Novel Therapeutic Targets in Neuropsychiatric Disorders

Dualistic Equilibrium in Neurotransmission and Beyond: Unraveling the Pathophysiology and Unlocking Novel Therapeutic Targets in Neuropsychiatric Disorders

Guest Editors

Masaru Tanaka
Simone Battaglia

MDPI

Basel • Beijing • Wuhan • Barcelona • Belgrade • Novi Sad • Cluj • Manchester

Guest Editors
Masaru Tanaka
HUN-REN-SZTE
Neuroscience Research Group
University of Szeged
(HUN-REN-SZTE)
Szeged
Hungary

Simone Battaglia
Department of Psychology
University of Bologna
Bologna
Italy

Editorial Office
MDPI AG
Grosspeteranlage 5
4052 Basel, Switzerland

This is a reprint of the Special Issue, published open access by the journal *Biomedicines* (ISSN 2227-9059), freely accessible at: https://www.mdpi.com/journal/biomedicines/special_issues/Neurotransmission.

For citation purposes, cite each article independently as indicated on the article page online and as indicated below:

Lastname, A.A.; Lastname, B.B. Article Title. *Journal Name* **Year**, *Volume Number*, Page Range.

ISBN 978-3-7258-4851-5 (Hbk)
ISBN 978-3-7258-4852-2 (PDF)
https://doi.org/10.3390/books978-3-7258-4852-2

Contents

About the Editors

Masaru Tanaka

Masaru Tanaka, M.D., Ph.D., is Senior Research Fellow at the Danube Neuroscience Research Laboratory, HUN-REN-SZTE Neuroscience Research Group, Hungarian Research Network, University of Szeged. His work bridges bench and bedside approaches to decode how affective, cognitive, and nociceptive circuits lose balance across depression, dementia, chronic pain, and their frequent comorbidity. Having authored more than 140 peer-reviewed papers, he sits in the D1 percentile of global publication impact; several of his articles rank within the top 99.9 citation percentile in the fields of neuroscience and psychiatry. His scholarship has earned the Best Paper, Hot Paper, and Most Cited Paper Awards, alongside recognition as Best Reviewer of the Month. Dr. Tanaka serves on the editorial boards of several journals, including *Biomedicines*, where he champions rigorous, translationally minded science that paves the way for precision neuropsychiatric interventions. He obtained a PhD in Medicine and an MD in general Medicine from the University of Szeged and a Bachelors' degree in Biophysics from the university of Illinois, Urbana-Champaign.

Simone Battaglia

Simone Battaglia, Ph.D., is an Assistant Professor in Cognitive Neuroscience at the Centre for Studies and Research in Cognitive Neuroscience, Department of Psychology, University of Bologna; Research Fellow at the Department of Psychology, University of Turin; and Clinician at the Cognitive Neuropsychology Center of Niguarda Hospital in Milan. His research experience focuses on investigating the functional interplay of different brain areas involved in emotional learning, action control and spatial representation, brain plasticity, decision-making, and a variety of cognitive tasks. To this end, his research activities primarily revolve around the utilization of non-invasive brain stimulation techniques such as transcranial magnetic stimulation (TMS) and transcranial direct current stimulation (tDCS), in addition to employing various neuroscientific techniques to record physiological measures, including EEG, SCR, HRV, and EMG. In his activities, he employs a multimodal approach that integrates behavioral assessments, electrophysiological measurements, and neurostimulation techniques. The aim of his research is to develop innovative therapeutic protocols, with a particular focus on utilizing the cortico–cortical paired associative stimulation (ccPAS) method to facilitate neuroplasticity and enhance functional recovery in the brain.

Preface

As Guest Editors of the Special Issue "Dualistic Equilibrium in Neurotransmission and Beyond: Unraveling the Pathophysiology and Unlocking Novel Therapeutic Targets in Neuropsychiatric Disorders", we set out to capture a simple yet profound idea; health in the brain—and by extension the body—relies on a finely balanced dialog between opposing biochemical forces. When that dialog falters, mood, cognition, and behavior unravel. Our purpose was to assemble evidence that travels the full arc from molecular binding sites to patient-level biomarkers and interventions, and to spotlight research paths that can restore equilibrium where it is lost.

The resulting Reprint gathers eight peer-reviewed articles that examine monoaminergic allostery, trace-amine and cannabinoid–serotonin crosstalk, orexin-guided stress adaptation, microRNA-driven neuroinflammation, and isoform-specific tau diagnostics, each illustrating how multiscale approaches can reshape prevention, diagnosis, and therapy. Our intended readership spans basic neuroscientists, clinical psychiatrists, pharmacologists, computational modelers, and policy makers seeking mechanistic clarity and translational traction.

We are indebted to the contributing authors for their rigorous scholarship, to the expert reviewers whose incisive feedback raised every manuscript's standard, and to the *Biomedicines* Editorial Office for seamless coordination throughout the call, peer review, and production phases.

May this Reprint serve as both a distilled reference and a launching pad for future consortia that aim to convert insights on dualistic neurotransmission into precision interventions for depression, dementia, chronic pain, and allied disorders. We invite readers to explore the chapters that follow and to join the collaborative effort toward a truly convergent neuropsychiatry.

Masaru Tanaka and Simone Battaglia
Guest Editors

biomedicines

MDPI

Editorial

Dualistic Dynamics in Neuropsychiatry: From Monoaminergic Modulators to Multiscale Biomarker Maps

Masaru Tanaka [1,*] and Simone Battaglia [2,3]

[1] Danube Neuroscience Research Laboratory, HUN-REN-SZTE Neuroscience Research Group, Hungarian Research Network, University of Szeged (HUN-REN-SZTE), Tisza Lajos krt. 113, H-6725 Szeged, Hungary
[2] Center for Studies and Research in Cognitive Neuroscience, Department of Psychology "Renzo Canestrari", Cesena Campus, Alma Mater Studiorum, University of Bologna, 47521 Bologna, Italy; simone.battaglia@unibo.it
[3] Department of Psychology, University of Turin, 10124 Turin, Italy
* Correspondence: tanaka.masaru.1@med.u-szeged.hu; Tel.: +36-62-342-847

1. Introduction: The Dualistic Lens

Neuropsychiatry lives at the crossroads of chemistry and cognition, where millisecond synaptic sparks sculpt decades-long stories of mood, memory, and identity [1–3]. The same organ then turns inward, making brain–body self-inquiry a central paradox now probed by advanced imaging, stimulation, and physiological modeling [4–6]. Modern data depict neurotransmission as a yin–yang choreography: glutamatergic bursts checked by gamma-aminobutyric acid (GABA) brakes and cortical volleys echoed by visceral afferents carrying gut, liver, and immune cues, while nanoscopic receptor tweaks reverberate through whole networks [7–9]. Mapping the harmonics of this loop may decode consciousness and its breakdown across neuropsychiatric and neurodegenerative disease, since equilibrium failure begets illness [10–12].

Within this framework, psychiatric and neurodegenerative disorders appear less like single-node breakdowns and more like systemic disequilibria [13–15]. When the delicate balance collapses, as in post-traumatic stress disorder (PTSD), dysregulated fear circuitry and hypothalamic–pituitary–adrenal (HPA) axis perturbations create neuroendocrine noise—cortisol volatility, monoaminergic surges, failed fear extinction, and intrusive memory loops [16–18]. Similarly, in Alzheimer's disease (AD) or Parkinson's disease, oxidative stress derails networks, yet antioxidant-rich diets and compounds modestly stabilize memory and action control in longitudinal human cohorts [17,19,20]. Complementing those longitudinal data, reviews show that phytocompounds—including polyphenols, alkaloids, and terpenoids—improve cognition and neuropsychiatric symptoms across AD and related disorders [21–23]. An expanding Topical Collection, "Neurodegeneration No More," now assembles cutting-edge diagnostics, therapeutic targets, and integrative care models aimed at reversing disease trajectories, underscoring the urgency of interdisciplinary collaboration for neurodegenerative disease management [24]. Reinforcing this perspective, an increasing amount of evidence maps how medicinal plants inhibit nuclear factor kappa-light-chain-enhancer of activated B cells (NF-κB), cyclooxygenase-2 (COX-2), and inducible nitric oxide synthase (iNOS) while activating nuclear factor erythroid 2-related factor 2 (Nrf2) signaling, detailing dose windows and translational gaps across progressive neurodegenerative disease [25–27]. Nonetheless, three enduring translational gaps impede the conversion of conceptual advances into clinical benefit. The first is the bench-to-bedside divide: antioxidant interventions that show efficacy in rodent models or in silico screens rarely advance to well-powered clinical trials that rigorously account for sex, age, lifestyle

 https://doi.org/10.3390/biomedicines13061456

factors, and comorbidities [27–29]. Second, a network-integration blind spot: investigations isolate single receptors, overlooking the multiplex cortisol–monoamine–immune crosstalk that governs resilience across organs and lifespan [30–32]. Third, the composite-biomarker vacuum: p-tau isoforms, circulating microRNAs, cortisol rhythms, or receptor-binding positron emission tomography (PET) signals remain unharmonized, limiting our ability to stratify patients, forecast trajectories, and personalize interventions [33–37].

This Special Issue, "Dualistic Equilibrium in Neurotransmission and Beyond," is curated to illuminate that landscape, bridge its chasms, and chart future routes "https://www.mdpi.com/journal/biomedicines/special_issues/Neurotransmission (accessed on 12 June 2025)". By uniting eight studies that journey from resveratrol-induced monoamine oxidase A (MAO-A) allostery and trace amine receptor agonism to orexin-orchestrated stress adaptation and isoform-specific tau diagnostics, the collection strives to translate basic insights, weave an empirically grounded system map, and lay scaffolds for next-generation composite biomarker panels. Together, these contributions aim to ignite interdisciplinary alliances spanning medicinal chemistry, network neuroscience, computational modeling, clinical psychiatry, policy makers, caregivers, and public health leaders worldwide, driving progress in basic science, clinical translation, and population health and steering lasting therapeutic innovation for patients across the globe.

2. Eight Windows on Equilibrium

Molecular docking, dynamics, and predator-stressed rats reveal resveratrol and its glucuronide occupy an allosteric pocket on MAO-A, dampening brain and liver enzyme activity and pointing dietary polyphenols toward anxiolytic monoaminergic therapy [38]. Shemiakova et al. synthesize evidence positioning trace amine-associated receptors (TAARs) as novel antidepressant targets [39] (Table 1). TAAR1–TAAR9 extend beyond smell, populating limbic circuits. The TAAR1 agonist ulotaront succeeds in phase 2/3 depression trials. Preclinical data show that TAAR2/TAAR5 shape emotion, monoamine signaling, and hippocampal neurogenesis, suggesting TAAR-targeted drugs could outpace monoamine therapies and cut side-effects in hard-to-treat depression populations.

Table 1. Thematic clustering of the eight contributions in the Special Issue "Dualistic Equilibrium in Neurotransmission and Beyond." The table groups each paper under a shared mechanistic theme, lists its concise title, and links to the corresponding reference segment. This layout spotlights how the collection spans monoaminergic modulation, serotonergic/peripheral stress circuits, symptom-level and molecular modulators in psychiatric disorders, and biomarker discovery for neurodegeneration.

Group/Topic	Shared Idea	Paper	Ref.
Monoaminergic Targets for Mood Regulation	MAO-A or TAARs rebalance monoamines	Resveratrol as MAO-A allosteric modulator	[38]
		TAARs as novel antidepressant targets	[39]
Serotonergic and Peripheral Stress Systems	5-HT, CB1, orexin in stress and organs	Perinatal 5-HT enhancers alter gut–liver axis	[40]
		CB1–5-HT1A in stress-induced analgesia	[41]
		Orexin system in stress vigilance	[42]
Symptom Dynamics in Brain Disorders	Clinical/microRNA modulators of symptoms	OCD symptoms worsen depression in schizophrenia	[43]
		miR-200b-3p antagonism reduces ADHD traits	[44]
Molecular Biomarkers for Neurodegeneration	Next-gen fluid markers for early AD diagnosis	Plasma p-tau217/231 differentiation of AD	[45]

AD, Alzheimer's disease; ADHD, attention-deficit/hyperactivity disorder; CB1, cannabinoid receptor type 1; 5-HT, 5-hydroxytryptamine; 5-HT1A, 5-hydroxytryptamine receptor type 1A; miR-200b-3p, microRNA 200b family subtype the 3′ strand; MAO-A, monoamine oxidase A; OCD, obsessive–compulsive disorder; p-tau217/231, phosphorylated tau protein at threonine 217 and threonine 231; TAARs, trace amine-associated receptors.

Perinatal exposure of rats to 5-hydroxytryptophan (5-HTP) or tranylcypromine induces adult-onset histomorphometric and metabolic alterations in the jejunum and liver, spotlighting how early hyperserotonemia imprints a persistent gut–liver serotonergic loop beyond the brain [40]. Pharmacological pairing of CB1 and 5-HT1A agonists or antagonists before versus after cold stress in rats showed serotonergic signaling maintains stress-induced analgesia pre-stress while cannabinoid modulation predominates post-stress, exposing time-specific crosstalk vital for designing anti-stress pain interventions [41]. A narrative review synthesizes evidence that orexin/hypocretin neurons act as master neuromodulators coupling vigilance with autonomic, endocrine, and behavioral stress responses; highlights their roles in fear, anxiety, and learning; and surveys emerging orexin-based pharmacotherapies for sleep and stress disorders [42].

In 111 outpatients with schizophrenia, higher disorganized and obsessive–compulsive symptom scores independently predicted greater depressive severity, whereas a longer duration of untreated psychosis paradoxically correlated with milder depression, indicating that early circuit disorganization, rather than demographic factors, is the primary driver of comorbid depressive burden [43]. Striatal injection of a miR-200b-3p antagomir in spontaneously hypertensive rats alleviated inattention, reduced pro-inflammatory cytokines, and elevated antioxidant enzymes, spotlighting miR-200b-3p as a promising therapeutic microRNA target for attention-deficit/hyperactivity disorder (ADHD) [44].

A narrative review of 85 original studies concludes that plasma and cerebrospinal fluid (CSF) p-tau217 and p-tau231 outperform p-tau181 in detecting preclinical Aβ pathology, track tau-tangle progression, and differentiate AD from other dementias, positioning these isoform-specific assays as front-line, minimally invasive biomarkers for early diagnosis and staging [45].

3. Bridging the Gaps: How These Papers Move the Needle

Bridging conceptual insights to clinical utility requires proof that discoveries travel the full distance from molecules to networks to patients. The following three subsections illustrate this trajectory, showing how preclinical candidates acquire translational momentum, how receptor-centric views expand into circuit logic, and how layered biomarkers converge into actionable precision panels.

3.1. *Translational Momentum of Rodent Leads*

Three rodent-based investigations within the Special Issue push molecular leads toward the clinic. In chronically predator-stressed rats, resveratrol and its glucuronide occupied a newly charted monoamine-oxidase-A allosteric pocket, halved cortical and hepatic enzyme activity, and attenuated anxiety-like behavior, suggesting that a safe nutritional polyphenol could be repurposed for affective disorders [38]. Complementing this single-compound result, a recent narrative review shows that phytochemicals—from curcumin to flavonoids and alkaloids—concurrently quell neuroinflammation, oxidative stress, and mitochondrial dysfunction, easing major-depression phenotypes in preclinical and clinical studies [46]. Systemic delivery of the selective trace amine receptor-1 agonist RO5263397 reversed immobility in forced-swim and tail-suspension tests, normalized hippocampal neurogenesis, and reduced peripheral corticosterone, mechanistic outcomes echoed by the clinical-stage compound ulotaront now in phase 2/3 trials for depression and anxiety [39]. Meanwhile, CRISPR/Cas9 knockout of kynurenine-aminotransferase genes in mice suppressed cerebellar and hippocampal oxidative phosphorylation, highlighting kynurenine aminotransferase-dependent kynurenic control of mitochondrial respiration and energy metabolism in vivo [47,48]. Extending that axis, a quinoline-focused narrative review shows how halogenation, esterification, and in silico screening refine tryptophan-derived metabolites into multi-target ligands that cross the blood–brain barrier and quell excitotoxic-immune cascades, steering rational design for next-generation quinoline-based mitochondrial therapeutics [49]. Finally, stereotaxic inhibition of striatal miR-200b-3p in spontaneously hypertensive rats restored attentional performance, suppressed interleukin (IL)-6 and tumor necrosis factor (TNF)-alpha (α), and boosted superoxide-dismutase activity, delineating a microRNA–inflammation axis ripe for biomarker-guided antisense therapies that are advancing into first-in-human safety assessments [44]. Collectively, these convergent results validate target engagement, demonstrate behavioral rescue across independent models, and furnish biochemical read-outs that align seamlessly with ongoing or planned human studies, thereby shortening the bench-to-bedside journey.

3.2. From Receptor Islands to Circuit Continents—System-Level Integration

Perinatal elevation of systemic serotonin through 5-HTP or tranylcypromine resculpted adult gut–liver physiology: villus shortening, crypt hyperplasia, suppressed enterochromaffin 5-HT staining, and altered hepatic 5-HT-metabolizing enzymes, establishing a persistent peripheral serotonin circuit poised to influence brain mood circuits via the portal vein and vagus [40]. In an acute cold-stress model, bidirectional pharmacology revealed time-stamped reciprocity between CB1 and 5-HT1A signaling: co-agonism before stress magnified analgesia, whereas the identical cocktail after stress dampened it; selective antagonist pairings confirmed serotonergic dominance in stress initiation and cannabinoid control during recovery, underscoring a dynamic receptor handshake across limbic, periaqueductal-gray, and HPA nodes [41]. Complementing these rodent data, a comprehensive review positions orexin neurons as master switches that broadcast stress salience through widespread projections, coordinating vigilance, autonomic, and endocrine outputs while modulating monoamines, endocannabinoids, and neuropeptides, thereby offering a top-down scaffold for multi-target drug design [42]. Collectively, these findings shift the narrative from single-receptor pharmacology to network neuroscience, illuminating organ-to-brain loops and temporal hierarchies that future therapeutics must respect. A recent synthesis highlights that age-related vascular dysfunction, sarcopenic muscle loss, and neurodegenerative cognitive decline constitute a pathophysiological triad unified by oxidative stress and chronic inflammation [50].

3.3. Toward Composite Precision Panels

The Special Issue showcases how disparate biomarker layers can converge into patient-stratifying toolkits. A narrative synthesis of 85 studies reports that plasma and CSF p-tau217 and p-tau231 consistently outclass p-tau181, flagging pre-amyloid pathology with >90% accuracy, tracking Braak staging, and cleanly separating AD from frontotemporal and vascular dementias [45]. In a rodent model of ADHD, stereotaxic silencing of striatal miR-200b-3p rescued working-memory deficits, lowered IL-6 and TNF-α, and restored superoxide-dismutase activity, positioning this microRNA as both a mechanistic node and a peripheral read-out for neuro-immune dysregulation in ADHD [44]. Complementing these fluid signatures, a clinical cohort of 111 individuals with schizophrenia showed that disorganized and obsessive–compulsive symptom clusters, rather than demographic variables, predicted depressive load, while a longer untreated psychosis interval paradoxically attenuated it, nominating symptom network topology as a low-cost behavioral biomarker [43]. Together, isoform-specific tau assays, actionable microRNAs, and data-driven symptom lattices foreshadow multiplex panels capable of early detection, mechanistic staging, and personalized therapeutic steering across neuropsychiatric spectra.

4. Future Frontiers

Translating the mechanistic advances documented in this Special Issue into clinically transformative applications demands an integrated research agenda. We therefore outline five strategic imperatives—ranging from multi-omics imaging convergence to ethical governance—that together promise to consolidate molecular discoveries, refine patient stratification across the lifespan, and guide the deployment of network-targeted interventions.

4.1. Multi-Omics Coupling with In Vivo Imaging

Next-generation discovery hinges on stitching lipidomic, metabolomic and receptor-specific PET readouts within individuals [51–53]. Chemo-connectome scans link arachidonic acid flux or phospholipid turnover to network fragility [54–57]. To deepen interpretability, pipelines should also track brain-autonomic synchrony, capturing covariation between cortical activity and cardiac deceleration, charting loops that tie emotions to autonomic outflow [4,52,55]. Delivering this vision will require hybrid scanners, biofluid taps, and cloud analytics that fuse terabytes of omics spectra with voxel-wise binding maps in time [58–60].

4.2. Longitudinal, Sex-Balanced Cohorts

Most existing datasets are cross-sectional snapshots or male-skewed rodent lines [61–63]. We need cradle-to-senescence cohorts, stratified by chromosomal and hormonal sex, that collect neuroimaging, multi-omics, immune read-outs, and detailed life-event chronologies at repeated milestones [64–66]. Tracking the same individuals from perinatal stages through puberty, reproductive transitions, and neurodegenerative risk windows will reveal when gut–liver–brain loops or monoaminergic balances hit irreversible tipping points—and whether those inflections differ by sex, ancestry, or socio-environmental load [67–71].

4.3. Digital Phenotyping and Artificial Intelligence (AI) Biomarker Fusion

Wearables, smartphones, and ambient sensors convert gait micro-variability, sleep architecture, voice prosody, and social-touch signatures into continuous phenomic streams, illustrating the field's pivot from serendipitous drug discovery toward precision mental health research [72–76]. Parallel conceptual work urges replacing categorical Diagnostic and Statistical Manual of Mental Disorders (DSM)/International Classification of Diseases (ICD) diagnoses with dimensional Hierarchical Taxonomy of Psychopathology (HiTOP) and Research Domain Criteria (RDoC) taxonomies, integrating these phenomic streams into empirically anchored, biologically informed nosology [77–81]. Coupled with federated artificial intelligence (AI) that simultaneously ingests PET-omics, microRNA panels, and symptom lattices, these data lakes could generate personalized risk curves updated hourly [82–86]. Key priorities include open ontologies for feature harmonization, self-supervised algorithms that learn across modalities with minimal labels, and privacy-preserving architectures that keep raw data on-device while sharing encrypted embeddings for population-level modeling [87,88].

4.4. Network-Level Interventions

Insights from circuit-centric papers invite therapies that modulate entire networks rather than single receptors [89–91]. Closed-loop deep-brain or vagus nerve stimulators, guided by real-time neurochemical sensors, could nudge maladaptive oscillations back into equilibrium [89–91]. On the peripheral front, liver-targeted MAO-A inhibitors or gut-restricted 5-HT modulators may recalibrate central affect without crossing the blood–brain barrier, reducing systemic side-effects [68,92,93]. Combinatorial designs—such as pairing orexin antagonists with anti-inflammatory microRNA mimics—should be tested in adaptive platform trials that can rapidly prune ineffective arms [94–97].

4.5. *Ethical and Regulatory Horizon-Scanning*

As datasets sprawl and interventions become closed-loop, guardrails must keep pace [98–100]. Regulators will need new guidelines for multi-omics companion diagnostics, AI-driven adaptive trials, and implantable devices that learn on the fly [101–103]. Equitable access requires subsidized genomic and imaging pipelines in low-resource settings and bias audits for machine learning models [100–102]. Finally, consent frameworks should allow participants granular control over which data layers—lipids, speech, location—enter shared repositories, ensuring progress does not outstrip public trust [98,99,103].

5. Conclusions: Toward a Convergent Neuropsychiatry

The studies collected in this Special Issue validate "dualistic equilibrium" as a unifying framework for neuropsychiatric science, showing that health depends on balanced interactions between excitation and inhibition, central and peripheral signaling, and molecular events and network dynamics. Each contribution shifts the discourse from isolated observations to a layered map that connects monoaminergic allostery, trace amine receptor pharmacology, orexin-regulated stress circuitry, microRNA-driven inflammation, and isoform-specific tau pathology. The resulting atlas is mechanistically precise, since it identifies actionable binding pockets, temporal receptor handshakes, and fluid biomarkers; translationally actionable, because several rodent leads already align with phase 2 or phase 3 trials; and ethically responsible, thanks to an explicit focus on sex-balanced cohorts, privacy-aware digital phenotyping, and equitable access to advanced diagnostics.

The next milestone is collective execution. Specialist silos must give way to consortia that integrate medicinal chemistry, imaging physics, multi-omics analytics, computational psychiatry, regulatory science, and patient advocacy. Shared protocols for hybrid PET–omics pipelines, harmonized outcome measures for adaptive trials, and interoperable data standards for wearable-derived phenomics will accelerate discovery while preventing duplication. Funding bodies should prioritize platforms that enroll cradle-to-senescence participants in diverse settings, ensuring that findings generalize across sex, ancestry, and socio-economic strata. Regulatory agencies can support this trajectory by creating pathways for composite biomarker approval and real-time neuromodulation devices.

Anchored in dualistic equilibrium, guided by a systems lens, and propelled by an ethic of inclusivity, the field is now positioned to transform fragmented mechanistic snapshots into integrated, patient-centered care paradigms. Progress will hinge not on isolated breakthroughs but on coordinated, transparent collaboration that keeps scientific ambition and societal responsibility in steady alignment.

Author Contributions: Conceptualization, M.T. and S.B.; methodology, M.T.; software, M.T.; validation, M.T. and S.B.; formal analysis, M.T. and S.B.; investigation, M.T. and S.B.; resources, M.T.; data curation, M.T.; writing—original draft preparation, M.T.; writing—review and editing, M.T. and S.B.; visualization, M.T.; supervision, M.T.; project administration, M.T. and S.B.; funding acquisition, M.T. All authors have read and agreed to the published version of the manuscript.

Funding: This work was supported by HUN-REN Hungarian Research Network funding to M.T. S.B. is supported by #NEXTGENERATIONEU (NGEU) and funded by the Ministry of University and Research (MUR), National Recovery and Resilience Plan (NRRP), project MNESYS (PE0000006)—a multiscale integrated approach to the study of the nervous system in health and disease (DN. 1553 11.10.2022)—and Bial Foundation, Portugal (235/22). The views and opinions expressed are solely those of the authors and do not necessarily reflect those of the European Union, nor can the European Union be held responsible for them.

Conflicts of Interest: The authors declare no conflicts of interest.

Abbreviations

The following abbreviations are used in this manuscript:

AD	Alzheimer's disease
ADHD	attention-deficit/hyperactivity disorder
AI	artificial intelligence
CB1	cannabinoid receptor type 1
CSF	cerebrospinal fluid
HPA	hypothalamic–pituitary–adrenal
5-HT	5-hydroxytryptamine
5-HT1A	5-hydroxytryptamine receptor type 1A
5-HTP	5-hydroxytryptophan
IL	interleukin
MAO-A	monoamine oxidase A
miR-200b-3p	microRNA 200b family subtype the 3′ strand
OCD	obsessive–compulsive disorder
PET	positron emission tomography
p-tau217/231	phosphorylated tau protein at threonine 217 and threonine 231
TAARs	trace amine-associated receptors
TNF	tumor necrosis factor

References

1. Rabl, M.; Clark, C.; Dayon, L.; Popp, J. Neuropsychiatric symptoms in cognitive decline and Alzheimer's disease: Biomarker discovery using plasma proteomics. *J. Neurol. Neurosurg. Psychiatry* **2025**, *96*, 370–382. [CrossRef] [PubMed]
2. Pontone, G.M.; Mills, K.A.; Smith, G.S. Molecular imaging in neuropsychiatry. *Int. Rev. Psychiatry* **2017**, *29*, 527–529. [CrossRef] [PubMed]
3. Milham, M.P.; Craddock, R.C.; Klein, A. Clinically useful brain imaging for neuropsychiatry: How can we get there? *Depress. Anxiety* **2017**, *34*, 578–587. [CrossRef] [PubMed]
4. Battaglia, S.; Servajean, P.; Friston, K.J. The paradox of the self-studying brain. *Phys. Life Rev.* **2025**, *52*, 197–204. [CrossRef]
5. Dary, Z.; Lenggenhager, B.; Lagarde, S.; Medina Villalon, S.; Bartolomei, F.; Lopez, C. Neural bases of the bodily self as revealed by electrical brain stimulation: A systematic review. *Hum. Brain Mapp.* **2023**, *44*, 2936–2959. [CrossRef]
6. Bradley, C.; Nydam, A.S.; Dux, P.E.; Mattingley, J.B. State-dependent effects of neural stimulation on brain function and cognition. *Nat. Rev. Neurosci.* **2022**, *23*, 459–475. [CrossRef]
7. Zuurbier, K.R.; Fonseca, R.S.; Arneaud, S.L.; Wall, J.M.; Kim, J.; Tatge, L.; Otuzoglu, G.; Bali, S.; Metang, P.; Douglas, P.M. Yin Yang 1 and guanine quadruplexes protect dopaminergic neurons from cellular stress via transmissive dormancy. *Nat. Commun.* **2024**, *15*, 10592. [CrossRef]
8. Gupta, R.; Advani, D.; Yadav, D.; Ambasta, R.K.; Kumar, P. Dissecting the Relationship Between Neuropsychiatric and Neurodegenerative Disorders. *Mol. Neurobiol.* **2023**, *60*, 6476–6529. [CrossRef]
9. Novellino, F.; Saccà, V.; Donato, A.; Zaffino, P.; Spadea, M.F.; Vismara, M.; Arcidiacono, B.; Malara, N.; Presta, I.; Donato, G. Innate Immunity: A Common Denominator between Neurodegenerative and Neuropsychiatric Diseases. *Int. J. Mol. Sci.* **2020**, *21*, 1115. [CrossRef]
10. Luppi, A.I.; Vohryzek, J.; Kringelbach, M.L.; Mediano, P.A.; Craig, M.M.; Adapa, R.; Carhart-Harris, R.L.; Roseman, L.; Pappas, I.; Peattie, A.R. Distributed harmonic patterns of structure-function dependence orchestrate human consciousness. *Commun. Biol.* **2023**, *6*, 117. [CrossRef]
11. Wamsley, B.; Geschwind, D.H. Functional genomics links genetic origins to pathophysiology in neurodegenerative and neuropsychiatric disease. *Curr. Opin. Genet. Dev.* **2020**, *65*, 117–125. [CrossRef] [PubMed]
12. Cummings, J. The Role of Neuropsychiatric Symptoms in Research Diagnostic Criteria for Neurodegenerative Diseases. *Am. J. Geriatr. Psychiatry* **2021**, *29*, 375–383. [CrossRef]
13. Finlay, S.; Rudd, D.; McDermott, B.; Sarnyai, Z. Allostatic load and systemic comorbidities in psychiatric disorders. *Psychoneuroendocrinology* **2022**, *140*, 105726. [CrossRef]
14. Du, X.; Pang, T.Y. Is Dysregulation of the HPA-Axis a Core Pathophysiology Mediating Co-Morbid Depression in Neurodegenerative Diseases? *Front. Psychiatry* **2015**, *6*, 32. [CrossRef]

15. Michopoulos, V.; Vester, A.; Neigh, G. Posttraumatic stress disorder: A metabolic disorder in disguise? *Exp. Neurol.* **2016**, *284*, 220–229. [CrossRef]
16. Battaglia, S.; Di Fazio, C.; Borgomaneri, S.; Avenanti, A. Cortisol imbalance and fear learning in PTSD: Therapeutic approaches to control abnormal fear responses. *Curr. Neuropharmacol.* **2025**, *23*, 835–846. [CrossRef]
17. Battaglia, S.; Nazzi, C.; Thayer, J.F. Genetic differences associated with dopamine and serotonin release mediate fear-induced bradycardia in the human brain. *Transl. Psychiatry* **2024**, *14*, 24. [CrossRef]
18. Algamal, M.; Pearson, A.J.; Hahn-Townsend, C.; Burca, I.; Mullan, M.; Crawford, F.; Ojo, J.O. Repeated unpredictable stress and social isolation induce chronic HPA axis dysfunction and persistent abnormal fear memory. *Prog. Neuropsychopharmacol. Biol. Psychiatry* **2021**, *104*, 110035. [CrossRef]
19. Battaglia, S.; Nazzi, C.; Di Fazio, C.; Borgomaneri, S. The role of pre-supplementary motor cortex in action control with emotional stimuli: A repetitive transcranial magnetic stimulation study. *Ann. N. Y. Acad. Sci.* **2024**, *1536*, 151–166. [CrossRef]
20. Veurink, G.; Perry, G.; Singh, S.K. Role of antioxidants and a nutrient rich diet in Alzheimer's disease. *Open Biol.* **2020**, *10*, 200084. [CrossRef]
21. de Lima, E.P.; Laurindo, L.F.; Catharin, V.C.S.; Direito, R.; Tanaka, M.; Jasmin Santos German, I.; Lamas, C.B.; Guiguer, E.L.; Araújo, A.C.; Fiorini, A.M.R. Polyphenols, Alkaloids, and Terpenoids Against Neurodegeneration: Evaluating the Neuroprotective Effects of Phytocompounds Through a Comprehensive Review of the Current Evidence. *Metabolites* **2025**, *15*, 124. [CrossRef] [PubMed]
22. Can, B.; Sanlier, N. Alzheimer, Parkinson, dementia, and phytochemicals: Insight review. *Crit. Rev. Food Sci. Nutr.* **2025**, *65*, 1706–1728. [CrossRef] [PubMed]
23. Solfrizzi, V.; Agosti, P.; Lozupone, M.; Custodero, C.; Schilardi, A.; Valiani, V.; Santamato, A.; Sardone, R.; Dibello, V.; Di Lena, L.; et al. Nutritional interventions and cognitive-related outcomes in patients with late-life cognitive disorders: A systematic review. *Neurosci. Biobehav. Rev.* **2018**, *95*, 480–498. [CrossRef] [PubMed]
24. Tanaka, M.; Battaglia, S.; Liloia, D. Navigating Neurodegeneration: Integrating Biomarkers, Neuroinflammation, and Imaging in Parkinson's, Alzheimer's, and Motor Neuron Disorders. *Biomedicines* **2025**, *13*, 1045. [CrossRef]
25. Barbalho, S.M.; Leme Boaro, B.; da Silva Camarinha Oliveira, J.; Patočka, J.; Barbalho Lamas, C.; Tanaka, M.; Laurindo, L.F. Molecular Mechanisms Underlying Neuroinflammation Intervention with Medicinal Plants: A Critical and Narrative Review of the Current Literature. *Pharmaceuticals* **2025**, *18*, 133. [CrossRef]
26. Lv, H.; Ren, W.; Zheng, Y.; Wang, L.; Lu, G.; Yi, P.; Ci, X. Tenuigenin exhibits anti-inflammatory activity via inhibiting MAPK and NF-κB and inducing Nrf2/HO-1 signaling in macrophages. *Food Funct.* **2016**, *7*, 355–363. [CrossRef]
27. Puppala, E.R.; Prasad, N.; Prakash, A.N.; Abubakar, M.; Syamprasad, N.P.; Gangasani, J.K.; Naidu, V.G.M. Mesua assamica (King & Prain) kosterm. bark ethanolic extract attenuates rheumatoid arthritis via down-regulating TLR4/NF-κB/COX-2/iNOS and activation of Nrf2/HO-1 pathways: A comprehensive study on in-vitro and in-vivo models. *J. Ethnopharmacol.* **2024**, *335*, 118671. [CrossRef]
28. Hanlon, P.; Butterly, E.W.; Shah, A.S.; Hannigan, L.J.; Lewsey, J.; Mair, F.S.; Kent, D.M.; Guthrie, B.; Wild, S.H.; Welton, N.J. Treatment effect modification due to comorbidity: Individual participant data meta-analyses of 120 randomised controlled trials. *PLoS Med.* **2023**, *20*, e1004176. [CrossRef]
29. Simu, S.Y.; Alam, M.B.; Kim, S.Y. The Activation of Nrf2/HO-1 by 8-Epi-7-deoxyloganic Acid Attenuates Inflammatory Symptoms through the Suppression of the MAPK/NF-κB Signaling Cascade in In Vitro and In Vivo Models. *Antioxidants* **2022**, *11*, 1765. [CrossRef]
30. Walker, F.R.; Pfingst, K.; Carnevali, L.; Sgoifo, A.; Nalivaiko, E. In the search for integrative biomarker of resilience to psychological stress. *Neurosci. Biobehav. Rev.* **2017**, *74*, 310–320. [CrossRef]
31. de Kloet, E.R.; Joëls, M. The cortisol switch between vulnerability and resilience. *Mol. Psychiatry* **2024**, *29*, 20–34. [CrossRef] [PubMed]
32. Boahen, A.; Hu, D.; Adams, M.J.; Nicholls, P.K.; Greene, W.K.; Ma, B. Bidirectional crosstalk between the peripheral nervous system and lymphoid tissues/organs. *Front. Immunol.* **2023**, *14*, 1254054. [CrossRef] [PubMed]
33. Sethi, S.; Brietzke, E. Omics-based biomarkers: Application of metabolomics in neuropsychiatric disorders. *Int. J. Neuropsychopharmacol.* **2016**, *19*, pyv096. [CrossRef]
34. Wesseling, H.; Mair, W.; Kumar, M.; Schlaffner, C.N.; Tang, S.; Beerepoot, P.; Fatou, B.; Guise, A.J.; Cheng, L.; Takeda, S.; et al. Tau PTM Profiles Identify Patient Heterogeneity and Stages of Alzheimer's Disease. *Cell* **2020**, *183*, 1699–1713.e1613. [CrossRef]
35. van den Berg, M.M.J.; Krauskopf, J.; Ramaekers, J.G.; Kleinjans, J.C.S.; Prickaerts, J.; Briedé, J.J. Circulating microRNAs as potential biomarkers for psychiatric and neurodegenerative disorders. *Prog. Neurobiol.* **2020**, *185*, 101732. [CrossRef]
36. Ryan, R.; Booth, S.; Spathis, A.; Mollart, S.; Clow, A. Use of Salivary Diurnal Cortisol as an Outcome Measure in Randomised Controlled Trials: A Systematic Review. *Ann. Behav. Med.* **2016**, *50*, 210–236. [CrossRef]
37. Fu, H.; Rong, J.; Chen, Z.; Zhou, J.; Collier, T.; Liang, S.H. Positron Emission Tomography (PET) Imaging Tracers for Serotonin Receptors. *J. Med. Chem.* **2022**, *65*, 10755–10808. [CrossRef]

38. Novak, J.; Tseilikman, O.B.; Shatilov, V.A.; Zhukov, M.S.; Shevyrin, V.A.; Khismatullina, Z.R.; Fedorova, A.M.; Patrikyan, G.N.; Khaibullin, T.L.; Tseilikman, V.E. Resveratrol and Its Metabolite as Potential Allosteric Regulators of Monoamine Oxidase A Activity in the Brain and Liver Under Chronic Predator Stress. *Biomedicines* **2025**, *13*, 1196. [CrossRef]
39. Shemiakova, T.S.; Efimova, E.V.; Gainetdinov, R.R. TAARs as Novel Therapeutic Targets for the Treatment of Depression: A Narrative Review of the Interconnection with Monoamines and Adult Neurogenesis. *Biomedicines* **2024**, *12*, 1263. [CrossRef]
40. Gračan, R.; Blažević, S.A.; Brižić, M.; Hranilovic, D. Beyond the Brain: Perinatal Exposure of Rats to Serotonin Enhancers Induces Long-Term Changes in the Jejunum and Liver. *Biomedicines* **2024**, *12*, 357. [CrossRef]
41. Nocheva, H.; Stoynev, N.; Vodenicharov, V.; Krastev, D.; Krastev, N.; Mileva, M. Cannabinoid and Serotonergic Systems: Unraveling the Pathogenetic Mechanisms of Stress-Induced Analgesia. *Biomedicines* **2024**, *12*, 235. [CrossRef] [PubMed]
42. Jászberényi, M.; Thurzó, B.; Bagosi, Z.; Vécsei, L.; Tanaka, M. The Orexin/Hypocretin System, the Peptidergic Regulator of Vigilance, Orchestrates Adaptation to Stress. *Biomedicines* **2024**, *12*, 448. [CrossRef]
43. Panov, G.; Dyulgerova, S.; Panova, P.; Stefanova, S. Untangling depression in schizophrenia: The role of disorganized and obsessive-compulsive symptoms and the duration of untreated psychosis. *Biomedicines* **2024**, *12*, 2646. [CrossRef] [PubMed]
44. Chang, T.-M.; Lin, H.-L.; Tzang, C.-C.; Liang, J.-A.; Hsu, T.-C.; Tzang, B.-S. Unraveling the Role of miR-200b-3p in Attention-Deficit/Hyperactivity Disorder (ADHD) and Its Therapeutic Potential in Spontaneously Hypertensive Rats (SHR). *Biomedicines* **2024**, *12*, 144. [CrossRef]
45. Jarek, D.J.; Mizerka, H.; Nuszkiewicz, J.; Szewczyk-Golec, K. Evaluating p-tau217 and p-tau231 as biomarkers for early diagnosis and differentiation of Alzheimer's Disease: A narrative review. *Biomedicines* **2024**, *12*, 786. [CrossRef]
46. Figueiredo Godoy, A.C.; Frota, F.F.; Araújo, L.P.; Valenti, V.E.; Pereira, E.d.S.B.M.; Detregiachi, C.R.P.; Galhardo, C.M.; Caracio, F.C.; Haber, R.S.; Fornari Laurindo, L. Neuroinflammation and Natural Antidepressants: Balancing Fire with Flora. *Biomedicines* **2025**, *13*, 1129. [CrossRef]
47. Juhász, L.; Spisák, K.; Szolnoki, B.Z.; Nászai, A.; Szabó, Á.; Rutai, A.; Tallósy, S.P.; Szabó, A.; Toldi, J.; Tanaka, M. The Power Struggle: Kynurenine Pathway Enzyme Knockouts and Brain Mitochondrial Respiration. *J. Neurochem.* **2025**, *169*, e70075. [CrossRef]
48. Tanaka, M.; Szabó, Á.; Vécsei, L. Redefining roles: A paradigm shift in tryptophan–kynurenine metabolism for innovative clinical applications. *Int. J. Mol. Sci.* **2024**, *25*, 12767. [CrossRef]
49. Tanaka, M.; Szatmári, I.; Vécsei, L. Quinoline Quest: Kynurenic Acid Strategies for Next-Generation Therapeutics via Rational Drug Design. *Pharmaceuticals* **2025**, *18*, 607. [CrossRef]
50. de Lima, E.P.; Tanaka, M.; Lamas, C.B.; Quesada, K.; Detregiachi, C.R.P.; Araújo, A.C.; Guiguer, E.L.; Catharin, V.M.C.S.; de Castro, M.V.M.; Junior, E.B. Vascular impairment, muscle atrophy, and cognitive decline: Critical age-related conditions. *Biomedicines* **2024**, *12*, 2096. [CrossRef]
51. Wang, R.; Li, B.; Lam, S.M.; Shui, G. Integration of lipidomics and metabolomics for in-depth understanding of cellular mechanism and disease progression. *J. Genet. Genom.* **2020**, *47*, 69–83. [CrossRef] [PubMed]
52. Yu, H.; Villanueva, N.; Bittar, T.; Arsenault, E.; Labonté, B.; Huan, T. Parallel metabolomics and lipidomics enables the comprehensive study of mouse brain regional metabolite and lipid patterns. *Anal. Chim. Acta* **2020**, *1136*, 168–177. [CrossRef] [PubMed]
53. Wang, J.; Zeng, Y.; Song, J.; Zhu, M.; Zhu, G.; Cai, H.; Chen, C.; Jin, M.; Song, Y. Perturbation of arachidonic acid and glycerolipid metabolism promoted particulate matter-induced inflammatory responses in human bronchial epithelial cells. *Ecotoxicol. Environ. Saf.* **2023**, *256*, 114839. [CrossRef]
54. Giovacchini, G.; Chang, M.C.; Channing, M.A.; Toczek, M.; Mason, A.; Bokde, A.L.; Connolly, C.; Vuong, B.-K.; Ma, Y.; Der, M.G. Brain incorporation of [11C] arachidonic acid in young healthy humans measured with positron emission tomography. *J. Cereb. Blood Flow. Metab.* **2002**, *22*, 1453–1462. [CrossRef]
55. Zhuo, C.; Hou, W.; Tian, H.; Wang, L.; Li, R. Lipidomics of the brain, retina, and biofluids: From the biological landscape to potential clinical application in schizophrenia. *Transl. Psychiatry* **2020**, *10*, 391. [CrossRef]
56. Arici, M.K.; Tuncbag, N. Unveiling hidden connections in omics data via pyPARAGON: An integrative hybrid approach for disease network construction. *Brief. Bioinform.* **2024**, *25*, bbae399. [CrossRef]
57. Wozniak, J.M.; Li, W.; Governa, P.; Chen, L.Y.; Jadhav, A.; Dongre, A.; Forli, S.; Parker, C.G. Enhanced mapping of small-molecule binding sites in cells. *Nat. Chem. Biol.* **2024**, *20*, 823–834. [CrossRef]
58. Evangelista, L.; Zattoni, F.; Cassarino, G.; Artioli, P.; Cecchin, D.; Dal Moro, F.; Zucchetta, P. PET/MRI in prostate cancer: A systematic review and meta-analysis. *Eur. J. Nucl. Med. Mol. Imaging* **2021**, *48*, 859–873. [CrossRef]
59. Gaca-Tabaszewska, M.; Bogusiewicz, J.; Bojko, B. Metabolomic and lipidomic profiling of gliomas—A new direction in personalized therapies. *Cancers* **2022**, *14*, 5041. [CrossRef]
60. Piazza, I.; Beaton, N.; Bruderer, R.; Knobloch, T.; Barbisan, C.; Chandat, L.; Sudau, A.; Siepe, I.; Rinner, O.; de Souza, N.; et al. A machine learning-based chemoproteomic approach to identify drug targets and binding sites in complex proteomes. *Nat. Commun.* **2020**, *11*, 4200. [CrossRef]

61. Karshikoff, B. Why PNI scientists need to engage in exploratory hypothesis-generating biomarker studies. *Brain Behav. Immun. Health* **2024**, *42*, 100904. [CrossRef] [PubMed]
62. Young, A.L.; Oxtoby, N.P.; Ourselin, S.; Schott, J.M.; Alexander, D.C. A simulation system for biomarker evolution in neurodegenerative disease. *Med. Image Anal.* **2015**, *26*, 47–56. [CrossRef] [PubMed]
63. van der Veen, R.; Bonapersona, V.; Joëls, M. The relevance of a rodent cohort in the Consortium on Individual Development. *Dev. Cogn. Neurosci.* **2020**, *45*, 100846. [CrossRef]
64. Fahlström, A.; Yu, Q.; Ulfhake, B. Behavioral changes in aging female C57BL/6 mice. *Neurobiol. Aging* **2011**, *32*, 1868–1880. [CrossRef]
65. Xie, L.; Das, S.R.; Li, Y.; Wisse, L.E.M.; McGrew, E.; Lyu, X.; DiCalogero, M.; Shah, U.; Ilesanmi, A.; Denning, A.E.; et al. A multi-cohort study of longitudinal and cross-sectional Alzheimer's disease biomarkers in cognitively unimpaired older adults. *Alzheimers Dement.* **2025**, *21*, e14492. [CrossRef]
66. Xu, Y.; Liu, S.; Zhou, Z.; Qin, H.; Zhang, Y.; Zhang, G.; Ma, H.; Han, X.; Liu, H.; Liu, Z. Integrated multi-omics analysis revealed the molecular networks and potential targets of cellular senescence in Alzheimer's disease. *Hum. Mol. Genet.* **2025**, *34*, 381–391. [CrossRef]
67. Gupta, H.; Suk, K.T.; Kim, D.J. Gut Microbiota at the Intersection of Alcohol, Brain, and the Liver. *J. Clin. Med.* **2021**, *10*, 541. [CrossRef]
68. Yan, M.; Man, S.; Sun, B.; Ma, L.; Guo, L.; Huang, L.; Gao, W. Gut liver brain axis in diseases: The implications for therapeutic interventions. *Signal Transduct. Target. Ther.* **2023**, *8*, 443. [CrossRef]
69. He, X.; Hu, M.; Xu, Y.; Xia, F.; Tan, Y.; Wang, Y.; Xiang, H.; Wu, H.; Ji, T.; Xu, Q.; et al. The gut-brain axis underlying hepatic encephalopathy in liver cirrhosis. *Nat. Med.* **2025**, *31*, 627–638. [CrossRef]
70. Bauer, E.E.; Shoeman, A.; Buhr, T.J.; Daniels, K.M.; Lyte, M.; Clark, P.J. Voluntary binge-patterned alcohol drinking and sex-specific influences on monoamine-related neurochemical signatures in the mouse gut and brain. *Alcohol. Clin. Exp. Res.* **2021**, *45*, 996–1012. [CrossRef]
71. Mohajeri, M.H.; La Fata, G.; Steinert, R.E.; Weber, P. Relationship between the gut microbiome and brain function. *Nutr. Rev.* **2018**, *76*, 481–496. [CrossRef] [PubMed]
72. Tanaka, M. From Serendipity to Precision: Integrating AI, Multi-Omics, and Human-Specific Models for Personalized Neuropsychiatric Care. *Biomedicines* **2025**, *13*, 167. [CrossRef] [PubMed]
73. Sheikh, M.; Qassem, M.; Kyriacou, P.A. Wearable, Environmental, and Smartphone-Based Passive Sensing for Mental Health Monitoring. *Front. Digit. Health* **2021**, *3*, 662811. [CrossRef] [PubMed]
74. Smith, D.G. Digital phenotyping approaches and mobile devices enhance CNS biopharmaceutical research and development. *Neuropsychopharmacology* **2018**, *43*, 2504–2505. [CrossRef]
75. Psaltos, D.; Chappie, K.; Karahanoglu, F.I.; Chasse, R.; Demanuele, C.; Kelekar, A.; Zhang, H.; Marquez, V.; Kangarloo, T.; Patel, S.; et al. Multimodal Wearable Sensors to Measure Gait and Voice. *Digit. Biomark.* **2019**, *3*, 133–144. [CrossRef]
76. Chen, S.; Lach, J.; Lo, B.; Yang, G.Z. Toward Pervasive Gait Analysis With Wearable Sensors: A Systematic Review. *IEEE J. Biomed. Health Inf.* **2016**, *20*, 1521–1537. [CrossRef]
77. Tanaka, M. Beyond the boundaries: Transitioning from categorical to dimensional paradigms in mental health diagnostics. *Adv. Clin. Exp. Med.* **2024**, *33*, 1295–1301. [CrossRef]
78. Kotov, R.; Krueger, R.F.; Watson, D. A paradigm shift in psychiatric classification: The Hierarchical Taxonomy Of Psychopathology (HiTOP). *World Psychiatry* **2018**, *17*, 24–25. [CrossRef]
79. Cuthbert, B.N. The RDoC framework: Facilitating transition from ICD/DSM to dimensional approaches that integrate neuroscience and psychopathology. *World Psychiatry* **2014**, *13*, 28–35. [CrossRef]
80. Lilienfeld, S.O.; Treadway, M.T. Clashing Diagnostic Approaches: DSM-ICD Versus RDoC. *Annu. Rev. Clin. Psychol.* **2016**, *12*, 435–463. [CrossRef]
81. McGorry, P.D.; Hickie, I.B.; Kotov, R.; Schmaal, L.; Wood, S.J.; Allan, S.M.; Altınbaş, K.; Boyce, N.; Bringmann, L.F.; Caspi, A.; et al. New diagnosis in psychiatry: Beyond heuristics. *Psychol. Med.* **2025**, *55*, e26. [CrossRef] [PubMed]
82. Ghosh, S.; Zhao, X.; Alim, M.; Brudno, M.; Bhat, M. Artificial intelligence applied to 'omics data in liver disease: Towards a personalised approach for diagnosis, prognosis and treatment. *Gut* **2025**, *74*, 295–311. [CrossRef] [PubMed]
83. Jiang, L.; Xu, C.; Bai, Y.; Liu, A.; Gong, Y.; Wang, Y.P.; Deng, H.W. Autosurv: Interpretable deep learning framework for cancer survival analysis incorporating clinical and multi-omics data. *NPJ Precis. Oncol.* **2024**, *8*, 4. [CrossRef]
84. Paolini, A.; Baldassarre, A.; Bruno, S.P.; Felli, C.; Muzi, C.; Ahmadi Badi, S.; Siadat, S.D.; Sarshar, M.; Masotti, A. Improving the Diagnostic Potential of Extracellular miRNAs Coupled to Multiomics Data by Exploiting the Power of Artificial Intelligence. *Front. Microbiol.* **2022**, *13*, 888414. [CrossRef]
85. Danek, B.P.; Makarious, M.B.; Dadu, A.; Vitale, D.; Lee, P.S.; Singleton, A.B.; Nalls, M.A.; Sun, J.; Faghri, F. Federated learning for multi-omics: A performance evaluation in Parkinson's disease. *Patterns* **2024**, *5*, 100945. [CrossRef]

86. Westerlund, A.M.; Hawe, J.S.; Heinig, M.; Schunkert, H. Risk Prediction of Cardiovascular Events by Exploration of Molecular Data with Explainable Artificial Intelligence. *Int. J. Mol. Sci.* **2021**, *22*, 10291. [CrossRef]
87. Yan, C.; Yan, H.; Liang, W.; Yin, M.; Luo, H.; Luo, J. DP-SSLoRA: A privacy-preserving medical classification model combining differential privacy with self-supervised low-rank adaptation. *Comput. Biol. Med.* **2024**, *179*, 108792. [CrossRef]
88. Sarmadi, A.; Fu, H.; Krishnamurthy, P.; Garg, S.; Khorrami, F. Privacy-Preserving Collaborative Learning Through Feature Extraction. *IEEE Trans. Dependable Secur. Comput.* **2022**, *21*, 486–498. [CrossRef]
89. Chen, M.; Guo, K.; Ding, Y.; Liu, W.; Yu, R.; Zhang, L.; Hu, Y.; Wu, Y.; Zhang, R. Vagus nerve stimulation modulating the directed brain network of patients with drug-resistant epilepsy. *Biomed. Signal Process. Control* **2024**, *95*, 106361. [CrossRef]
90. Ryvlin, P.; Rheims, S.; Hirsch, L.J.; Sokolov, A.; Jehi, L. Neuromodulation in epilepsy: State-of-the-art approved therapies. *Lancet Neurol.* **2021**, *20*, 1038–1047. [CrossRef] [PubMed]
91. Gouveia, F.V.; Warsi, N.M.; Suresh, H.; Matin, R.; Ibrahim, G.M. Neurostimulation treatments for epilepsy: Deep brain stimulation, responsive neurostimulation and vagus nerve stimulation. *Neurotherapeutics* **2024**, *21*, e00308. [CrossRef] [PubMed]
92. McVey Neufeld, K.A.; Bienenstock, J.; Bharwani, A.; Champagne-Jorgensen, K.; Mao, Y.; West, C.; Liu, Y.; Surette, M.G.; Kunze, W.; Forsythe, P. Oral selective serotonin reuptake inhibitors activate vagus nerve dependent gut-brain signalling. *Sci. Rep.* **2019**, *9*, 14290. [CrossRef]
93. Hwang, Y.K.; Oh, J.S. Interaction of the Vagus Nerve and Serotonin in the Gut-Brain Axis. *Int. J. Mol. Sci.* **2025**, *26*, 1160. [CrossRef]
94. Kaizer, A.M.; Hobbs, B.P.; Koopmeiners, J.S. A multi-source adaptive platform design for testing sequential combinatorial therapeutic strategies. *Biometrics* **2018**, *74*, 1082–1094. [CrossRef]
95. Coalition, A.P.T. Adaptive platform trials: Definition, design, conduct and reporting considerations. *Nat. Rev. Drug Discov.* **2019**, *18*, 797–807. [CrossRef]
96. Li, J.; Chen, L.; Sun, H.; Zhan, M.; Laurent, R.; Mignani, S.; Majoral, J.P.; Shen, M.; Shi, X. Cationic phosphorus dendron nanomicelles deliver microRNA mimics and microRNA inhibitors for enhanced anti-inflammatory therapy of acute lung injury. *Biomater. Sci.* **2023**, *11*, 1530–1539. [CrossRef]
97. Clarke, N.W.; James, N.D. How to Compose Platform Trials. *Eur. Urol. Focus.* **2023**, *9*, 715–718. [CrossRef]
98. Misra, B.B.; Langefeld, C.D.; Olivier, M.; Cox, L.A. Integrated Omics: Tools, Advances, and Future Approaches. *J. Mol. Endocrinol.* **2018**, *62*, R21–R45. [CrossRef]
99. Chen, T.; Abadi, A.; Cao, K.; Tyagi, S. multiomics: A user-friendly multi-omics data harmonisation R pipeline. *F1000Research* **2021**, *10*, 538. [CrossRef]
100. Santra, S.; Kukreja, P.; Saxena, K.; Gandhi, S.; Singh, O.V. Navigating regulatory and policy challenges for AI enabled combination devices. *Front. Med. Technol.* **2024**, *6*, 1473350. [CrossRef] [PubMed]
101. Exley, A.R.; Rantell, K.; McBlane, J. Clinical development of cell therapies for cancer: The regulators' perspective. *Eur. J. Cancer* **2020**, *138*, 41–53. [CrossRef] [PubMed]
102. Liu, X.; Cruz Rivera, S.; Moher, D.; Calvert, M.J.; Denniston, A.K. Reporting guidelines for clinical trial reports for interventions involving artificial intelligence: The CONSORT-AI extension. *Lancet Digit. Health* **2020**, *2*, e537–e548. [CrossRef] [PubMed]
103. Ehidiamen, A.; Oladapo, O. Enhancing ethical standards in clinical trials: A deep dive into regulatory compliance, informed consent, and participant rights protection frameworks. *World J. Biol. Pharm. Health Sci.* **2024**, *20*, 309–320. [CrossRef]

biomedicines

MDPI

Article

Unraveling the Role of miR-200b-3p in Attention-Deficit/Hyperactivity Disorder (ADHD) and Its Therapeutic Potential in Spontaneously Hypertensive Rats (SHR)

Tung-Ming Chang [1], Hsiu-Ling Lin [2], Chih-Chen Tzang [3], Ju-An Liang [4], Tsai-Ching Hsu [4,5,6,*] and Bor-Show Tzang [4,5,6,7,*]

1 Pediatric Neurology, Changhua Christian Children's Hospital, Changhua Christian Hospital, Changhua 500, Taiwan; 128658@cch.org.tw
2 Cardiac Function Examination Room, Chung Shan Medical University Hospital, Taichung 402, Taiwan; echolin01@gmail.com
3 School of Medicine, College of Medicine, National Taiwan University, Taipei City 100, Taiwan; jerrytzang@gmail.com
4 Institute of Medicine, Chung Shan Medical University, Taichung 402, Taiwan; 994103aajj@gmail.com
5 Immunology Research Center, Chung Shan Medical University, Taichung 402, Taiwan
6 Department of Clinical Laboratory, Chung Shan Medical University Hospital, Taichung 402, Taiwan
7 Department of Biochemistry, School of Medicine, Chung Shan Medical University, Taichung 402, Taiwan
* Correspondence: htc@csmu.edu.tw (T.-C.H.); bstzang@csmu.edu.tw (B.-S.T.); Tel.: +886-4-3609-8964 (T.-C.H.); +886-4-3609-7585 (B.-S.T.)

Abstract: Attention-deficit/hyperactivity disorder (ADHD) is a prevalent neurodevelopmental disorder in children with unknown etiology. Impaired learning ability was commonly reported in ADHD patients and has been associated with dopamine uptake in the striatum of an animal model. Another evidence also indicated that micro-RNA (miR)-200b-3p is associated with learning ability in various animal models. However, the association between miR-200b-3p and ADHD–related symptoms remains unclear. Therefore, the current study investigated the role of miR-200b-3p in ADHD-related symptoms such as inattention and striatal inflammatory cytokines. To verify the influence of miR-200b-3p in ADHD-related symptoms, striatal stereotaxic injection of miR-200b-3p antagomir (AT) was performed on spontaneously hypertensive rats (SHR). The antioxidant activity and expressions of miR-200b-3p, slit guidance ligand 2 (Slit2), and inflammatory cytokines in the striatum of SHR were measured using quantitative real-time polymerase chain reaction (RT-qPCR), immunohistochemistry (IHC), immunoblotting, and enzyme-linked immunosorbent assay (ELISA). The spontaneous alternation of SHR was tested using a three-arm Y-shaped maze. The administration of miR-200b-3p AT or taurine significantly decreased striatal tumor necrosis factor (TNF)-α, interleukin (IL)-1β, and IL-6 in SHR, along with increased super-oxide dismutase (SOD) and glutathione peroxidase (GSH-Px) activities and significantly higher spontaneous alternation. In this paper, we show that miR-200b-3p AT and taurine alleviates ADHD-related symptoms in SHR. These findings provide insights into ADHD's molecular basis and suggest miR-200b-3p as a potential therapeutic target. Concurrently, this study also suggests broad implications for treating neurodevelopmental disorders affecting learning activity such as ADHD.

Keywords: taurine; attention deficit hyperactivity disorder (ADHD); neuropsychiatric disorder; microRNA (miR)-200b-3p; striatum; spontaneously hypertensive rats (SHR); inflammatory factors; spontaneous alternations

1. Introduction

According to the latest Diagnostic and Statistical Manual of Mental Disorders, fifth edition (DSM-5), attention-deficit/hyperactivity disorder (ADHD) is classified as neurodevelopmental disorders (NDDs). Notably, ADHD is known as a global neuropsychiatric deficit that accounts for approximately 8–12% of all children [1]. Although the etiology of ADHD is complicated and still unclear, neurodevelopmental theory indicates that disruptions in normal brain development during early life can lead to neuropsychiatric symptoms in later life, impacting disorders such as autism spectrum disorder, ADHD, schizophrenia, bipolar disorder, and obsessive compulsive disorder [2]. Additionally, inattentiveness and hyperactivity/impulsiveness are known as the main symptoms of ADHD that lead to various conditions such as depression, epilepsy, and learning deficits [3]. Substantial evidence has reported that gene variants and environmental triggers are the main possible causes of ADHD [4]. Hence, the conventional treatment of ADHD involves a multimodal approach by addressing various aspects of the condition such as cognitive behavioral therapy (CBT), behavioral interventions, exercise, psychoeducation, and medication [1].

MicroRNAs (miRNAs), first discovered in 1993, are known as noncoding RNAs that exhibit pivotal roles in modulating gene expression [5,6]. MiRNAs exist in all animal systems, and some miRNAs are reported to be highly conserved in various species [7,8], which regulate gene expression by binding 3′UTR specific regions of target messenger ribonucleic acid (mRNA) to silence gene expression and promotor-specific regions of target mRNA to induce transcription [9,10]. MiRNAs have gained significant recognition for their roles in neuropsychiatric disorders, with extensive research in recent decades focusing on their impacts on neurodevelopmental conditions like ADHD, autism, and Alzheimer's disease. These studies primarily explore the influences of miRNAs on cognitive, behavioral, memory, and learning deficits [11–13]. Notably, a recent study indicated that the miRNA expression profile, including miR-4516, miR-6090, miR-4763-3p, miR-4281, and miR-4466, has great diagnostic accuracy and specificity in assessing ADHD [14]. A similar result was also reported, where the expression levels of miR-126-5p, miR-140-3p, and miR-30e-5p in total white blood cells (WBCs) revealed great clinical potential as diagnostic and therapeutic biomarkers for ADHD [15]. Although these miRNAs change significantly in ADHD patients as compared to healthy individuals, the precise roles of each miRNA and their interactions in the development of ADHD are still unclear. However, the application of miRNAs aids in pinpointing potential targets for therapy and paves the way for the possibility of genetic mRNA treatments.

Taurine, known as a free β-amino acid, is a very abundant neurotransmitter in the human nervous system that exhibits diverse physiological roles such as a regulator of calcium transport and homeostasis, an osmolyte, and a trophic factor in the development of central nervous system [16–19]. Taurine has been demonstrated to have therapeutic potential in a broad range of disorders, including neurodegenerative diseases such as Alzheimer's disease, Parkinson's disease, epilepsy [20], muscle atrophy [21], congestive heart failure [22,23], rheumatoid arthritis [24], thrombosis [25], and lipid metabolism disorders [26]. Additionally, taurine exhibits neuroprotective properties through its ability to stabilize cell membranes, inhibits reactive oxygen species (ROS)-producing enzymes, and indirectly acts as an antioxidant by maintaining cellular redox balance, effectively safeguarding neuronal health [27]. Recent evidence revealed that amino acid supplementation may influence genetic expression through epigenetic mechanisms such as DNA hypermethylation, potentially altering the outcomes of NDDs [28]. Maternal protein restriction during gestation in spontaneously hypertensive rats (SHR), a well-documented ADHD animal model for investigating the treatment of ADHD [29], led to a positive correlation between DNA hypermethylation at the CpG island of the renal prostaglandin E receptor 1 (Ptger1) gene and increased Ptger1 mRNA expression in offsprings. Interestingly, the study also found that post-weaning dietary adjustments, either to a low-protein or high-protein diet, could modify the Ptger1 DNA hypermethylation caused by fetal malnutrition [28]. These findings revealed that nutritional supplements like taurine may influence genetic expressions through epigenetic mechanisms like DNA hypermethylation, potentially altering the outcomes of NDDs.

Compared with the controls, SHR receiving high-dose taurine (45 mmol/kg) for four weeks revealed significantly decreased hyperactive behavior by reducing inflammatory cytokines, functional connectivity (FC) signal, and the mean amplitude of low-frequency fluctuation (mALFF) in the bilateral hippocampus [30]. Additionally, the administration of high-dose taurine reduced the dopamine uptake in striatal synaptosomes of SHR and increased the spontaneous alternation of SHR [31]. Although these findings suggested the ameliorating effects of taurine on ADHD-like symptoms in SHR, the mechanism of taurine in improving the symptoms of ADHD is still unclear. Adding to this, recent studies have linked the expression of miR-200b-3p with learning ability in various disease models [32,33]. Building on this evidence, the current study explores the role of miR-200b-3p in SHR, aiming to evaluate its therapeutic potential for ADHD. Therefore, the current study investigated the role of miR-200b-3p in SHR to assess its therapeutic potential in ADHD. We hypothesized that the administration of either taurine or miR-200b-3p antagomir (AT) positively influences the neurobiological and behavioral symptoms associated with ADHD in the SHR. Specifically, taurine or miR-200b-3p AT will lead to a reduction in the miR-200b-3p level and an increase in its target, Slit2, expression in the striatum of SHR, accompanied by a reduction in oxidative stress in the striatum and improved inattention behavior.

2. Materials and Methods

This study was designed based on previous publications [31,34] and explored the effects of taurine and miR-200b-3p AT on ADHD-related symptoms using spontaneously hypertensive rats (SHR), a model for ADHD. The research involved dividing rats into groups for various treatments and control conditions, administering taurine diets, stereotaxic injections of miR-200b-3p antagomir, and conducting behavioral, molecular, and biochemical analyses. Techniques such as RT-qPCR, ELISA, immunohistochemistry, and immunoblotting were used to assess mRNA expression, inflammatory cytokines, antioxidant enzyme levels, and protein expression as described elsewhere [35–37]. Additionally, the study evaluated working memory using a Y-maze test and employed statistical analysis to interpret the data [38].

2.1. Animals and Experimental Procedure

To investigate the influence of taurine and miR-200b-3p antagomir on ADHD-related symptoms, the spontaneously hypertensive rat (SHR/NCrlCrlj; SHR), a valid ADHD animal model, and the Wistar Kyoto rat (WKY/NCrlCrlj; WKY), control rats for SHR, were adopted in this study [34]. All rats were obtained at three weeks old from the National Laboratory Animal Center, Taipei, Taiwan, and separated into five groups (five rats/group), including the Control, Taurine, Sham, miR ATNC (miR-200b-3p antagomir negative control), and miR AT (miR-200b-3p antagomir) groups. The animals were kept in a facility at 22 ± 2 °C with a 12/12 h light–dark cycle. Experimental handling was approved and supervised by the Institutional Animal Care and Use Committee at Chung Shan Medical University (IACUC approval number: 2136). The taurine dose used in this study was 45 mmol/kg diet according to our previous publication [30,31]. At four weeks of age, rats from the taurine group were administered a taurine diet, while those rats from the other groups were fed a standard chow diet until they reached eight weeks of age. Stereotaxic injection surgery was performed on rats from the Sham, miR ATNC, and miR AT groups at five weeks of age. The Y-maze test was conducted for all rats one day prior to their sacrifice by CO_2 asphyxiation at eight weeks of age. The striatum tissue of rats from each group was resected and kept in a −80 °C freezer before analysis.

2.2. MicroRNA and Striatal Stereotaxic Injection

To assess the impacts of blocking striatum miR-200b-3p expression in SHR, rat miR-200b-3p antagomir (AT) and the antagomir-negative control (ATNC) were purchased (BioLion Technology Co., Ltd., Taipei, Taiwan). Five nmol miR-200b-3p AT and ATNC in 1 μL PBS were mixed with 1 μL HiPerFect transfection reagent (Cat. #: 301705, Qiagen, Germantown, MA, USA) prior to injection into the striatum of SHR. The striatal stereo-taxic injection was performed as described elsewhere [35]. Briefly, SHR were intraperitoneally injected with urethane (1.25 g/kg) to anesthetize them, and they were placed on an animal heating pad. Next, the rats were fixed in a stereotactic apparatus, and a hole was drilled in the skull. The mixed solution was then injected (1 μL/min) into the left striatum of rats using a 10 μL Hamilton syringe (Sigma-Aldrich, St. Louis, MO, USA) connected to a microinfusion pump (Stoelting Co., Wood Dale, IL, USA). The skin was sutured after injection.

2.3. Quantitative Real-Time PCR (RT-qPCR)

To detect the mRNA expression in the striatum of rats, RT-qPCR analysis was performed based on a previous study [33]. Total RNA was extracted from the left striatum of rats using miRNeasy Kits (Cat. #: 217604, Qiagen, Germantown, MA, USA) and subsequently reversed to complementary DNA (cDNA) using miRCURY LNA RT Kit (Cat. #: 339340, Qiagen, Germantown, MA, USA). Quantitative real-time PCR (RT-qPCR) was completed using miRCURY LNA SYBR® Green PCR Kits (Cat. #: 339345, Qiagen, Germantown, MA, USA) and analyzed using Applied Biosystems StepOne Plus Real-Time PCR System. The specific primers used in this study are shown in Table 1. The relative gene expression was analyzed as described elsewhere [36].

Table 1. Primers for quantitative real-time PCR (qRT-PCR).

Gene	Forward Primer	Reverse Primer
Slit2	5′-CGCCAAAGGGATTCAAGTGT-3′	5′-CACTGGCATATTGGTTCATTCA-3′
β-actin	5′-CCCATCTATGAGGGTTACGC-3′	5′-TTTAATGTCACGCACGATTTC-3′
TNF-α	5′-TCAGCCGATTTGCCATTTCAT-3′	5′-ACACGCCAGTCGCTTCACAGA-3′
IL-1β	5′-GTCCTTTCACTTGCCCTCAT-3′	5′-CAAACTGGTCACAGCTTTCGA-3′
IL-6	5′-AATGCCTCGTGCTGTCTGACC-3′	5′-GGTGGGTGTGCCGTCTTTCATC-3′

Slit2: Slit guidance ligand 2; *TNF*: Tumor necrosis factor; *IL*: Interleukin.

2.4. Enzyme-Linked Immunosorbent Assay (ELISA)

To detect the levels of inflammatory cytokines and the activity of antioxidant enzymes, ELISA tests were performed. The striatum tissues were homogenized, and the supernatants were collected after centrifugation. The levels of superoxide dismutase (SOD) and glutathione peroxidase (GSH-Px) in rat striatum were measured using ELISA kits purchased from MyBioSource (Cat. #: MBS266897, MyBioSource, San Diego, CA, USA; Cat. #: MBS032696, MyBioSource, San Diego, CA, USA). The contents of tumor necrosis factor-α (TNF-α), interleukin-1β (IL-1β), and interleukin-6 (IL-6) were also measured using ELISA kits obtained from Invitrogen (Cat. #: KRC3011, Invitrogen, Thermo Fisher Scientific, Waltham, MA, USA; Cat. #: BMS630 Invitrogen, Thermo Fisher Scientific, Waltham, MA, USA; Cat. #: ERA31RB, Invitrogen, Thermo Fisher Scientific, Waltham, MA, USA).

2.5. Immunohistochemistry (IHC)

To detect the expression of the Slit2 protein in the striatum of SHR, immunohistochemistry (IHC) was performed as described elsewhere [37]. Animals were euthanized by carbon dioxide. The striatum tissues were excised, soaked in 10% formalin, and subsequently embedded with paraffin wax. The embedded tissues were sectioned into 5 μm slices and incubated overnight with antibodies against rat Slit2 (Cat. #: ab7665, Abcam, Waltham, MA, USA). Finally, the sections were observed and quantified using the automated Tissue-FAXS PLUS system (TISSUE GNOSTICS, Vienna, Austria).

2.6. Immunoblotting

To detect the Slit2 protein expression in the striatum tissue of SHR with different treatments, immunoblot was conducted as described in our previous study [31]. Total proteins were extracted from the striatal tissues in PRO-PREP™ buffer (iNtRON Bio-technology, Inc.,

Seongnam, Republic of Korea), and the concentrations of protein were measured according to a modified Bradford's assay using a spectrophotometer (Hitachi U3000, Tokyo, Japan) at 595 nm. The proteins were separated into a sodium dodecyl sulfate polyacrylamide gel electrophoresis (SDS-PAGE) via electrophoresis and then transferred onto a nitrocellulose membrane (Amersham Biosciences, Piscataway, NJ, USA). After blocking the membrane with 5% nonfat dry milk, antibodies against rat Slit2 (Cat. #:ab7665, Abcam, Waltham, MA, USA), or β-actin (Cat. #: MAB1501, Merck Millipore, Burlington, MA, USA), they were incubated for 2 h with mild shaking. Subsequent incubation of horseradish peroxidase (HRP) conjugated secondary antibody for another hour was performed. For detecting the antigen–antibody complexes, Immobilon Western Chemiluminescent HRP Substrate (Millipore, Burlington, MA, USA) and an imaging analyzer (GE ImageQuant TL 8.1, GE Healthcare Life Sciences, Pittsburgh, PA, USA) were used.

2.7. Spontaneous Alternation

The working memory of the rats was assessed according to a previous method described elsewhere [31,38]. Briefly, a three-arm Y-shaped maze with 200 lx illumination was used to test the spontaneous alternation. The three arms are angled 120° to each other, and each arm is 20 inches long, 4 inches wide, and 15 inches high. A rat is considered to have entered the arm when its four paws are in the arm. Spontaneous alternation was defined as the entry of all three arms in consecutive choices in triplet sets overlapped, and the percentage of spontaneous alternation was shown as (actual alternations/maximal alternations) ×100. The maximum number of alternations was defined as the total number of arm entries minus two.

2.8. Statistical Analysis

GraphPad Prism 5.0 software was used to analyze the experimental data. The data were presented as mean ± S.D. Two-way ANOVA with Bonferroni's post hoc test for multiple comparisons was used to analyze the effects of rat type and treatment, as well as the interaction of these two factors. One-way ANOVA with Tukey's multiple comparisons post hoc test was performed to determine the significance of different treatments of SHR. A p-value less than 0.05 ($p < 0.05$) was considered as statistically significant.

3. Results

3.1. Effect of High-Dose Taurine on Expressions of miR-200b-3p and Silt2 in the Striatum of WKY and SHR

We first employed RT-qPCR and immunoblotting to assess the expression levels of miR-200b-3p and Slit2 in the striatum of both WKY and SHR. As shown in Figure 1A, the expression of miR-200b-3p was significantly higher in the striatum of SHR as compared to WKY rats. No significant difference in miR-200b-3p expression was observed between the WKY rats administered high-dose taurine and those on a control diet. A significantly decreased miR-200b-3p level was detected in SHR treated with high-dose taurine compared to the SHR controls (Figure 1A). No significant difference in the expressions of Slit2 mRNA, a target gene of miR-200b-3p, and Slit2 protein was observed in the striatum of WKY rats treated with high-dose taurine (Figure 1B,C). Notably, significantly upregulated levels of both Slit2 mRNA and Slit2 protein were detected in the striatum of SHR treated with high-dose taurine compared to the SHR controls (Figure 1B,C).

3.2. Effects of miR-200b-3p Antagomir on miR-200b-3p and Slit2 Protein Expressions in Striatum of SHR

The expressions of miR-200b-3p and Slit2 protein in the striatum of SHR were detected using RT-qPCR and immunoblotting analysis, respectively. Compared with the controls, the level of miR-200b-3p was significantly decreased in the striatum of SHR treated with high-dose taurine as well as those rats treated with miR-200b-3p antagomir (Figure 2A). Additionally, a significantly increased expression of Slit2 protein was detected in the striatum of SHR treated with high-dose taurine and miR-200b-3p antagomir, respectively

(Figure 2B). Immunohistochemistry (IHC) was also performed to confirm the expressions of the Slit2 protein in the striatum of SHR with different treatments. A significantly higher Slit2 protein level was detected in the striatum of SHR treated with high-dose taurine and miR-200b-3p antagomir, respectively, compared with the controls (Figure 3A,B).

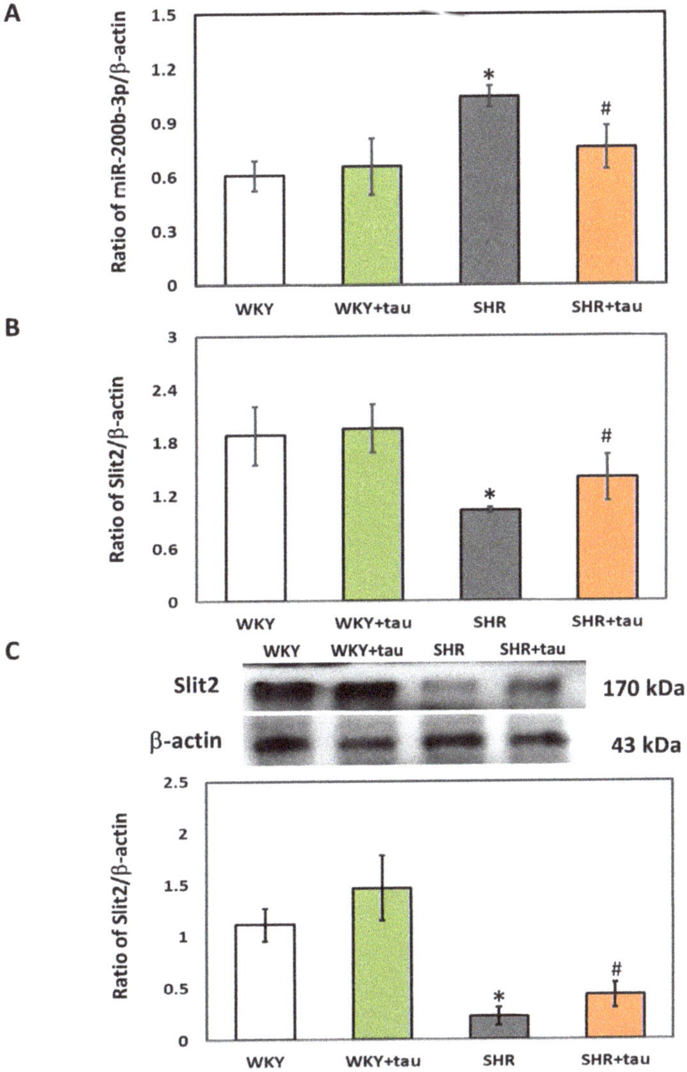

Figure 1. Comparison of miR-200b-3p and Slit2 expressions in the striatum of WKY and SHR. (**A**) miR-200b-3p, (**B**) Slit2 mRNA, and (**C**) Slit2 protein in the striatum of WKY and SHR from different groups ($n = 5$ per group). Data are shown as mean ± S.D. The symbols, * $p < 0.05$ and # $p < 0.05$, indicate significant differences compared with the WKY group and SHR group, respectively, using two-way ANOVA with Bonferroni's post hoc test. WKY (fed with Cho diet); WKY + tau (fed with 45 mM taurine); SHR (fed with Cho diet); SHR + tau (fed with 45 mM taurine).

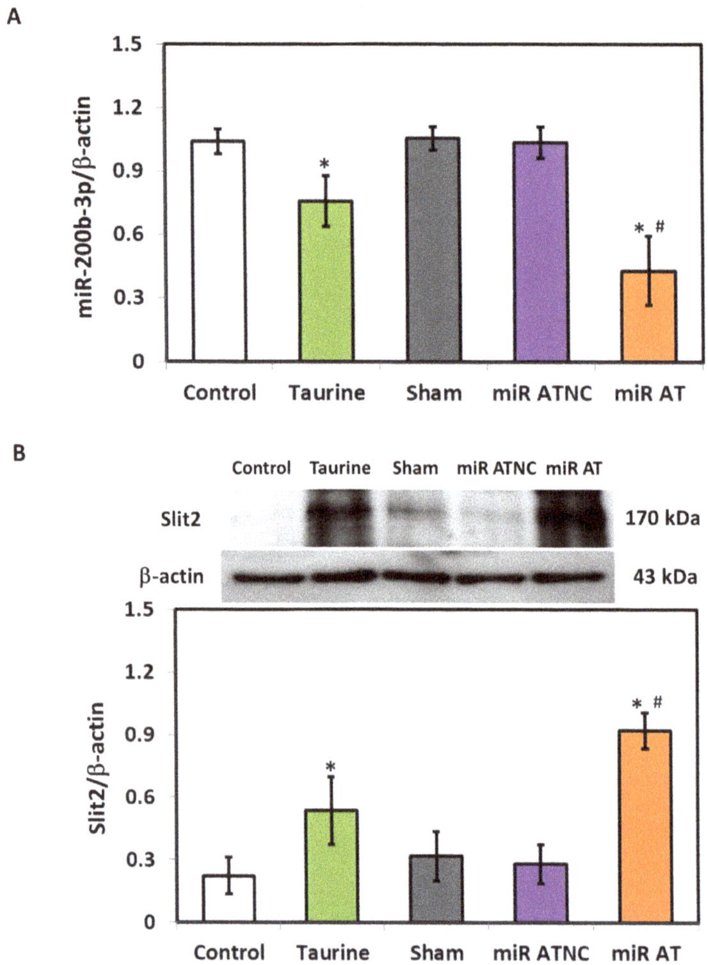

Figure 2. Expression of miR-200b-3p and Slit2 protein in SHR treated with miR-200b-3p antagomir. (**A**) miR-200b-3p and (**B**) Slit2 protein in the striatum of SHR from different groups ($n = 5$ per group). Data are shown as mean ± S.D. The symbols, * $p < 0.05$, and # $p < 0.05$, indicate significant differences compared with the Control group and Sham group, respectively, using one-way ANOVA with Tukey's multiple comparisons post hoc test. Control (fed with Cho diet); Taurine (fed with 45 mM taurine); Sham (fed with Cho diet); miR ATNC (injection of miR-200b-3p antagomir negative-control); miR AT (injection of miR-200b-3p antagomir).

3.3. MiR-200b-3p Antagomir Attenuated the Expressions of Inflammatory Cytokines and Increased the Activity of Antioxidant Enzymes

To verify the effects of miR-200b-3p antagomir on inflammation-related factors, the expressions of TNF-α, IL-1β, and IL-6 in the striatum of SHR were measured. Significantly lower levels of TNF-α, IL-1β, and IL-6 mRNA and their protein expressions were observed in the striatum of SHR treated with high-dose taurine and miR-200b-3p antagomir, respectively, compared to the controls (Figure 4A,B). Additionally, a significantly higher activity of GSH-Px and SOD was detected in the striatum of SHR treated with high-dose taurine and miR-200b-3p antagomir, respectively (Figure 5A,B).

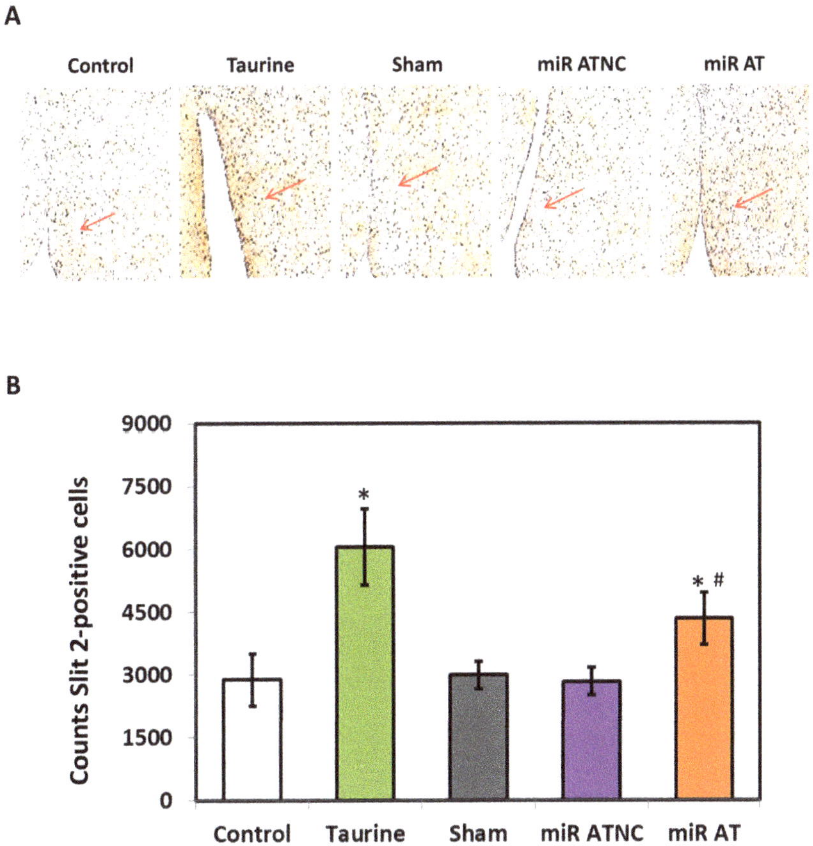

Figure 3. Immunohistological stainings for Slit2 proteins. (**A**) Representative images of the striatal section with immunohistological stainings of SHR with different treatments ($n = 5$ per group). The arrow indicates the expression of Slit2 proteins. (**B**) Quantified results for Slit2 protein expression. The symbol, * $p < 0.05$, and # $p < 0.05$, indicate significant differences compared with the Control group and Sham group, respectively, using one-way ANOVA with Tukey's multiple comparisons post hoc test. Control (fed with Cho diet); Taurine (fed with 45 mM taurine); Sham (fed with Cho diet); miR ATNC (injection of miR-200b-3p antagomir negative-control); miR AT (injection of miR-200b-3p antagomir).

3.4. MiR-200b-3p Antagomir Improves Working Memory in SHR

To verify the effects of miR-200b-3p antagomir on working memory in SHR, arm entries, and spontaneous alternation tests were performed with a three arms Y-maze test (Figure 6A). A significantly lower total number of arm entries was observed in SHR treated with high-dose taurine compared to those of the control group. A similar result was also detected in SHR treated with miR-200b-3p antagomir as compared with those from the Sham and miR ATNC groups, respectively (Figure 6B). Additionally, a significantly higher percentage of spontaneous alternation was detected in SHR treated with high-dose taurine and miR-200b-3p antagomir compared to the control groups (Figure 6C).

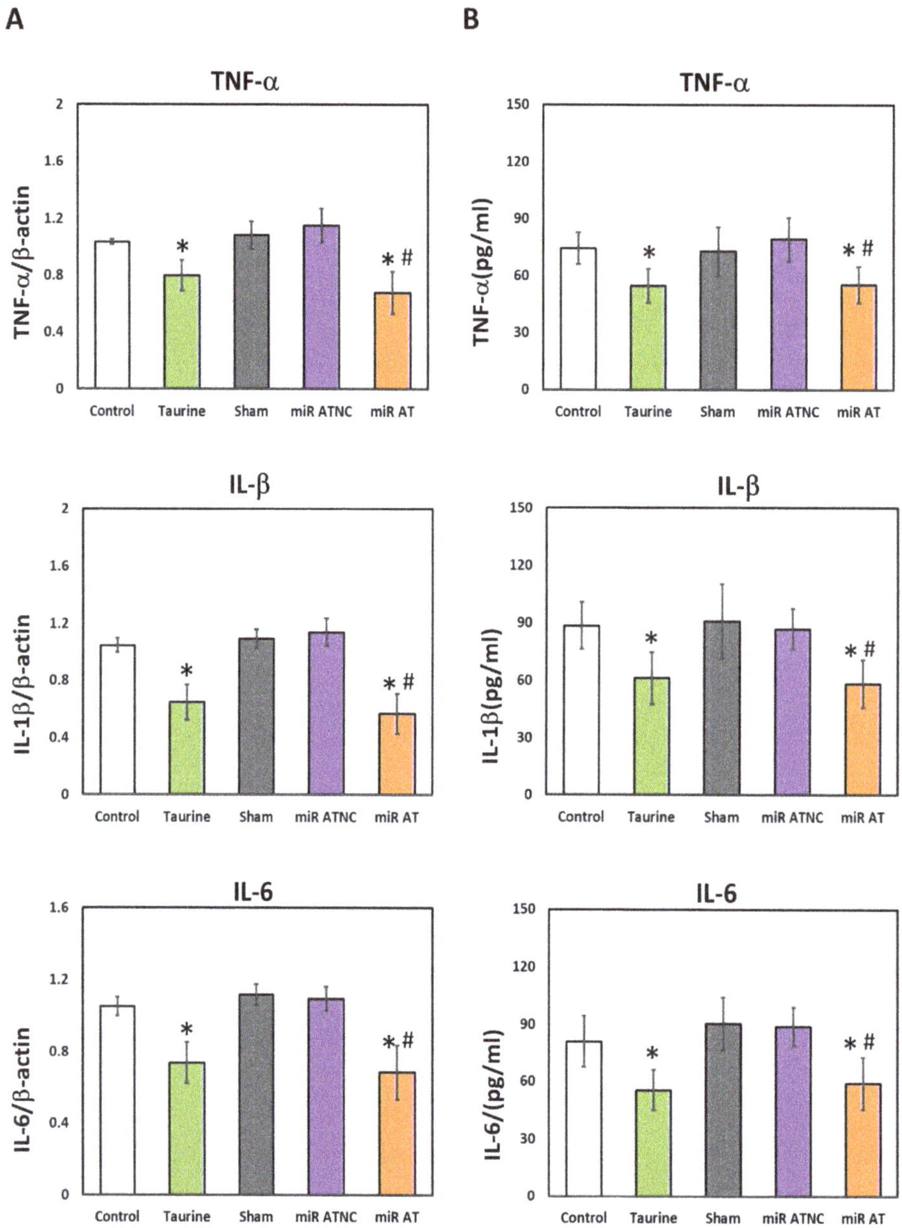

Figure 4. Levels of inflammatory cytokines in the striatum of SHR treated with miR-200b-3p antagomir. (**A**) Relative mRNA expression of TNF-α, IL-1β, and IL-6 and (**B**) concentrations of TNF-α, IL-1β, and IL-6 in the striatum of SHR from different groups ($n = 5$ per group). Data are shown as mean ± S.D. The symbol, * $p < 0.05$, and # $p < 0.05$, indicate significant differences compared with the Control group and Sham group, respectively, using one-way ANOVA with Tukey's multiple comparisons post hoc test. Control (fed with Cho diet); Taurine (fed with 45 mM taurine); Sham (fed with Cho diet); miR ATNC (injection of miR-200b-3p antagomir negative-control); miR AT (injection of miR-200b-3p antagomir).

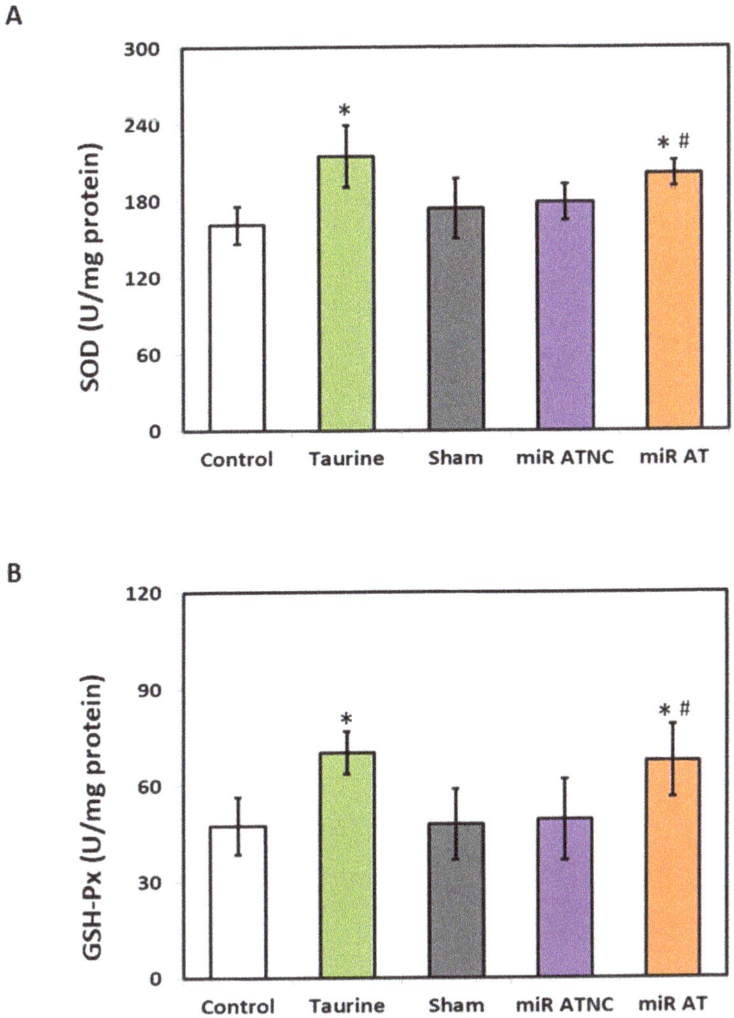

Figure 5. The levels of SOD and GSH-Px in the striatum of rats treated with miR-200b-3p antagomir. The activity of (**A**) SOD and (**B**) GSH-Px in the striatum of SHR from different groups ($n = 5$ per group). Data are shown as mean ± S.D. The symbol, * $p < 0.05$, and # $p < 0.05$, indicate significant differences compared with the Control group and Sham group, respectively, using one-way ANOVA with Tukey's multiple comparisons post hoc test. Control (fed with Cho diet); Taurine (fed with 45 mM taurine); Sham (fed with Cho diet); miR ATNC (injection of miR-200b-3p antagomir negative-control); miR AT (injection of miR-200b-3p antagomir).

In summary, our experimental results revealed that the administration of taurine or miR-200b-3p AT significantly ameliorates the striatal proinflammatory cytokines, including TNF-α, IL-1β, and IL-6, and increases the activity of anti-oxidant enzyme activity, including SOD and GSH-Px, in SHR. Concurrently, a significant increase in spontaneous alternation was detected in SHR treated with taurine or miR-200b-3p AT.

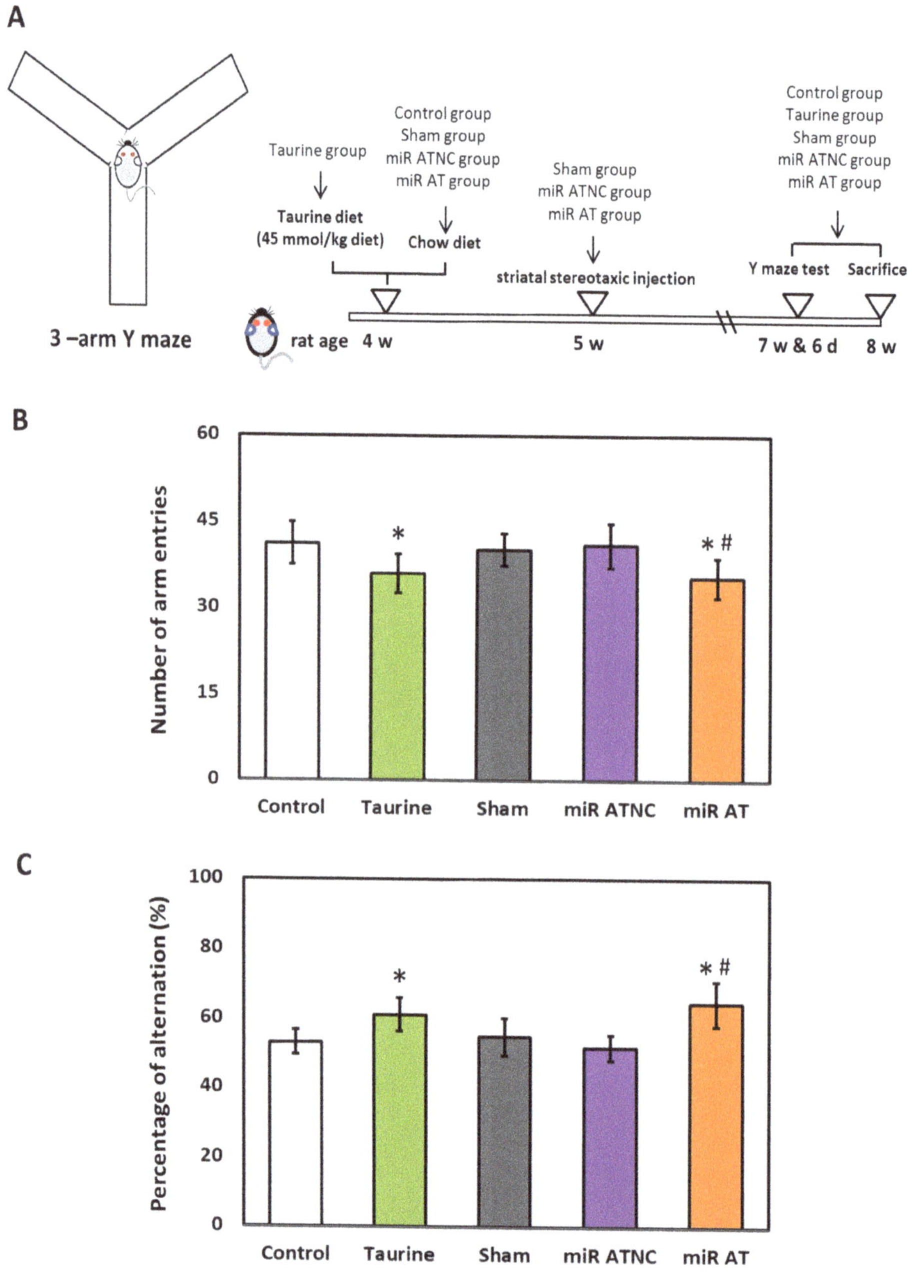

Figure 6. Effects of miR-200b-3p antagomir on inattention of SHR. (**A**) Schematic diagram of 3-arm Y-maze device and experimental design. (**B**) Total arm entries and (**C**) spontaneous alternation behavior in SHR from different groups ($n = 5$ per group). Data are shown as mean ± S.D. The symbol, * $p < 0.05$, and # $p < 0.05$, indicate significant differences compared with the Control group and Sham group, respectively, using one-way ANOVA with Tukey's multiple comparisons post hoc test. Control (fed with Cho diet); Taurine (fed with 45 mM taurine); Sham (fed with Cho diet); miR ATNC (injection of miR-200b-3p antagomir negative-control); miR AT (injection of miR-200b-3p antagomir).

4. Discussion

MicroRNAs (miRNAs) are known as a family of untranslated single-stranded RNAs with approximately 22 nucleotides in length [39]. Although the detailed mechanism of miRNAs is still not fully understood, the function of most miRNAs in mammals is thought to inhibit the target gene translation by mRNA degradation, which plays an essential role in controlling cell division, differentiation, and death [40]. In recent decades, miRNAs have been versatile, being used in the diagnosis, prognosis, and as therapeutic targets in many diseases, including cancers, CNS disorders, hepatic diseases, autoimmune disorders, and cardiovascular diseases [41–45]. Although increasing studies have been focused on investigating the miRNAs in attention-deficit/hyperactivity disorder (ADHD) [15], the roles and applications of miRNAs in ADHD are still very limited. For the first time, we reported that high-dose taurine significantly attenuated the level of miR-200b-3p along with increased Slit2 protein in the striatum of SHR, leading to attenuated expressions of inflammatory cytokines, elevated activity of antioxidants, and increased spontaneous alternations. These findings indicated the involvement and regulatory roles of miR-200b-3p in ADHD-like symptoms and suggested miR-200b-3p as a therapeutic target for ADHD-like symptoms.

MiR-200b-3p is a member of miR-200b family, which contains miR-200a, miR-200b, miR-200c, miR-429, and miR-141. Although most studies investigating miR-200b-3p are related to its regulation and mechanism on malignant phenotype tumors [46], miR-200b-3p also exhibits modulatory roles in many physiological and pathological processes, including the formation of insulin-producing cells [47], fetal cartilage differentiation [48], preeclampsia [49], wound healing [50], and neuropathological disorders [51]. However, very limited information is known about the roles of miR-200b-3p in ADHD-like symptoms. Recently, upregulated miR-200b-3p was reported to be associated with the development of brain arteriovenous malformations [52]. Another study also indicated that miR-200b-3p antagomir improved spatial and learning memory loss in hypoxia-ischemia animals [53]. These findings indicated that the decline of miR-200b-3p expression may reveal a protective effect on brain development as well as improved spatial and learning memory, which may provide a possible explanation for the effects of the downregulated miR-200b-3p level in the striatum of SHR treated with high-dose taurine. However, more investigations are still required to verify the precise mechanism of miR-200b-3p in the pathological processes of ADHD and its related symptoms.

The current study reported the decreased expressions of proinflammatory cytokines and the increased activity of antioxidant enzymes in the striatum of SHR receiving high-dose taurine. However, information about the role of miR-200b-3p on the expression of proinflammatory cytokines and antioxidant enzyme activity is still unclear. Notably, the enhancement of various inflammatory cytokines by miR-200b-3p was reported in an avian model [54]. A recent study indicated that upregulation of gga-miR-200b-3p promotes macrophage differentiation and enhances the expressions of proinflammatory cytokines such as TNF-α, IL-1β, IL-6, and IL-12 by directly targeting monocyte to macrophage differentiation-associated (MMD) [54]. This finding indicated evidence that miR-200b-3p directly regulates the expressions of various proinflammatory cytokines. Although no direct evidence indicated the act of miR-200b-3p on antioxidant enzymes such as superoxide dismutase (SOD) and glutathione peroxidases (GPxs), a recent review study indicated the association between ROS and the miR-200 family [55]. Notably, compelling evidence has indicated the existence of a reciprocal connection between antioxidant enzyme activity and the miR-200b family that maintains the cellular redox balance [56]. Apart from the findings mentioned above, the downregulated inflammatory cytokines and upregulated antioxidant activity may also be caused by the action of taurine [57], which also provides another rationale for the findings in this study.

In this study, SHR fed with high-dose taurine revealed significantly decreased miR-200b-3p in the striatum. In fact, current research on taurine-regulated miRs and their related mechanisms is still very limited. Therefore, very little information is known about the regulatory mechanism of taurine on miR-200b-3p expression. Interestingly, in an ex vivo study of adaptive osmotic response under hypertonic stress, significantly upregulated Na+/Cl−-taurine transporter, a hypertonic responsive gene, was due to the downregulated levels of miR-29b-3p and miR-200b-3p [58]. As taurine and the taurine transporter are known to play essential roles in the modulation of neuron osmosis and neurotransmitter balance [19], this finding may provide a possible explanation for the mechanism of the regulatory role of taurine on the miR-200b-3p level. Further investigations are required to verify the detailed network of how taurine downregulates the level of miR-200b-3p.

Although there are various animal models for investigating ADHD, SHR are currently recognized as the most appropriate animal model for ADHD. Various studies have reported that attention-deficit/hyperactivity disorder (ADHD) is linked to changes in encoding processes, specifically in working or short-term memory [59]. Interestingly, the spontaneously hypertensive rats (SHR) displays certain dysfunctional domains associated with ADHD [60,61]. Indeed, spontaneously hypertensive rats (SHR) exhibit symptoms related to hypertension [62] and ADHD-like syndromes such as inattention, hyperactivity, and impulsivity [60]. Moreover, the dysregulation of dopamine signaling between the frontal cortex and the striatum is known as an important occurrence associated with behavioral changes in ADHD [63]. Notably, similar deficits in energy metabolism, dopaminergic signaling, and neural development are also reported in the striatum of SHR [31,64]. Therefore, in this study, SHR were the appropriate animal model to investigate the effects of taurine and miR-200b-3p AT on ADHD-related symptoms.

In order to assess clinical relevance, it is essential to compare the doses administered to animals in this study with those necessary for humans. Previous evidence has suggested that the taurine intake from daily food consumption is approximately 58 mg [65], aligning with the taurine concentration (30 to 160 mg) found in a standard 100 g taurine-rich food like fish, beef, or pork [66]. However, high-dose taurine has been demonstrated as nontoxic to humans [67] and has been applied in different pathophysiological conditions such as skeletal muscle disorders and heart failure [21,68]. For the clinical treatment of congestive heart failure [69], hypertension [70], and dystrophic myotonia [71], taurine is used at doses as high as 6 g per day or more. Notably, the highest tolerable dose of taurine was identified as 21 g per day in a clinical trial aimed at managing epilepsy [72]. These findings suggest that high-dose taurine intake is well tolerated for the treatment of various human pathological conditions. The taurine dose used in this study was 45 mmol taurine/kg diet (5.6 g taurine/kg diet), which is equivalent to a dose of 0.9 g taurine/kg diet in humans [73]. The dose of taurine used in this study is much lower than that used for various diseases mentioned above [72], which provides rational support for ADHD treatment.

Certain concerns within this study require further emphasis. First, there are some issues that need to be raised in the animal behavior experiment of this study. Since only the striatum was measured, this study is still limited in interpreting the experimental results of taurine and miR-200b-3p antagomir affecting animal behavior. Additionally, the test of spontaneous alternation alone may not provide a comprehensive assessment of ADHD symptoms or working memory. Therefore, other tests such as a locomotion test, Morris water maze test, open field test, and Barnes maze test may be merited to clarify the effects of taurine and miR-200b-3p antagomir on learning and cognition in SHR in the future [74,75]. Additionally, this study shows that the elevated miR-200b-3p levels in the striatum of SHR were reduced by the administration of taurine, resulting in improved attention. However, it is worth noting that taurine is known to influence a broad range of miRNAs involved in various physiological and pathological processes, including CNS development, hormone metabolism, inflammation, and cognitive function [76–80]. Therefore, further investigations are warranted to better understand the specific regulatory network of miRNAs modulated by taurine, particularly in the context of improving ADHD-like symptoms in SHR. Moreover, it is important to acknowledge that microRNA-based therapy faces several limitations and challenges that must be addressed before translating these findings into clinical applications. Notably, issues such as immunotoxic reactions and suboptimal delivery systems have been identified as significant hurdles in recent research [81,82]. Hence, the development of miRNA therapies with low toxicity, high effectiveness, and precise targeting is essential for advancing miRNA-based drug development.

5. Conclusions

Irregular dopamine signaling between the frontal cortex and the striatum is recognized as a noteworthy phenomenon associated with behavioral changes in ADHD [63,83]. Therefore, in this study, we investigated the effects of taurine supplementation on the striatum of SHR. As shown in Figure 7, SHR fed with taurine exhibited a noteworthy reduction in miR-200b-3p expression in the striatum of the brain, accompanied by diminished expressions of inflammatory cytokines, including TNF-α, IL-1β, and IL-6, and heightened antioxidant enzyme activity, including SOD and GSH-Px. Intriguingly, SHR treated with the miR-200b-3p antagomir also displayed reduced expressions of inflammation-related cytokines and increased antioxidant enzyme activity in the striatum of the brain. Furthermore, regardless of whether the SHR were administered taurine or injected with the miR-200b-3p antagomir, a significant improvement in their working memory was observed. These findings suggest that the miR-200b-3p antagomir reveals a similar function to taurine and highlights its potential as a therapeutic target for ADHD treatment.

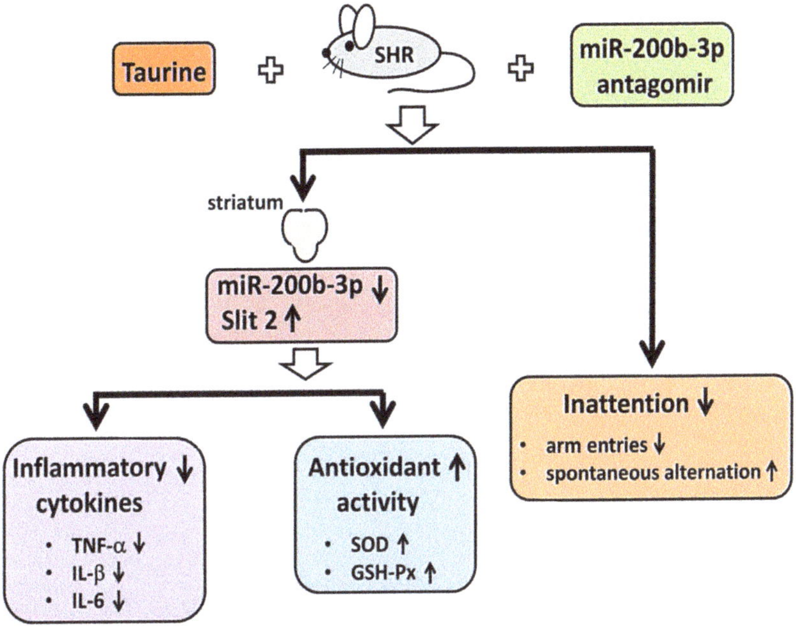

Figure 7. Graphical abstract of the effects of both taurine and miR-200b-3p antagomir on striatum of SHR and inattention.

Author Contributions: Conceptualization, T.-M.C., H.-L.L., C.-C.T., J.-A.L., T.-C.H. and B.-S.T.; Data curation, T.-M.C., H.-L.L., C.-C.T., J.-A.L., T.-C.H. and B.-S.T.; Formal analysis, T.-M.C., H.-L.L., C.-C.T., J.-A.L., T.-C.H. and B.-S.T.; Funding acquisition, T.-M.C. and B.-S.T.; Methodology, B.-S.T.; Project administration, T.-M.C., T.-C.H. and B.-S.T.; Resources, B.-S.T.; Supervision, B.-S.T.; Writing—original draft, C.-C.T., T.-C.H. and B.-S.T.; Writing—review and editing, T.-M.C., H.-L.L., C.-C.T., J.-A.L., T.-C.H. and B.-S.T. All authors have read and agreed to the published version of the manuscript.

Funding: This study was supported by the funding from Ministry of Science and Technology (MOST 108-2320-B-040-024-MY3), Taiwan, and the cooperative project from Chung Shan Medical University and Changhua Christian Hospital (CSMU-CCH-112-04), Taiwan.

Institutional Review Board Statement: The animal study protocol was approved by the Institutional Animal Care and Use Committee of Chung Shan Medical University, Taiwan (approval number: 2136).

Informed Consent Statement: Not applicable.

Data Availability Statement: The data presented in this study are available upon request from the corresponding author.

Conflicts of Interest: The authors declare no conflicts of interest.

References

1. Danielson, M.L.; Bitsko, R.H.; Ghandour, R.M.; Holbrook, J.R.; Kogan, M.D.; Blumberg, S.J. Prevalence of parent-reported ADHD diagnosis and associated treatment among U.S. children and adolescents, 2016. *J. Clin. Child Adolesc. Psychol.* **2018**, *53*, 199–212. [CrossRef] [PubMed]
2. Tanaka, M.; Spekker, E.; Szabó, Á.; Polyák, H.; Vécsei, L. Modelling the neurodevelopmental pathogenesis in neuropsychiatric disorders. Bioactive kynurenines and their analogues as neuroprotective agents-in celebration of 80th birthday of Professor Peter Riederer. *J. Neural Transm.* **2022**, *129*, 627–642. [CrossRef] [PubMed]
3. Biederman, J.; Mick, E.; Faraone, S.V. Age-dependent decline of symptoms of attention deficit hyperactivity disorder: Impact of remission definition and symptom type. *Am. J. Psychiatry* **2000**, *157*, 816–818. [CrossRef]
4. Asherson, P.; IMAGE Consortium. Attention-Deficit Hyperactivity Disorder in the post-genomic era. *Eur. Child Adolesc. Psychiatry* **2004**, *13* (Suppl. S1), 150–170. [CrossRef]
5. Lee, R.C.; Feinbaum, R.L.; Ambros, V. The *C. elegans* heterochronic gene lin-4 encodes small RNAs with antisense complementarity to lin-14. *Cell* **1993**, *75*, 843–854. [CrossRef]
6. Wightman, B.; Ha, I.; Ruvkun, G. Posttranscriptional regulation of the heterochronic gene lin-14 by lin-4 mediates temporal pattern formation in *C. elegans*. *Cell* **1993**, *75*, 855–862. [CrossRef] [PubMed]
7. Li, S.C.; Chan, W.C.; Hu, L.Y.; Lai, C.H.; Hsu, C.N.; Lin, W.C. Identification of homologous microRNAs in 56 animal genomes. *Genomics* **2010**, *96*, 1–9. [CrossRef] [PubMed]
8. Friedlander, M.R.; Lizano, E.; Houben, A.J.; Bezdan, D.; Banez-Coronel, M.; Kudla, G.; Mateu-Huertas, E.; Kagerbauer, B.; González, J.; Chen, K.C.; et al. Evidence for the biogenesis of more than 1000 novel human microRNAs. *Genome Biol.* **2014**, *15*, R57. [CrossRef] [PubMed]
9. Forman, J.J.; Legesse-Miller, A.; Coller, H.A. A search for conserved sequences in coding regions reveals that the let-7 microRNA targets Dicer within its coding sequence. *Proc. Natl. Acad. Sci. USA* **2008**, *105*, 14879–14884. [CrossRef] [PubMed]
10. Dharap, A.; Pokrzywa, C.; Murali, S.; Pandi, G.; Vemuganti, R. MicroRNA miR-324-3p induces promoter-mediated expression of RelA gene. *PLoS ONE* **2013**, *8*, e79467. [CrossRef] [PubMed]
11. Juvale, I.I.A.; Che Has, A.T. The Potential Role of miRNAs as Predictive Biomarkers in Neurodevelopmental Disorders. *J. Mol. Neurosci.* **2021**, *71*, 1338–1355. [CrossRef] [PubMed]
12. Abdolahi, S.; Zare-Chahoki, A.; Noorbakhsh, F.; Gorji, A. A Review of Molecular Interplay between Neurotrophins and miRNAs in Neuropsychological Disorders. *Mol. Neurobiol.* **2022**, *59*, 6260–6280. [CrossRef] [PubMed]
13. Tanaka, M.; Szabó, Á.; Vécsei, L.; Giménez-Llort, L. Emerging Translational Research in Neurological and Psychiatric Diseases: From In Vitro to In Vivo Models. *Int. J. Mol. Sci.* **2023**, *24*, 15739. [CrossRef] [PubMed]
14. Zhu, P.; Pan, J.; Cai, Q.Q.; Zhang, F.; Peng, M.; Fan, X.L.; Ji, H.; Dong, Y.W.; Wu, X.Z.; Wu, L.H. MicroRNA profile as potential molecular signature for attention deficit hyperactivity disorder in children. *Biomarkers* **2022**, *27*, 230–239. [CrossRef]
15. Wang, L.J.; Kuo, H.C.; Lee, S.Y.; Huang, L.H.; Lin, Y.; Lin, P.H.; Li, S.C. MicroRNAs serve as prediction and treatment-response biomarkers of attention-deficit/hyperactivity disorder and promote the differentiation of neuronal cells by repressing the apoptosis pathway. *Transl. Psychiatry* **2022**, *12*, 67. [CrossRef] [PubMed]
16. Davison, A.N.; Kaczmarek, L.K. Taurine—A possible neurotransmitter? *Nature* **1971**, *234*, 107–108. [CrossRef]
17. Wu, J.Y.; Prentice, H. Role of taurine in the central nervous system. *J. Biomed. Sci.* **2010**, *17* (Suppl. S1), S1. [CrossRef]
18. Kumari, N.; Prentice, H.; Wu, J.Y. Taurine and its neuroprotective role. In *Taurine 8, 18th International Taurine Meeting, Marrakech, Morocco, 7–13 April 2012*; Advances in Experimental Medicine and Biology; Springer: New York, NY, USA, 2013; Volume 775, pp. 19–27. [CrossRef]
19. Jakaria, M.; Azam, S.; Haque, M.E.; Jo, S.H.; Uddin, M.S.; Kim, I.S.; Choi, D.K. Taurine and its analogs in neurological disorders: Focus on therapeutic potential and molecular mechanisms. *Redox Biol.* **2019**, *24*, 101223. [CrossRef]
20. Chung, M.C.; Malatesta, P.; Bosquesi, P.L.; Yamasaki, P.R.; Santos, J.L.; Vizioli, E.O. Advances in drug design based on the amino Acid approach: Taurine analogues for the treatment of CNS diseases. *Pharmaceuticals* **2012**, *5*, 1128–1146. [CrossRef] [PubMed]
21. De Luca, A.; Pierno, S.; Camerino, D.C. Taurine: The appeal of a safe amino acid for skeletal muscle disorders. *J. Transl. Med.* **2015**, *13*, 243. [CrossRef]
22. Ito, T.; Schaffer, S.; Azuma, J. The effect of taurine on chronic heart failure: Actions of taurine against catecholamine and angiotensin II. *Amino Acids.* **2014**, *46*, 111–119. [CrossRef] [PubMed]
23. Schaffer, S.; Kim, H.W. Effects and Mechanisms of Taurine as a Therapeutic Agent. *Biomol. Ther.* **2018**, *26*, 225–241. [CrossRef]

24. Malek Mahdavi, A.; Javadivala, Z. A systematic review of preclinical studies on the efficacy of taurine for the treatment of rheumatoid arthritis. *Amino Acids* **2021**, *53*, 783–800. [CrossRef] [PubMed]
25. Roşca, A.E.; Vlădăreanu, A.M.; Mirica, R.; Anghel-Timaru, C.M.; Mititelu, A.; Popescu, B.O.; Căruntu, C.; Voiculescu, S.E.; Gologan, Ş.; Onisâi, M.; et al. Taurine and Its Derivatives: Analysis of the Inhibitory Effect on Platelet Function and Their Antithrombotic Potential. *J. Clin. Med.* **2022**, *11*, 666. [CrossRef]
26. Kp, A.D.; Martin, A. Recent insights into the molecular regulators and mechanisms of taurine to modulate lipid metabolism: A review. *Crit. Rev. Food Sci. Nutr.* **2022**, *18*, 6005–6017. [CrossRef] [PubMed]
27. Surai, P.F.; Earle-Payne, K.; Kidd, M.T. Taurine as a Natural Antioxidant: From Direct Antioxidant Effects to Protective Action in Various Toxicological Models. *Antioxidants* **2021**, *10*, 1876. [CrossRef]
28. Jia, H.; Miyoshi, M.; Li, X.; Furukawa, K.; Otani, L.; Shirahige, K.; Miura, F.; Ito, T.; Kato, H. The Epigenetic Legacy of Maternal Protein Restriction: Renal Ptger1 DNA Methylation Changes in Hypertensive Rat Offspring. *Nutrients* **2023**, *15*, 3957. [CrossRef]
29. Sagvolden, T.; Russell, V.A.; Aase, H.; Johansen, E.B.; Farshbaf, M. Rodent models of attention-deficit/hyperactivitydisorder. *Biol. Psychiatry* **2005**, *57*, 1239–1247. [CrossRef]
30. Chen, V.C.; Hsu, T.C.; Chen, L.J.; Chou, H.C.; Weng, J.C.; Tzang, B.S. Effects of taurine on resting-state fMRI activity in spontaneously hypertensive rats. *PLoS ONE* **2017**, *12*, e0181122. [CrossRef]
31. Chen, V.C.; Chiu, C.C.; Chen, L.J.; Hsu, T.C.; Tzang, B.S. Effects of taurine on striatal dopamine transporter expression and dopamine uptake in SHR rats. *Behav. Brain Res.* **2018**, *348*, 219–226. [CrossRef]
32. Sim, M.S.; Soga, T.; Pandy, V.; Wu, Y.S.; Parhar, I.S.; Mohamed, Z. MicroRNA expression signature of methamphetamine use and addiction in the rat nucleus accumbens. *Metab. Brain Dis.* **2017**, *32*, 1767–1783. [CrossRef] [PubMed]
33. Hsu, H.W.; Rodriguez-Ortiz, C.J.; Lim, S.L.; Zumkehr, J.; Kilian, J.G.; Vidal, J.; Kitazawa, M. Copper-Induced Upregulation of MicroRNAs Directs the Suppression of Endothelial LRP1 in Alzheimer's Disease Model. *Toxicol. Sci.* **2019**, *170*, 144–156. [CrossRef]
34. Regan, S.L.; Williams, M.T.; Vorhees, C.V. Review of rodent models of attention deficit hyperactivity disorder. *Neurosci. Biobehav. Rev.* **2022**, *132*, 621–637. [CrossRef]
35. Dabrowska, S.; Andrzejewska, A.; Kozlowska, H.; Strzemecki, D.; Janowski, M.; Lukomska, B. Neuroinflammation evoked by brain injury in a rat model of lacunar infarct. *Exp. Neurol.* **2021**, *336*, 113531. [CrossRef] [PubMed]
36. Livak, K.J.; Schmittgen, T.D. Analysis of relative gene expression data using real-time quantitative PCR and the $2^{-\Delta\Delta CT}$ method. *Methods* **2001**, *25*, 402–408. [CrossRef]
37. Chou, Y.H.; Liu, Y.L.; Hsu, T.C.; Yow, J.L.; Tzang, B.S.; Chiang, W.H. Tumor acidity-responsive polymeric nanoparticles to promote intracellular delivery of zoledronic acid by PEG detachment and positive charge exposure for enhanced antitumor potency. *J. Mater. Chem. B* **2022**, *10*, 4363–4374. [CrossRef] [PubMed]
38. Katz, R.J.; Schmaltz, K. Dopaminergic involvement in attention. A novel animal model. *Prog. Neuropsychopharmacol.* **1980**, *4*, 585–590. [CrossRef]
39. Pasquinelli, A.E. MicroRNAs: Deviants no longer. *Trends Genet.* **2002**, *18*, 171–173. [CrossRef]
40. Miska, E.A. How microRNAs control cell division, differentiation and death. *Curr. Opin. Genet. Dev.* **2005**, *15*, 563–568. [CrossRef]
41. Iguchi, H.; Kosaka, N.; Ochiya, T. Versatile applications of microRNA in anti-cancer drug discovery: From therapeutics to biomarkers. *Curr. Drug Discov. Technol.* **2010**, *7*, 95–105. [CrossRef]
42. Long, J.M.; Lahiri, D.K. Advances in microRNA experimental approaches to study physiological regulation of gene products implicated in CNS disorders. *Exp. Neurol.* **2012**, *235*, 402–418. [CrossRef]
43. Gehrau, R.C.; Mas, V.R.; Maluf, D.G. Hepatic disease biomarkers and liver transplantation: What is the potential utility of microRNAs? *Expert. Rev. Gastroenterol. Hepatol.* **2013**, *7*, 157–170. [CrossRef]
44. Harris, V.K.; Sadiq, S.A. Biomarkers of therapeutic response in multiple sclerosis: Current status. *Mol. Diagn. Ther.* **2014**, *18*, 605–617. [CrossRef] [PubMed]
45. De Gonzalo-Calvo, D.; Vea, A.; Bär, C.; Fiedler, J.; Couch, L.S.; Brotons, C.; Llorente-Cortes, V.; Thum, T. Circulating non-coding RNAs in biomarker-guided cardiovascular therapy: A novel tool for personalized medicine? *Eur. Heart J.* **2019**, *40*, 1643–1650. [CrossRef] [PubMed]
46. Chen, S.; Tu, Y.; Yuan, H.; Shi, Z.; Guo, Y.; Gong, W.; Tu, S. Regulatory functions of miR-200b-3p in tumor development (Review). *Oncol. Rep.* **2022**, *47*, 96. [CrossRef]
47. Chen, W.; Jiang, W.; Dong, J.; Wang, J.; Wang, B. miR-200b-3p Induces the Formation of Insulin-Producing Cells from Umbilical Cord Mesenchymal Stem Cells by Targeting ZEB2. *Crit. Rev. Eukaryot. Gene Expr.* **2022**, *32*, 33–46. [CrossRef] [PubMed]
48. Zhang, Z.; He, C.; Bao, C.; Li, Z.; Jin, W.; Li, C.; Chen, Y. MiRNA Profiling and Its Potential Roles in Rapid Growth of Velvet Antler in Gansu Red Deer (*Cervus elaphus kansuensis*). *Genes* **2023**, *14*, 424. [CrossRef]
49. Liu, H.; Wang, X. MiR-200b-3p is upregulated in the placental tissues from patients with preeclampsia and promotes the development of preeclampsia via targeting profilin 2. *Cell Cycle* **2022**, *21*, 1945–1957. [CrossRef]
50. Huang, W.; Chen, J.; Xu, E.; Zhu, T.; Cai, X. KCNQ1OT1 mediates keratinocyte migration to promote skin wound healing through the miR-200b-3p/SERP1 axis. *Burns* **2022**, *49*, 415–424. [CrossRef]
51. Zheng, Y.L.; Su, X.; Chen, Y.M.; Guo, J.B.; Song, G.; Yang, Z.; Chen, P.J.; Wang, X.Q. microRNA-Based Network and Pathway Analysis for Neuropathic Pain in Rodent Models. *Front. Mol. Biosci.* **2022**, *8*, 780730. [CrossRef]

52. Florian, I.A.; Buruiana, A.; Timis, T.L.; Susman, S.; Florian, I.S.; Balasa, A.; Berindan-Neagoe, I. An Insight into the microRNAs Associated with Arteriovenous and Cavernous Malformations of the Brain. *Cells* **2021**, *10*, 1373. [CrossRef] [PubMed]
53. Zhang, N.; Yang, L.; Meng, L.; Cui, H. Inhibition of miR-200b-3p alleviates hypoxia-ischemic brain damage via targeting Slit2 in neonatal rats. *Biochem. Biophys. Res. Commun.* **2020**, *523*, 931–938. [CrossRef] [PubMed]
54. Lin, W.; Zhou, L.; Liu, M.; Zhang, D.; Yan, Y.; Chang, Y.F.; Zhang, X.; Xie, Q.; Luo, Q. gga-miR-200b-3p Promotes Macrophage Activation and Differentiation via Targeting Monocyte to Macrophage Differentiation-Associated in HD11 Cells. *Front. Immunol.* **2020**, *11*, 563143. [CrossRef] [PubMed]
55. Kozak, J.; Jonak, K.; Maciejewski, R. The function of miR-200 family in oxidative stress response evoked in cancer chemotherapy and radiotherapy. *Biomed. Pharmacother.* **2020**, *125*, 110037. [CrossRef]
56. Lin, Y.; Liu, X.; Cheng, Y.; Yang, J.; Huo, Y.; Zhang, C. Involvement of MicroRNAs in hydrogen peroxide-mediated gene regulation and cellular injury response in vascular smooth muscle cells. *J. Biol. Chem.* **2009**, *284*, 7903–7913. [CrossRef]
57. Kim, C.; Cha, Y.N. Taurine chloramine produced from taurine under inflammation provides anti-inflammatory and cytoprotective effects. *Amino Acids* **2014**, *46*, 89–100. [CrossRef]
58. Ng, H.M.; Ho, J.C.H.; Nong, W.; Hui, J.H.L.; Lai, K.P.; Wong, C.K.C. Genome-wide analysis of MicroRNA-messenger RNA interactome in ex-vivo gill filaments, *Anguilla japonica*. *BMC Genom.* **2020**, *21*, 208. [CrossRef]
59. Kofler, M.J.; Singh, L.J.; Soto, E.F.; Chan, E.S.M.; Miller, C.E.; Harmon, S.L.; Spiegel, J.A. Working memory and short-term memory deficits in ADHD: A bifactor modeling approach. *Neuropsychology* **2020**, *34*, 686–698. [CrossRef]
60. Meneses, A.; Perez-Garcia, G.; Ponce-Lopez, T.; Tellez, R.; Gallegos-Cari, A.; Castillo, C. Spontaneously hypertensive rat (SHR) as an animal model for ADHD: A short overview. *Rev. Neurosci.* **2011**, *22*, 365–371. [CrossRef]
61. Lee, W.S.; Yoon, B.E. Necessity of an Integrative Animal Model for a Comprehensive Study of Attention-Deficit/Hyperactivity Disorder. *Biomedicines* **2023**, *11*, 1260. [CrossRef]
62. Yoshida, M.; Watanabe, Y.; Yamanishi, K.; Yamashita, A.; Yamamoto, H.; Okuzaki, D.; Shimada, K.; Nojima, H.; Yasunaga, T.; Okamura, H.; et al. Analysis of genes causing hypertension and stroke in spontaneously hypertensive rats: Gene expression profiles in the brain. *Int. J. Mol. Med.* **2014**, *33*, 887–896. [CrossRef] [PubMed]
63. Arnsten, A.F. Toward a new understanding of attention-deficit hyperactivity disorder pathophysiology: An important role for prefrontal cortex dysfunction. *CNS Drugs* **2009**, *23*, 33–41. [CrossRef] [PubMed]
64. Womersley, J.S.; Dimatelis, J.J.; Russell, V.A. Proteomic analysis of maternal separation-induced striatal changes in a rat model of ADHD: The spontaneously hypertensive rat. *J. Neurosci. Methods* **2015**, *252*, 64–74. [CrossRef]
65. Rana, S.K.; Sanders, T.A.B. Taurine concentrations in the diet, plasma, urine and breast milk of vegans compared with omnivores. *Br. J. Nutr.* **1986**, *56*, 17–27. [CrossRef] [PubMed]
66. Purchas, R.W.; Rutherfurd, S.M.; Pearce, P.D.; Vather, R.; Wilkinson, B.H. Concentrations in beef and lamb of taurine, carnosine, coenzyme Q(10), and creatine. *Meat Sci.* **2004**, *66*, 629–637. [CrossRef] [PubMed]
67. Kontro, P. Interactions of taurine and dopamine in the striatum. In *The Biology of Taurine*; Advances in Experimental Medicine and Biology; Springer: Boston, MA, USA, 1987; Volume 217, pp. 347–355. [CrossRef]
68. Ahmadian, M.; Roshan, V.D.; Aslani, E.; Stannard, S.R. Taurine supplementation has anti-atherogenic and anti-inflammatory effects before and after incremental exercise in heart failure. *Ther. Adv. Cardiovasc. Dis.* **2017**, *11*, 185–194. [CrossRef]
69. Azuma, J.; Sawamura, A.; Awata, N.; Ohta, H.; Hamaguchi, T.; Harada, H.; Takihara, K.; Hasegawa, H.; Yamagami, T.; Ishiyama, T.; et al. Therapeutic effect of taurine in congestive heart failure: A double-blind crossover trial. *Clin. Cardiol.* **1985**, *8*, 276–282. [CrossRef] [PubMed]
70. Fujita, T.; Ando, K.; Noda, H.; Ito, Y.; Sato, Y. Effects of increased adrenomedullary activity and taurine in young patients with borderline hypertension. *Circulation* **1987**, *75*, 525–532. [CrossRef]
71. Durelli, L.; Mutani, R.; Fassio, F. The treatment of myotonia: Evaluation of chronic oral taurine therapy. *Neurology* **1983**, *33*, 599–603. [CrossRef]
72. Bergamini, L.; Mutani, R.; Delsedime, M.; Durelli, L. First clinical experience on the antiepileptic action of taurine. *Eur. Neurol.* **1974**, *11*, 261–269. [CrossRef]
73. Nair, A.B.; Jacob, S. A simple practice guide for dose conversion between animals and human. *J. Basic Clin. Pharm.* **2016**, *7*, 27–31. [CrossRef] [PubMed]
74. Saré, R.M.; Lemons, A.; Smith, C.B. Behavior Testing in Rodents: Highlighting Potential Confounds Affecting Variability and Reproducibility. *Brain Sci.* **2021**, *11*, 522. [CrossRef] [PubMed]
75. Améndola, L.; Weary, D.; Zobel, G. Effects of personality on assessments of anxiety and cognition. *Neurosci. Biobehav. Rev.* **2022**, *141*, 104827. [CrossRef]
76. Oenarto, J.; Karababa, A.; Castoldi, M.; Bidmon, H.J.; Görg, B.; Häussinger, D. Ammonia-induced miRNA expression changes in cultured rat astrocytes. *Sci. Rep.* **2016**, *6*, 18493. [CrossRef] [PubMed]
77. Shi, X.; Qiu, Z.; Inam-U-Llah; Zhang, M.; Li, K.; Wu, P.; Suleman, R.; Aadil, R.M.; Piao, F. The microRNAs Expression Profile in Sciatic Nerves of Diabetic Neuropathy Rats After Taurine Treatment by Sequencing. In *Taurine 11, Proceedings of the 21st International Taurine Meeting, Shenyang, China, 20–26 May 2018*; Advances in Experimental Medicine and Biology; Springer: Singapore, 2019; Volume 1155, pp. 935–947. [CrossRef]

78. Nabi, A.A.; Atta, S.A.; El-Ahwany, E.; Elzayat, E.; Saleh, H. Taurine Upregulates miRNA-122-5p Expression and Suppresses the Metabolizing Enzymes of Glycolytic Pathway in Hepatocellular Carcinoma. *Mol. Biol. Rep.* **2021**, *48*, 5549–5559. [CrossRef] [PubMed]
79. Li, L.; Lu, C.; Zhang, D.; Liu, H.; Cui, S. Taurine promotes estrogen synthesis by regulating microRNA-7a2 in mice ovarian granulosa cells. *Biochem. Biophys. Res. Commun.* **2022**, *626*, 129–134. [CrossRef]
80. Song, Q.; Guo, J.X.; Ma, Y.X.; Ou, T.; Zhang, J.; Li, H.Z.; Mi, S.Q.; Zhang, Y.Z.; Oda, H.; Chen, W. Taurine alleviated hepatic steatosis in oleic acid-treated-HepG2 cells and rats fed a high-fat diet. *Heliyon* **2023**, *9*, e16401. [CrossRef]
81. Grodzka, O.; Procyk, G.; Gąsecka, A. The Role of MicroRNAs in Myocarditis-What Can We Learn from Clinical Trials? *Int. J. Mol. Sci.* **2022**, *23*, 16022. [CrossRef]
82. Zhai, W.; Zhao, M.; Zhang, G.; Wang, Z.; Wei, C.; Sun, L. MicroRNA-Based Diagnosis and Therapeutics for Vascular Cognitive Impairment and Dementia. *Front. Neurol.* **2022**, *13*, 895316. [CrossRef]
83. Cools, R.; Froböse, M.; Aarts, E.; Hofmans, L. Dopamine and the motivation of cognitive control. *Handb. Clin. Neurol.* **2019**, *163*, 123–143. [CrossRef]

biomedicines

MDPI

Article

Cannabinoid and Serotonergic Systems: Unraveling the Pathogenetic Mechanisms of Stress-Induced Analgesia

Hristina Nocheva [1], Nikolay Stoynev [1], Vlayko Vodenicharov [2], Dimo Krastev [3], Nikolay Krastev [4] and Milka Mileva [5,*]

1 Department of Physiology and Pathophysiology, Medical Faculty, Medical University, 2 Zdrave Str., 1431 Sofia, Bulgaria; hndimitrova@medfac.mu-sofia.bg (H.N.); nstoynev@medfac.mu-sofia.bg (N.S.)
2 Department of Epidemiology and Hygiene, Medical Faculty, Medical University, 2 Zdrave Str., 1431 Sofia, Bulgaria; v.vodenicharov@medfac.mu-sofia.bg
3 Department of Anatomy and Physiology, South-West University "Neofit Rilski", Blagoevgrad, 66, Ivan Mihaylov Str., 2700 Blagoevgrad, Bulgaria; dimo_krustev@mail.bg
4 Department of Anatomy, Faculty of Medicine, Medical University, 2, Zdrave Str., 1431 Sofia, Bulgaria; dr.krustev.dm@gmail.com
5 Institute of Microbiology "Stephan Angeloff", Bulgarian Academy of Sciences, 26, Acad. Georgi Bonchev Str., 1113 Sofia, Bulgaria
* Correspondence: milkamileva@gmail.com

Abstract: The perception of „stress" triggers many physiological and behavioral responses, collectively called the stress response. Such a complex process allows for coping with stress and also triggers severe pathology. Because of the multidirectional effect of stress on the body, multiple systems participate in its pathogenesis, with the endogenous cannabinoid and the serotoninergic ones among them. These two systems also take part in the pain perception decrease, known as stress-induced analgesia (SIA), which can then be taken as an indirect indicator of the stress response. The aim of our study was to study the changes in cold SIA (c-SIA) resulting from the exogenous activation of cannabinoid receptor type 1 (CB1) and 5-hydroxytryptamine (5-HT, serotonin) receptor type 1_A (5-HT1A). Various combinations of agonists and/or antagonists of CB1 and 5-HT1A, before or after 1 h of cold exposure, were applied, since we presumed that the exogenous activation of the receptors before the cold exposure would influence the pathogenesis of the stress response, while their activation after the stressful trigger would influence the later development. Our results show that the serotonergic system "maintained" c-SIA in the pre-stress treatment, while the cannabinoids' modulative effect was more prominent in the post-stress treatment. Here, we show the interactions of the two systems in the stress response. The interpretation and understanding of the mechanisms of interaction between CB1 and 5-HT1A may provide information for the prevention and control of adverse stress effects, as well as suggest interesting directions for the development of targeted interventions for the control of specific body responses.

Keywords: pain perception; cannabinoid receptor CB1; 5-HT receptor 1A; cold stress-induced analgesia; stress-response

1. Introduction

As things have become increasingly complex and hectic, stress seems to be a ubiquitous aspect of life. Confrontation with adverse circumstances, perceived as „stress", triggers in both humans and animals a cascade of intricate physiological and behavioral responses, collectively referred to as the stress response. At the heart of such a response, a range of coordinated events orchestrates a network of afferent and efferent projections, starting with the activation of the autonomic nervous system (ANS) and the hypothalamic-pituitary–adrenal (HPA) axis, and culminating in the release of glucocorticoids from the adrenal cortex. The ANS is responsible for the immediate reactions to the stressor—the activation of the sympathetic nervous system underlines the "fight or flight" response, enabling the body to defend itself, while the parasympathetic nervous system aims at restoring the balance when the stressor has been answered. The hypothalamus is a crucial player, acting as a central coordinator of the stress response. The activation of the HPA finally leads to cortisol release, which exerts widespread effects on metabolism, immune function, and inflammation. Stress changes the biochemistry of the brain, involving other specific areas, such as the limbic system and brainstem nuclei. Glucocorticoid feedback along the HPA axis is regulated at the level of the hypothalamus by a diverse group of afferent and efferent projections to the limbic lobe of the brain, brainstem nuclei, and projections along the spinal cord [1].

The main evolutionary purpose of the stress response is to provide an opportunity for the organism to optimally cope with a specific adverse situation, increasing its adaptation and the chance to survive. But this complex process, driving the homeostasis to a thoroughly different level, can also trigger specific (stress-)induced pathology [2,3]. A complex series of biochemical reactions disrupt the body's homeostasis leading to changes in behavioral responses. A growing number of studies in this direction indicate that a stressful lifestyle (acute or chronic exposure to stress) is associated with increased arterial pressure, endothelial dysfunction, disturbances in the lipid profile, and metabolic deviations, which in turn are the basis of significant social pathology: leading causes of mortality (such as cardiovascular disease, diabetes, cancer), decreasing quality of life (obesity), or other unfavorable consequences (reproductive problems).

Given the negative consequences of stress, many studies have tried to reveal its underlying pathogenetic mechanisms. Understanding the molecular mechanisms of the stress response is crucial since that would make it possible to determine specific practical approaches and strategies to limit or at least mitigate the pathological effects. The difficulty in studying stress is largely related to the subjective nature of the experience. The perception of a specific situation such as „stress" by the specific individual depends on factors such as attitude, value system, motivation, and others, which can hardly be objective; the individual perception of the predictability and controllability of the stressful situation also plays a role [4]. In order to track the influence of specific impacts on the stress-reaction, the use of an objective indicator is required that can be relatively easily measured and serve to objectify changes over time. During the stress response, many physiological parameters of the organism change with the aim of optimal adaptation to the specific situation, adequate response, and the possibility of survival. In this context, the perception of pain, which is basically defined as protective (since it includes reflexes aimed at preserving the health and life of the individual), in the specifics of the stress response, appears unfavorable. A kind of paradox arises—pain perception would limit the organism's ability to overcome stress. Therefore, it seems logical that pain perception decreases during the stressful situation, thus eliminating its paralyzing effect on the body.

The first information about the decrease in pain perception in stressful situations was provided by Beecher, who observed wounded soldiers during the World War II. He noted that wounds, which under other circumstances were felt as very painful, caused a weak sensation of pain [5–7]. In fact, this built-in mammalian pain-suppressing response has a defensive purpose—making it possible to focus more effectively on the stressful (fearful) stimulus, thus better coping with the stress [8]. SIA is a complex process, although endogenous opioids play a key role in mediating endogenous analgesia [9], several mediating systems have also been proved to be involved [10]. As for the anatomical substrate of SIA, some subcortical areas, such as the periaqueductal gray, the amygdala, and the rostral ventromedial medulla, seem critical for the descending inhibitory pain pathways [10–12]. The dependence of SIA on stress itself allows an increase in the pain threshold during the stress-dominated period to be taken as a relatively objective indicator of the body's stress reaction.

Given the multidirectional effect of stress on the body, multiple systems are implicated in its pathogenesis, and one in particular has been demonstrated to participate in the mechanism of SIA [13]. In recent decades, the endocannabinoid system (ECS) has been the focus of many studies due to its participation in both physiological and pathophysiological reactions [14,15]. The ECS is a neuromodulatory system consisting of (i) a complex network of G-protein-coupled cannabinoid receptors type 1 (CB1) and 2 (CB2) [15], widely distributed in the central and peripheral nervous systems [16]; (ii) their endogenous ligands—endocannabinoids: anandamide (N-arachidonoyl ethanolamine, AEA) and 2-arachidonylglycerol (2-AG); and (iii) an enzyme system engaged in their biosynthesis and subsequent metabolisms [15]. However, there may also be additional "players" such as the transient receptor potential vanilloid 1 (TRPV1) [17] and several putative CB1 receptor antagonist peptides [15]. The cannabinoid CB1 receptors are highly expressed in several limbic brain regions (i.e., hippocampus, amygdala, prefrontal cortex), and involved in the HPA axis [18,19] and adrenal gland regulation [20]. The CB2 receptors have been detected in glial cells, and, to a much lesser extent, in neurons of several brain regions such as the amygdala, hippocampus, cerebral cortex, hypothalamus, and cerebellum [21,22]. For the moment, the overall evidence indicates the pivotal role of CB1, and not CB2, in HPA axis regulation following stress exposure [23,24].

As a lipid signaling system whose components are expressed widely across the body, the ECS plays a key role in the regulation of a wide array of physiological processes including metabolism, mood, motor function, appetite, cardiovascular control, gastrointestinal tract function, developmental biology, cell fate, immune and inflammatory response, endocrine function, neurotransmission, and pain [25]. It appears that the ECS plays an important role in the regulation of stress-related behavior [26], with its role appearing to be aimed at modulating the stress-response in order to "spare" the organism. The system continues to be the focus of many studies in the attempt to "rehabilitate" exogenous cannabinoids and enable their wider use given their many positive effects on the body. Research mostly focuses on several directions: (a) evaluating the pharmacology of cannabinoids and endocannabinoid system modulators; (b) evaluating cannabinoids' effects in different animal models of pathological or injury-related persistent pain; (c) describing the pharmacokinetics of cannabinoids in humans. Some cannabis-based medicines (CBMs) have proven to be efficient in reducing chronic pain [27,28]. In addition to pain, the therapeutic use of cannabis reduces stress, distress, and anxiety in both experimental animals and humans [29]. The results from animal studies have shown that the pharmacological blockade of CB1 receptors alters stress-induced behavior [30,31] and models conditioned fear responses [32]. The pharmacological enhancement of ECS signaling, by the blockade of endocannabinoids' metabolism and/or uptake, reduces stress-related behavior and facilitates the extinction of stress-conditioned responses [33]. At the same time, proof exists that the chronic use of cannabis has the opposite effect, leading to an increase in mental and somatic symptoms, including anxiety and panic attacks [29,34]. It is the observed adverse side effects that fuel the reserves of the ECS's opponents.

In the last decade, our team has also focused on the ECS during stress. It is not the only system involved in the stress response: behavioral responses to stress are similar in humans and animals, and this complex response includes different neurotransmitters—catecholamines, serotonin, dopamine, dynorphin, 5-HT, acetylcholine, nitric oxide, and, of course, endocannabinoids [2]. This encouraged us to evaluate the interactions of ECS with other mediator systems—adrenergic [35] and nitric oxide [36], as well as the joint effects of cannabinoids with the Tyr-MIF-1 family of peptides [37]. Our observations substantiated the need for further investigation into ECS signaling under various stressogens, and ECS's interrelation with the serotonergic system seemed to be a promising candidate [38,39].

Serotonin (5-hydroxytryptamine, 5-HT) is one of the key neurotransmitters involved in a wide variety of behavioral and cognitive responses. 5-HT-releasing neurons are vastly distributed in the central nervous system, which is the primary target of nociceptive information. Such neurons can regenerate and their activation under various stressful conditions is associated with depression, anxiety, and cognitive impairment. Serotonin is released in association with pain-related behaviors, manifesting both pro- and antinociceptive effects [40–42].

The investigations of Marks et coauthors (2009), as well as Chae et al. (2020), also support the theory of the interaction between cannabinoid and serotonergic systems in the brain [43–45]. Additionally, there are shreds of evidence indicating that interplays between the two systems are also involved in the stress-response development [46]. SIA is a relatively easy indicator to be determined. On the other hand, it could be used to objectify the stress response, as numerous studies show the relationship between the two of them. In this regard, there is evidence that certain parameters' changes during stress invariably and specifically affect pain sensitivity and, accordingly, cause SIA—e.g., the increase in endogenous opioid levels [47], the activation of the sympathetic nervous system [48], or the potentiation of the descending control of spinal nociception [49]. Taking the level of SIA as an indirect indicator of the degree of the stress response, we decided to evaluate the changes in the pain thresholds of rats exposed to one hour of cold environment.

The healing effects of cold on the body were already known to the ancient Egyptians and Greeks. They used cold water immersion to treat various ailments and pain symptoms [50].

In modern clinical practice for pain reduction, cryotherapy is a widely used modality for pain relief, which is practiced in a wide range of medical fields and produces analgesic effects. Specialist clinicians classify it as the so-called non-pharmacological approaches to achieve pain control and an analgesic effect in which the threshold of pain sensitivity is increased [51,52].

In a previous study of our team, we evaluated the effects of cannabinoids and the nitric oxide-ergic system on the modulation of stress response before and after restraint stress—the results showed interesting differences in the effect of cannabinoid-nitric oxide interaction on restraint-SIA before and after stress [53]. Such findings encouraged us to hypothesize that exogenous factors would have different effects if administered before or after the stressful impact: in the first case they would be involved in the pathogenesis of the stress reaction, while in the second in its modulation. On the other hand, both the endogenous cannabinoid and the serotonergic systems are known to be involved in the body's stress-response but also take part in SIA. Acute stress has been proved to exert an analgesic effect by activating the serotonergic system [54]; 2-arachidonoylglycerol and anandamide increase in the midbrain after acute stress has been demonstrated, pointing at an endocannabinoid mechanism involved in stress-induced analgesia [13]. Considering the evidence for the involvement of the two systems in the stress response and the development of cold SIA, in the present study, we aimed to investigate the interaction between cannabinoids and the serotoninergic system through the exogenous activation of cannabinoid receptor type 1 (CB1) and 5-hydroxytryptamine (5-HT, serotonin) receptor type 1A (5-HT1A). To further refine the involvement of each of the systems in the reported effects, we provided additional treatments with the appropriate antagonists of both receptor types. The analysis of the combined results of the agonists' effect, on the one hand, compared with the results obtained after antagonizing one receptor type with the simultaneous activation of the other, on the other hand, would allow us to better specify the importance of each of the systems for their joint effect.

The benefit of research on the mechanisms of stress can be seen in several directions. To begin with the medical and psychological influences of post-traumatic disorders, depressive, anxiety disorders, etc., preventive strategies could also be developed based on interventions to mitigate stress impact. Specifically, regarding the ECS, investigating its involvement in the stress response and the potential benefits of its activation or suppression may provide interesting directions for the development of targeted interventions and medications that modulate specific body responses.

2. Materials and Methods

2.1. General Study Design

The aim of this study was to determine the joint effect of the cannabinoid and the serotonergic systems on cold SIA. The effect of both systems was followed by administration of cannabinoid (CB1) and serotonin (5-HT1A) receptor agonists before and after one hour of cold stress.

Further clarification of the degree of involvement of each of the systems in the reported effect was achieved by injecting the animals with combinations of an agonist of one receptor and an antagonist of the other, again before and after the stressogenic impact.

Cold stress method has been described long ago, and among the first to use it were E. Zeisberger [55] and Z. Wiesenfeld and R. G. Hallin in 1981 [56]. The method has evolved into cold water immersion, cold water swim, repetitive cold stress, chronic cold stress. In our experiments, we aimed to induce not cold stress itself but cold stress-induced analgesia, and for such purposes, we needed an acute stress method. It should also be a stress method that is easy to induce and is effective at the same time to activate the HPA axis without causing permanent physical or psychological disorders in the experimental animals. Our previous experiments [36,57] showed that one hour of cold environment (4 °C) exposure provoked stress analgesia—experimental animals' paw pressure thresholds were statistically higher than control animals' ones. In addition, substantial studies have confirmed the effects of cold stress on memory and behavior, as well as its implication in some cognitive changes and anxiety disorders [58].

To determine analgesia, we chose the Randal Selitto Paw Pressure test method—it allows repeated determination of the pain threshold without negative consequences for the experimental animals, as well as without causing significant discomfort, which makes it suitable according to the ethical criteria for working with laboratory animals [59].

2.2. Animals

Adult male Wistar rats, 250–300 g body weight (BW), were kept in plastic cages under a 12 h light:12 h darkness cycle (light onset at 08.00 h), at 24 ± 1 °C; a standard diet and tap water were available ad libitum [60]. All experimental protocols (regarding the number of animals in the experimental groups and the respective treatments) were approved by our institutional animal care committee—the Bulgarian Food Safety Association (BFSA)—Permission Protocol № 314/06.10.2021.

2.3. Methodology

Since we hypothesized that the interaction between CB1- and 5HTA1-agonists could have a different outcome if the receptors were activated before or after the stressful impact, the animals were treated with a combination of CB1- and 5-HT1A-agonists before or after cold environment exposure. An eventual decrease in pain thresholds would point to an anti-stress effect, while the increase in the pain thresholds should be regarded as an indicator of increased activity in the body's stress systems.

In the pre-stress experimental set-up, the measurement of pain thresholds began 10 min after the end of the cold exposure.

In the post-stress experimental set-up, the measurement of pain thresholds started 10 min after the injection of the substances.

2.4. Experimental Groups

Group 1 (Controls)—the animals (n = 8) in this group were injected with 1 mL of saline;

Group 2 (AEA+DPAT+1 h CS)—the animals (n = 8) in this group were injected with CB1-agonist (anandamide, AEA) and 5-HT1A- receptors' agonist (8-Hydroxy-DPAT hydrobromide, DPAT) BEFORE being subjected to 1 h of cold stress;

Group 3 (1 h CS+AEA+DPAT)—the animals (n = 8) in this group were injected with agonists of both receptors (AEA and DPAT) AFTER being subjected to 1 h of cold stress;

Group 4 (AEA+NAN+1 h CS)—the animals ($n = 8$) in this group were injected with CB1 receptors' agonist AEA and 5-HT1A receptors' antagonist (NAN-190 hydrobromide, NAN) BEFORE being subjected to 1 h of cold stress;

Group 5 (1 h CS+AEA+NAN)—the animals ($n = 8$) in this group were injected with CB1 receptors' agonist AEA and 5-HT1A receptors' antagonist NAN AFTER being subjected to 1-h of cold stress;

Group 6 (DPAT+AM+1 h CS)—the animals ($n = 8$) in this group were injected with the 5-HT1A receptors' agonist DPAT and CB1 receptor's antagonist AM251 BEFORE being subjected to 1 h of cold stress;

Group 7 (1 h CS+DPAT+AM)—the animals ($n = 8$) in this group were injected with of the 5-HT1A receptors' agonist DPAT and CB1 receptors' antagonist AM251 AFTER being subjected to 1 h of cold stress.

2.5. Acute Model of Cold Stress

Acute cold stress was induced by placing the animals at a low environmental temperature (4 °C) for 1 h. During the time of cold exposure, no food and water were allowed; the rats could move freely, allocated in individual cages without sawdust.

2.6. Drugs

All the drugs were purchased from Sigma (Sigma Chem. Co., St. Louis, MO, USA). The CB1-agonist N-arachidonoyl-ethanolamine (AEA, 1 mg/kg BW); the CB1-antagonist N-(Piperidin-1-yl)-5-(4-iodophenyl)-1-(2,4-dichlorophenyl)-4-methyl-1H-pyrazole-3-carboxamide (AM251, 1.25 mg/kg BW); the 5HT1A-agonist (R)-(+)-8-Hydroxy-DPAT hydrobromide (DPAT, 1 mg/kg BW); and the 5HT1A-antagonist NAN-190 hydrobromide (NAN, 1 mg/kg BW), dissolved in vehicle [61,62] were intraperitoneally administered in different combinations before or after stress exposure.

2.7. Nociceptive Test

Paw-pressure test (PP; Randall–Selitto test): The changes in the mechanical nociceptive thresholds of the rats were measured using an analgesimeter (Ugo Basile, Gemonio, Italy). The pressure was applied to the rat hind-paw and the pressure required for eliciting a nociceptive response, such as a squeak or struggle, was taken as the mechanical nociceptive threshold (paw-pressure thresholds, PPT—represented in arbitrary units, AU, according to the scale of the analgesimeter). A cut-off value of 500 g was observed to prevent damage in the paw [63].

2.8. Statistical Analysis

Results were statistically assessed using a General Linear Model for repeated measures (mixed model ANOVA), and one-way analysis of variance (ANOVA at each time point followed by Newman–Keuls post hoc comparison test. Values were presented as mean ± S.E.M and $p < 0.05$ was considered to indicate statistical significance.

3. Results

In the present study, we investigated the interaction between exogenously administered cannabinoid (AEA) and serotonin receptor (DPAT) agonists, and their joint effect on cold stress-induced analgesia, determined by measuring the paw pressure threshold (PPT).

The co-administration of the substances was before or after exposure of the experimental animals to one-hour of cold (4 °C).

3.1. Antinociceptive Effect of AEA and DPAT before and after 1 h of Cold Exposure

For our experiment, we chose the doses as follows: the CB1-agonist N-arachidonoylethanolamine (anandamide, AEA, 1 mg/kg BW); the CB1-antagonist N-(Piperidin-1-yl)-5-(4-iodophenyl)-1-(2,4-chlorophenyl)-4-methyl-1H-pyrazole-3-carboxamide (AM251, 1.25 mg/kg BW); the 5HT1A-agonist (R)-(+)-8-Hydroxy-DPAT hydrobromide (DPAT, 1 mg/kg BW);

and the 5HT1A-antagonist NAN-190 hydrobromide (NAN, 1 mg/kg BW), dissolved in the vehicle.

Figure 1 shows the paw pressure thresholds (PPT) of the experimental animals after 1 h of exposure at 4 °C (1 h of cold stress, 1 h CS). In the 1h CS group, we observed an increase in PPT values compared with those of the control animals. One-way ANOVA showed a significant effect—*p*-values were <0.00001 (F = 2749.61972 on the 10th min; F = 1375.5814 on the 20th min; F = 1962.33333 on the 30th min; F = 2373.71795 on the 40th min) for the whole time estimated (Figure 1).

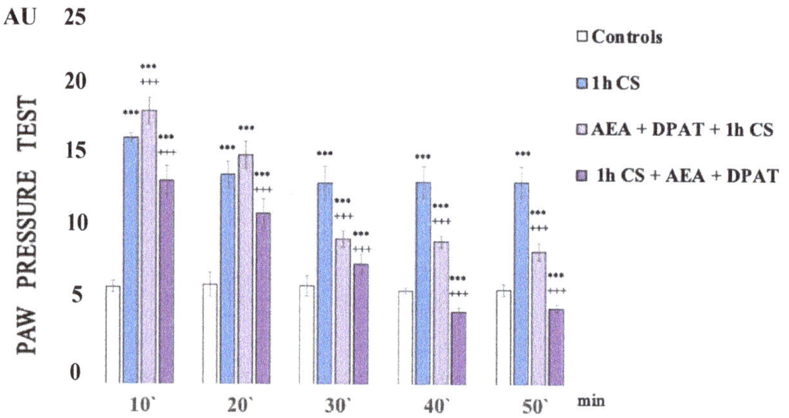

Figure 1. Effect on cold-SIA after administration of CB1 agonist (anandamide, AEA) and 5HT1A-agonist DPAT before or after stress exposure. Pain thresholds are presented as mean values ± S.E.M. in arbitrary units (AU). *** $p < 0.001$, vs. controls; +++ $p < 0.001$. AEA—exogenously administered anandamide; DPAT—5-HT1A-agonist; 1 h CS—1 h of cold stress.

At the very beginning of the experiments, the control values of the pain thresholds were determined using the paw pressure method (our long-term practice shows that, if we work with properly handled animals, there is no statistically significant difference between the paw pressure thresholds, PPT, of animals injected with a physiological solution and intact animals).

One hour of cold exposure (1 h of cold stress, 1 h CS) produced a sustained and statistically significant increase in paw pressure thresholds (PPT) in the experimental group compared with the control one. The results of the experiments were analyzed using one-way ANOVA.

A statistically relevant potentiation of cold-SIA (c-SIA) was observed at the 10th min after AEA and DPAT pretreatment (p = 000021, F = 38.98676), while a decrease in PPT followed the administration of the same combination (AEA+DPAT) after stress exposure (Figure 1).

3.2. *Effects of Agonist/Antagonist Co-Administration before and after Cold Exposure on Cold-SIA*

To better elucidate the contribution of each of the two systems to the effects described, we chose an approach in which each one of the agonists was co-administered with the antagonist of the other receptor.

The administration of the CB1 agonist AEA together with the 5HT1A-antagonist NAN before exposure to stress completely abolished the development of c-SIA. The obtained results showed that the PPT of the experimental animals were similar to the controls and even showed a tendency towards hyperalgesia at the 50th minute of the experiment (AEA+NAN+1 h CS, Figure 2A).

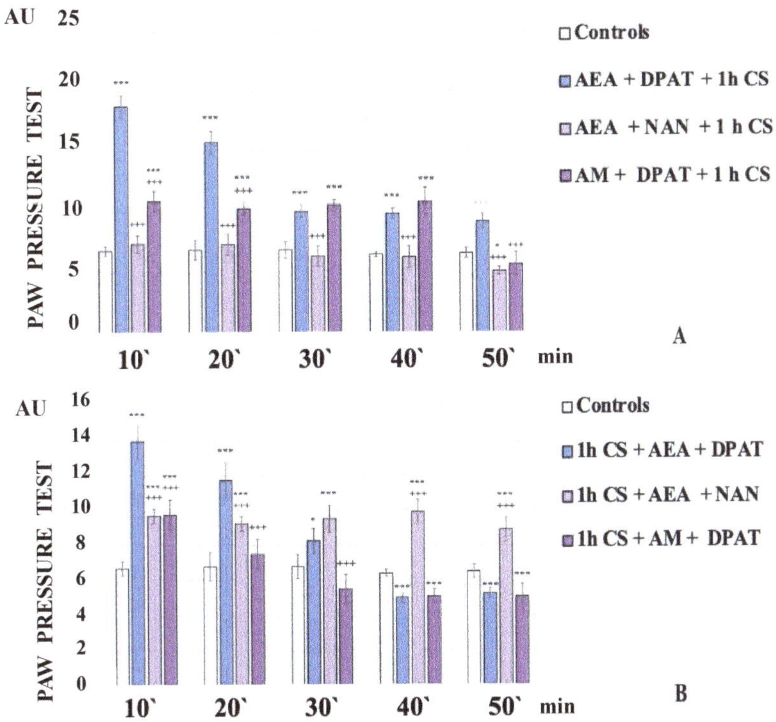

Figure 2. CB1- or 5HT1A-antagonization before (**A**) and after (**B**) stress exposure—effect on 1 h cold-SIA. Pain thresholds are presented as mean values ± S.E.M. in arbitrary units (AU). *** $p < 0.001$, * $p < 0.05$ vs. controls; +++ $p < 0.001$ vs. AEA+DPAT+1 h CS (**A**)/1 h CS+AEA+DPAT (**B**). AEA—exogenously administered anandamide; DPAT—5-HT1A-agonist; NAN—5-HT1A-antagonist; AM—CB1-antagonist; 1 h CS—1 h of cold stress.

AEA+NAN-administration after 1 h CS led to a constant level of c-SIA. The PPT of 1 h CS+AEA+NAN-animals were lower than the 1 h CS+AEA+DPAT-animals' ones at the 10th and 20th min but they exceeded them from the 30th min until the 50th min of the experiment (Figure 2B).

The administration of 5HT1A-agonist DPAT along with the CB1-antagonist AM251 before stress exposure led to a constant level of c-SIA for the first 40 min, followed by a brisk decrease at the 50th min of the experiment. The PPT of AM+DPAT+1 h CS-animals were lower than AEA+DPAT+1 h CS-animals' ones at the 10th and 20th min, while at the 30th and 40th min, they were comparable to them (Figure 2A).

AM+DPAT-administration after 1 h CS decreased PPT at the 10th min compared with 1 h CS+AEA+DPAT-animals' ones, with no c-SIA detected at the 20th min, and a tendency toward hyperalgesia from the 30th min to the end of the experiment (1 h CS+AM+DPAT, Figure 2B).

The analysis of the data obtained from the different experimental setups allowed us to confirm our hypothesis about the joint effect of the exogenous activation of the cannabinoid and serotonergic systems. The results obtained pointed that the two systems impacted on c-SIA, decreasing it, but they participated differently in the pathogenesis of the stress reaction and in the modulation of an already activated stress response of the body. In a more general context, the results should be considered in terms of the individual and joint importance of the systems in the body's stress response, pain perception, and the possibility of including them in therapeutic schemes approfittating of their positive influence.

4. Discussion

The exogenous manipulation of cannabinoid and serotonin receptors by means of agonists and antagonists allowed us to draw different conclusions regarding the joint effect of the two systems on c-SIA.

In first place, cold exposure led to statistically higher PPT in experimental animals compared with control ones, allowing us to conclude that stress-analgesia was induced. The results were concordant with the literature data about cold stress as a factor inducing stress analgesia, including our previous findings [36,64].

In second place, we found that the exogenous administration of CB1- and 5HT1A-agonists together, before or after stress, generally influenced c-SIA in rats, and the changes in PPTs differed before and after stress exposure. Our findings are summarized in Table 1, and additionally illustrated in Figure 3.

Table 1. Summarizes the most important points of the results.

	Before 1 h Cold Stress	After 1 h Cold Stress
AEA+DPAT	• transient potentiating of c-SIA on the 10th min; • tendency to decrease c-SIA after the 10th min; • stable level of c-SIA from the 30th min until the end of the time estimated.	• tendency to decrease c-SIA from the 10th min; • control values are reached soon after the 30th min; • tendency to hyperalgesia on 40th min until the end of the experiment.
AEA+NAN	• total abolishment of c-SIA	• time-constant c-SIA
AM+DPAT	• stable level of c-SIA	• reduced c-SIA to the control values after the 20th min

AEA—exogenously administered anandamide; DPAT—5-HT1A-agonist; NAN—5-HT1A-antagonist; AM—CB1-antagonist.

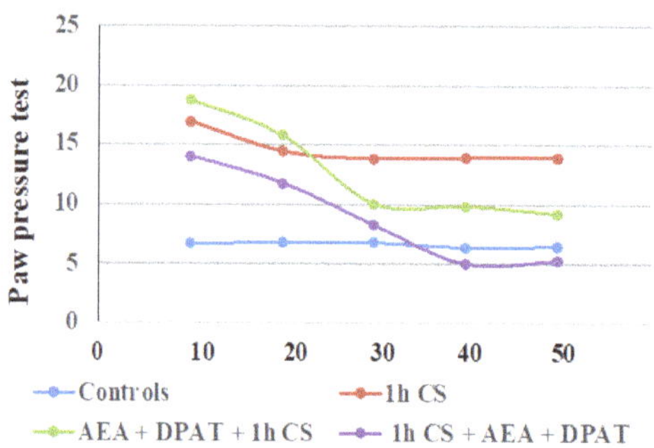

Figure 3. Effect on cold-SIA after administration of CB1 agonist (AEA) and 5HT1A-agonist DPAT before or after stress exposure—the results are presented as tendencies over time. AEA—exogenously administered cannabinoid; DPAT—5HT1A-agonist; AM—CB1-antagonist, CS—1 h of cold stress.

The results are consistent with the literature data on the involvement of ECS in analgesia. At the supraspinal level, cannabinoids have been proved to exert analgesic action in the periaqueductal gray [65,66], the thalamus [67], the rostral ventromedial medulla [68,69], and the amygdala [32,70]. Cannabinoids suppress behavioral responses to noxious stimulation and decrease nociceptive processing through the activation of cannabinoid CB1 and CB2 receptor subtypes [71]. At the spinal level, an endocannabinoid modulative effect on nociception has been documented in behavioral [72,73], electrophysiological [74–76], and neurochemical [77,78] studies. The endocannabinoid analgesic effect has also been proved at the peripheral level in several animal models [79–81]. Such multi-level involvement of the ECS in the mechanisms of analgesia probably accounts for the observed maintenance of some level of analgesia until the end of the follow-up period in the pre-treatment trials. The effects from cannabinoids and serotonin agonists' administration before cold exposure imply that the corresponding receptors participate in a specific way in the mechanisms of development (i.e., in the pathogenesis) of the body's stress response. Since we assume that the changes in the PPTs of animals exposed to stress, compared with those of animals without stress (controls), are an indirect indicator of the level of the stress-reaction of the organism, we could conclude that the exogenous administration of both agonists modulates the stress-response with an initial activation followed by a moderate decrease in activity. The results also support the idea that the serotonergic system is relatively more important than the ECS in "maintaining" c-SIA in pre-treated animals, while in the case of post-treatment, analgesia depends, to a relatively higher degree, on the activity of the cannabinoid system. Our conclusions have been additionally illustrated in Figure 4A,B.

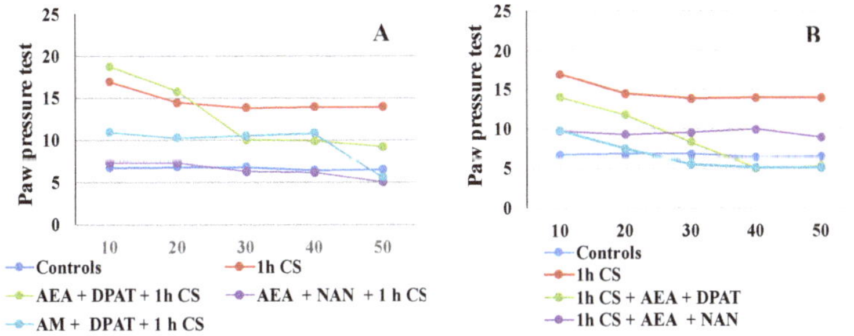

Figure 4. CB1- or 5HT1A-antagonization before (**A**) and after (**B**) cold stress exposure and effect on 1 h cold-SIA—the results are presented as tendencies over time. AEA—exogenously administered anandamide; DPA—5-HT1A-agonist; NAN—5-HT1A-antagonist; AM—CB1-antagonist, 1 h CS—1 h of cold stress.

The statistically significant decrease in c-SIA level described in our study after the exogenous administration of both cannabinoid- and 5-HT1A-receptors' agonists after the stressor, could be explained by the endocannabinoids' modulation of the neuroendocrine function through the HPA axis [82]. The decrease in its activity is probably important for the better adaptation and survival of animals when exposed to stressful stimuli. In the conditions where the experimental animals have already been exposed to cold, and therefore c-SIA has already been induced, the subsequent introduction of the combination of cannabinoid and serotonin receptors' agonists suggests that the interaction between both receptors modulates c-SIA—decreasing it, but not thoroughly abolishing it.

Our results indicate that the interaction between the two systems has opposing effects before and after the stressogenic impact. Moreover, the activation of serotonin receptors prior to stress appears to be a necessary condition for the onset of c- SIA as well as its duration, thus the interaction follows the "all or nothing" principle. Conversely, once c-SIA has already been induced, antagonizing the 5HTA1-receptors contributes to its duration. Our research shows that interactions between mediator systems differ in non-stress and post-stress conditions, and the outcome of these different interactions differentially affects the stress response itself. It is logical to expect that not only the systems we have investigated are subject to different relationships, but as are all other mediator systems. This suggests that the prophylactic and therapeutic protocols of influencing the stress-response, resp. stress-induced pathology, should take such differences into account. On the other hand, from the obtained results, and in particular from the overtime tendencies illustrated in Figures 3 and 4, it can be seen that the effect of the interactions between the systems varies over time. This is logical, insofar as the timely and effective activation of stress-response mechanisms favors adaptation, but at the same time, their timely shutdown favors the restoration of balance and homeostasis. Such logic supports the multidirectional effect we have demonstrated of the interaction between endocannabinoids and the serotonin system.

A known limitation in the interpretation of the in vivo effects described above is the lack of indications about specific changes in receptors' expression. In a previous study, we performed an in vivo determination of the analgesic activity of administered substances coupled with the in vitro immunohistochemical determination of the expression of cannabinoid receptors. Interesting data were obtained on changes in the CB1 receptors' expression in rat brainstem after the introduction of cannabinoids and peptides of the Tyr-MIF-1 family against a background of heat stress. The parallel reporting of in vivo effects and specific in vitro changes in the expression of a given receptor would enable more precise conclusions regarding the role of the receptor, and the mediator system, respectively, for the observed effects. It would be interesting to track possible receptor changes (up-/downregulation, conformation shifts, etc.) under conditions of chronic (cold or other type of) stress. Furthermore, since receptors' affinity is also important for the obtained effects, the determination of specific changes could enable a more thorough and detailed interpretation of the in vivo results.

Our research involves mainly acute trials. In the longer term, it would be interesting to follow up on the in vivo effect of exposing the animals to chronic stress. Various chronic stress setups have been described in the literature, and we also have some as yet unpublished data from the exposure of animals to repetitive swimming stress. Our preliminary results are concordant with the literature data that acute and chronic stress can differently affect some parameters [83,84]. On the other hand, studies on the effects of chronic stress are of particular interest, due to their clear connection with neurodegenerative diseases—dementia, Alzheimer's disease, etc. [85–87]. Another interesting direction would be to establish the effect of another type of stress—in this sense, there is evidence that restraint stress in rats can be considered as the equivalent of psychosocial stress in humans [88], and other suitable models would be learned helplessness, social defeat, and social isolation [89]. Tracking the interactions between the cannabinoid and other mediator systems, e.g., dopaminergic and GABA-ergic, is also among our future, given the involvement of D1- and $GABA_A$- receptors in the development of depressive behavior [90].

Our research was primarily aimed at the interpretation of the stress response, but the analysis of the literature data carried out in connection with a previous publication [53] suggested that the findings could be useful in the drug development field [91,92]. Both systems represent targets for pharmaceutical development: several agonist drugs are known [93,94] for both the cannabinoid and the serotonin receptors, since both the up- and downregulation of ECS-/5-HT-mediated signaling are desired in specific pathophysiological conditions [91,95]. Other drugs (e.g., opioids) antagonize the serotonin transporter and increase serotonin levels, causing so-called serotonin toxicity [96]. It is also important that CB receptors exhibit constitutive activity [97,98], meaning that their ligands' intrinsic activities vary from agonist, through partial agonist and antagonist, to inverse agonist. Moreover, they exhibit biased signaling, thus structurally diverse agonists stabilize different ranges of active conformations of the receptors, consequently allowing the activation of different biochemical pathways [99]. Knowing the outcome of the exogenous antagonization/potentiation of a certain type of receptor, as well as the possible interactions between the different types, would provide certain guidelines for the therapeutic effect of the developed chemical structures. Also, the availability of data on specific interactions between individual receptors should be considered in view of possible adverse drug effects [95].

The potential clinical significance of this type of research is determined by the two systems—the cannabinoid and the serotoninergic themselves. Cannabinoids have been known about since ancient times, but their modern presence in medical practice is compromised by evidence of adverse effects [100]. At the same time, a large-scale campaign for their "rehabilitation" is underway, considering the beneficial effects of cannabinoids in the reduction of chronic pain treatment [101], chemotherapy-induced nausea and vomiting [102], and for some other medical conditions [103]. With this in mind, any study involving ECS contributes to elucidating its involvement in physiological and pathophysiological responses, thereby confirming or refuting the health benefits of cannabinoid-based substances. On the other hand, in recent years, the serotoninergic system has been the focus of numerous studies with the discovery of the kynurenine pathway [104]. In 2020,

Savitz produced a rather interesting title [105], raising the question of the relationship of this system with major depressive disorder, bipolar disorder, and schizophrenia. The relationship between the serotonin and the kynurenine systems lies in the fact that they have a common precursor—tryptophan, and the development of mood disorders is associated with serotonin depletion. Therefore, any research on the interactions of the serotoninergic system with other systems can provide useful data and new perspectives to explore.

An additional benefit of our study is the thermal factor—in recent years, our team has investigated changes in the stress response at different environmental temperatures, and the results [37,38], as well as some not yet published, show that high and low temperatures differently affect stress reaction, which should be taken into consideration in the field of occupational medicine and health promotion programs for temperature-challenged workplaces.

We hope that the present study contributes to a better understanding of the role of the endogenous cannabinoid and the serotonergic systems interacting in both the pathogenesis and mediation of the stress response. Since both types of receptors (cannabinoid and serotonin) are widely distributed in the human body and, at the same time, represent valuable targets for the pharmacological influencing of a number of pathological conditions, we believe that the proposed information could provide interesting directions for different fields of science.

In conclusion, we have found a different type of interaction between the ECS and the serotoninergic system before and after stress. We assume that the potentiation of c-SIA (observed in the pre-stress treatment) is due to a higher degree of the effect of the serotonergic system that "maintains" analgesia, while the c-SIA (observed in the post-stress treatment) is more the result of the cannabinoids' modulative effect on the HPA axis.

Author Contributions: Conceptualization, H.N.; methodology, H.N. and N.S.; software, H.N. and V.V.; validation, H.N., V.V. and N.S.; formal analysis, H.N.; investigation, H.N., V.V., N.S., N.K. and D.K.; resources, H.N.; data curation, M.M., D.K. and N.K.; writing—original draft preparation, H.N., D.K. and M.M.; writing—review and editing, H.N., D.K. and M.M.; visualization, H.N., V.V., M.M. and N.S.; supervision, H.N.; project administration, H.N.; funding acquisition, H.N. All authors have read and agreed to the published version of the manuscript.

Funding: The research has been funded by a Grant 85/04.06.2021 from the Council of Medical Science, MU-Sofia. The authors take this opportunity to thank the Council of Medical Science, MU-Sofia, for the financial support of their project.

Institutional Review Board Statement: All experimental protocols were approved by Bulgarian institutional animal care committee—the Bulgarian Food Safety Association (BFSA)—Permission Protocol № 314/06.10.2021.

Informed Consent Statement: Not applicable.

Data Availability Statement: The protocols for the experiments carried out on the project are stored in the personal database of the leading researcher Hristina Nocheva, whom the Grant 85/04.06.2021, as well as the Permission Protocol from BFSA, were awarded.

Acknowledgments: All authors express their heartfelt gratitude to the Rector's Board of Southwestern University "Neofit Rilski"—Blagoevgrad, for the financial support for the publication of this article and for encouraging our future scientific developments.

Conflicts of Interest: The authors declare no conflicts of interest.

References

1. Smith, S.M.; Vale, W.W. The role of the hypothalamic-pituitary-adrenal axis in neuroendocrine responses to stress. *Dialogues Clin. Neurosci.* **2022**, *8*, 367–381. [CrossRef] [PubMed]
2. Lee, R.S. The physiology of stress and the human body's response to stress. In *Epigenetics of Stress and Stress Disorders*; Academic Press: Cambridge, MA, USA, 2022; Volume 31, pp. 1–18. [CrossRef]
3. Oh, J.; Lee, H.Y.; Khuong, Q.L.; Markuns, J.F.; Bullen, C.; Barrios, O.E.A.; Hwang, S.S.; Suh, Y.S.; McCool, J.; Kachur, S.P.; et al. Mobility restrictions were associated with reductions in COVID-19 incidence early in the pandemic: Evidence from a real-time evaluation in 34 countries. *Sci. Rep.* **2021**, *11*, 13717. [CrossRef] [PubMed]

4. Koolhaas, J.M.; Bartolomucci, A.; Buwalda, B.; de Boer, S.F.; Flügge, G.; Korte, S.M.; Meerlo, P.; Murison, R.; Olivier, B.; Palanza, P.; et al. Stress revisited: A critical evaluation of the stress concept. *Neurosci. Biobehav. Rev.* **2011**, *35*, 1291–1301. [CrossRef] [PubMed]
5. Beecher, H.K. Pain in men wounded in battle. *Ann. Surg.* **1946**, *123*, 96–105. [CrossRef] [PubMed]
6. Ford, G.K.; Finn, D.P. Clinical correlates of stress-induced analgesia: Evidence from pharmacological studies. *Pain* **2008**, *140*, 3–7. [CrossRef] [PubMed]
7. Willer, J.C.; Dehen, H.; Cambier, J. Stress-induced analgesia in humans: Endogenous opioids and naloxone-reversible depression of pain reflexes. *Science* **1981**, *212*, 689–691. [CrossRef]
8. Butler, R.K.; Finn, D.P. Stress-induced analgesia. *Prog. Neurobiol.* **2009**, *88*, 184–202. [CrossRef]
9. Calcagnetti, D.J.; Helmstetter, F.J.; Fanselow, M.S. Quaternary naltrexone reveals the central mediation of conditional opioid analgesia. *Pharmacol. Biochem. Behav.* **1987**, *27*, 529–531. [CrossRef]
10. Watkins, L.R.; Mayer, D.J. Multiple endogenous opiate and non-opiate analgesia systems: Evidence of their existence and clinical implications. *Ann. N. Y. Acad. Sci.* **1986**, *467*, 273–299. [CrossRef]
11. Helmstetter, F.J.; Landeira-Fernandez, J. Conditional hypoalgesia is attenuated by naltrexone applied to the periaqueductal gray. *Brain Res.* **1990**, *537*, 88–92. [CrossRef]
12. Helmstetter, F.J. The amygdala is essential for the expression of conditional hypoalgesia. *Behav. Neurosci.* **1992**, *106*, 518–528. [CrossRef] [PubMed]
13. Hohmann, A.G.; Suplita, R.L.; Bolton, N.M.; Neely, M.H.; Fegley, D.; Mangieri, R.; Krey, J.F.; Walker, J.M.; Holmes, P.V.; Crystal, J.D.; et al. An endocannabinoid mechanism for stress-induced analgesia. *Nature* **2005**, *435*, 1108–1112. [CrossRef] [PubMed]
14. Woodhams, S.G.; Chapman, V.; Finn, D.P.; Hohmann, A.G.; Neugebauer, V. The cannabinoid system and pain. *Neuropharmacology* **2017**, *124*, 105–120. [CrossRef] [PubMed]
15. Micale, V.; Drago, F. Endocannabinoid system, stress and HPA axis. *Eur. J. Pharmacol.* **2018**, *834*, 230–239. [CrossRef] [PubMed]
16. Rothner, A.; Gov, T.; Hinden, L.; Nemirovski, A.; Tam, J.; Rosenzweig, B. Systemic Changes in Endocannabinoids and Endocannabinoid-like Molecules in Response to Partial Nephrectomy-Induced Ischemia in Humans. *Int. J. Mol. Sci.* **2023**, *24*, 4216. [CrossRef] [PubMed]
17. Immke, D.C.; Gavva, N.R. The TRPV1 receptor and nociception. *Semin. Cell Dev. Biol.* **2006**, *17*, 582–591. [CrossRef]
18. Herkenham, M.; Lynn, A.B.; Little, M.D.; Johnson, M.R.; Melvin, L.S.; de Costa, B.R.; Rice, K.C. Cannabinoid receptor localization in brain. *Proc. Natl. Acad. Sci. USA* **1990**, *87*, 1932–1936. [CrossRef]
19. Herkenham, M.; Lynn, A.; Johnson, M.R.; Melvin, L.; de Costa, B.; Rice, K. Characterization and localization of cannabinoid receptors in rat brain: A quantitative in vitro autoradiographic study. *J. Neurosci.* **1991**, *11*, 563–583. [CrossRef]
20. Ziegler, C.G.; Mohn, C.; Lamounier-Zepter, V.; Rettori, V.; Bornstein, S.R.; Krug, A.W.; Ehrhart-Bornstein, M. Expression and Function of Endocannabinoid Receptors in the Human Adrenal Cortex. *Horm. Metab. Res.* **2009**, *42*, 88–92. [CrossRef]
21. Van Sickle, M.D.; Duncan, M.; Kingsley, P.J.; Mouihate, A.; Urbani, P.; Mackie, K.; Stella, N.; Makriyannis, A.; Piomelli, D.; Davison, J.S.; et al. Identification and Functional Characterization of Brainstem Cannabinoid CB2 Receptors. *Science* **2005**, *310*, 329–332. [CrossRef]
22. Gong, J.-P.; Onaivi, E.S.; Ishiguro, H.; Liu, Q.-R.; Tagliaferro, P.A.; Brusco, A.; Uhl, G.R. Cannabinoid CB2 receptors: Immunohistochemical localization in rat brain. *Brain Res.* **2006**, *1071*, 10–23. [CrossRef]
23. Wang, M.; Hill, M.N.; Zhang, L.; Gorzalka, B.B.; Hillard, C.J.; Alger, B.E. Acute restraint stress enhances hippocampal endocannabinoid function via glucocorticoid receptor activation. *J. Psychopharmacol.* **2011**, *26*, 56–70. [CrossRef] [PubMed]
24. Cota, D.; Steiner, M.-A.; Marsicano, G.; Cervino, C.; Herman, J.; Grübler, Y.; Stalla, J.; Pasquali, R.; Lutz, B.; Stalla, G.K.; et al. Requirement of Cannabinoid Receptor Type 1 for the Basal Modulation of Hypothalamic-Pituitary-Adrenal Axis Function. *Endocrinology* **2007**, *148*, 1574–1581. [CrossRef] [PubMed]
25. Finn, D.P.; Haroutounian, S.; Hohmann, A.G.; Krane, E.; Soliman, N.; Rice, A.S.C. Cannabinoids, the endocannabinoid system and pain: A review of preclinical studies. *Pain* **2021**, *162*, S5–S25. [CrossRef] [PubMed]
26. Viveros, M.P.; Marco, E.M.; File, S.E. Endocannabinoid system and stress and anxiety responses. *Pharmacol. Biochem. Behav.* **2005**, *81*, 331–342. [CrossRef] [PubMed]
27. Aviram, J.; Samuelly-Leichtag, G. Efficacy of Cannabis-Based Medicines for Pain Management: A Systematic Review and Meta-Analysis of Randomized Controlled Trials. *Pain Physician* **2017**, *20*, E755–E796. PMID: 28934780. [CrossRef] [PubMed]
28. Petzke, F.; Tölle, T.; Fitzcharles, M.A.; Häuser, W. Cannabis-Based Medicines and Medical Cannabis for Chronic Neuropathic Pain. *CNS Drugs* **2022**, *36*, 31–44. [CrossRef]
29. Tournier, M.; Sorbara, F.; Gindre, C.; Swendsen, J.D.; Verdoux, H. Cannabis use and anxiety in daily life: A naturalistic investigation in a non-clinical population. *Psychiatry Res.* **2003**, *118*, 1–8. [CrossRef]
30. Arevalo, C.; De Miguel, R.; Hernandez-Tristan, R. Cannabinoid effects on anxiety-related behaviors and hypothalamic neurotransmitters. *Pharmacol. Biochem. Behav.* **2001**, *70*, 123–131. [CrossRef]
31. Haller, J.; Varga, B.; Ledent, C.; Barna, I.; Freund, T. Context-dependent effects of CB1 cannabinoid gene disruption on anxiety-like and social behavior in mice. *Eur. J. Neurosci.* **2004**, *16*, 1906–1912. [CrossRef]
32. Marsicano, G.; Wotjak, C.T.; Azad, S.C.; Bisogno, T.; Rammes, G.; Cascio, M.G.; Hermann, H.; Tang, J.; Hofmann, C.; Zieglgänsberger, W.; et al. The endogenous cannabinoid system controls extinction of aversive memories. *Nature* **2002**, *418*, 530–534. [CrossRef]

33. Kathuria, S.; Gaetani, S.; Fegley, D.; Valino, F.; Duranti, A.; Tontini, A.; Mor, M.; Tarzia, G.; La Rana, G.; Calignano, A.; et al. Modulation of anxiety through blockade of anandamide hydrolysis. *Nat. Med.* **2003**, *9*, 76–81. [CrossRef] [PubMed]
34. Hall, W.; Solowij, N. Adverse effects of cannabis. *Lancet* **1998**, *352*, 1611–1616. [CrossRef] [PubMed]
35. Nocheva, H.H.; Encheva-Stoykova, E.N.; Grigorov, E.E. Interaction between endocannabinoids and the adrenergic system before and after stress-exposure. *Pharmacia* **2021**, *69*, 249–254. [CrossRef]
36. Nocheva, H.; Encheva-Stoykova, E.N.; Bogdanov, G.; Tashev, R.; Nikolov, R. The endogenous cannabinoid system and nitric oxide interact in modulation of cold stress-induced analgesia. *CR Acad. Bulg. Sci.* **2022**, *75*, 1672–1679. [CrossRef]
37. Nocheva, H.H.; Tashev, R.E.; Bocheva, A.I.; Atanasova, D.Y.; Dandov, A.D.; Lazarov, N.E. Interactions between the endogenous cannabinoid system and the peptides of the Tyr-MIF-1 family modulate heat stress-induced analgesia. *Biomed. Rev.* **2020**, *31*, 91–103. [CrossRef]
38. Donner, N.C.; Siebler, P.H.; Johnson, D.T.; Villarreal, M.D.; Mani, S.; Matti, A.J.; Lowry, C.A. Serotonergic systems in the balance: CRHR1 and CRHR2 differentially control stress-induced serotonin synthesis. *Psychoneuroendocrinology* **2015**, *63*, 178–190. [CrossRef]
39. Leonard, B. The HPA and immune axes in stress: The involvement of the serotonergic system. *Eur. Psychiatry* **2005**, *20*, S302–S306. [CrossRef]
40. Marks, D.; Shah, M.; Patkar, A.; Masand, P.; Park, G.-Y.; Pae, C.-U. Serotonin-Norepinephrine Reuptake Inhibitors for Pain Control: Premise and Promise. *Curr. Neuropharmacol.* **2009**, *7*, 331–336. [CrossRef]
41. Chae, J.W.; Kang, D.H.; Li, Y.; Kim, S.H.; Lee, H.G.; Choi, J.I.; Yoon, M.H.; Kim, W.M. Antinociceptive effects of nefopam modulating serotonergic, adrenergic, and glutamatergic neurotransmission in the spinal cord. *Neurosci. Lett.* **2020**, *731*, 135057. [CrossRef]
42. Nunes-de-Souza, R.L.; Canto-de-Souza, A.; da-Costa, M.; Fornari, R.V.; Graeff, F.G.; Pela, I.R. Anxiety-induced antinociception in mice: Effects of systemic and intra-amygdala administration of 8-OH-DPAT and midazolam. *Psychopharmacology* **2000**, *150*, 300–310. [CrossRef] [PubMed]
43. Haj-Dahmane, S.; Shen, R.-Y. Modulation of the serotonin system by endocannabinoid signaling. *Neuropharmacology* **2011**, *61*, 414–420. [CrossRef] [PubMed]
44. Häring, M.; Marsicano, G.; Lutz, B.; Monory, K. Identification of the cannabinoid receptor type 1 in serotonergic cells of raphe nuclei in mice. *Neuroscience* **2007**, *146*, 1212–1219. [CrossRef] [PubMed]
45. Jahanshahi, A.; Le Maitre, E.; Temel, Y.; Lanfumey, L.; Hamon, M.; Lesch, K.-P.; Tordera, R.M.; Del Río, J.; Aso, E.; Maldonado, R.; et al. Altered expression of neuronal tryptophan hydroxylase-2 mRNA in the dorsal and median raphe nuclei of three genetically modified mouse models relevant to depression and anxiety. *J. Chem. Neuroanat.* **2011**, *41*, 227–233. [CrossRef] [PubMed]
46. McLaughlin, R.J.; Hill, M.N.; Gorzalka, B.B. Monoaminergic neurotransmission contributes to cannabinoid-induced activation of the hypothalamic-pituitary-adrenal axis. *Eur. J. Pharmacol.* **2009**, *624*, 71–76. [CrossRef] [PubMed]
47. Coderre, T.J.; Rollman, G.B. Stress analgesia: Effects of PCPA, yohimbine, and naloxone. *Pharmacol. Biochem. Behav.* **1984**, *21*, 681–686. [CrossRef]
48. Schlereth, T.; Birklein, F. The sympathetic nervous system and pain. *Neuromolecular Med.* **2008**, *10*, 141–147. [CrossRef]
49. Heinricher, M.M.; Tavares, I.; Leith, J.L.; Lumb, B.M. Descending control of nociception: Specificity, recruitment and plasticity. *Brain Res. Rev.* **2009**, *60*, 214–225. [CrossRef]
50. Saeki, Y. Effect of local application of cold or heat for relief of pricking pain. *Nurs. Health Sci.* **2002**, *4*, 97–105. [CrossRef]
51. Ernst, E.; Fialka, V. Ice freezes pain? A review of the clinical effectiveness of analgesic cold therapy. *J. Pain Symptom Manag.* **1994**, *9*, 56–59. [CrossRef]
52. Choi, J.C.; Park, H.J.; Park, J.A.; Kang, D.R.; Choi, Y.S.; Choi, S.; Lee, H.G.; Choi, J.H.; Choi, I.H.; Yoon, M.; et al. The increased analgesic efficacy of cold therapy after an unsuccessful analgesic experience is associated with inferior parietal lobule activation. *Sci. Rep.* **2022**, *12*, 14687. [CrossRef] [PubMed]
53. Nocheva, H.; Krastev, N.S.; Krastev, D.S.; Mileva, M. The Endogenous Cannabinoid and the Nitricoxidergic Systems in the Modulation of Stress Responses. *Int. J. Mol. Sci.* **2023**, *24*, 2886. [CrossRef] [PubMed]
54. Miczek, K.A.; Thompson, M.L.; Shuster, L. Opioid-like analgesia in defeated mice. *Science* **1982**, *215*, 1520–1522. [CrossRef] [PubMed]
55. Zeisberger, E. Interdependence of peripheral and central noradrenaline action in thermal adaption. *J. Physiol.* **1978**, *284*, 41P. [PubMed]
56. Wiesenfeld, Z.; Hallin, R.G. Influence of nerve lesions, strain differences and continuous cold stress on chronic pain behavior in rats. *Physiol. Behav.* **1981**, *27*, 735–740. [CrossRef] [PubMed]
57. Nocheva, H.; Kochev, D.; Krastev, D.; Bocheva, A. Cold stress-induced analgesia. Interactions between the Tyr-MIF-1 family of peptides and the endocannabinoid system. *CR Acad. Bulg. Sci.* **2013**, *66*, 1639–1644.
58. Marzouki, H.; Aboussaleh, Y.; Najimi, M.; Chigr, F.; Ahami, A. Effect of Cold Stress on Neurobehavioral and Physiological Parameters in Rats. *Front. Physiol.* **2021**, *12*, 660124. [CrossRef] [PubMed]
59. Kayser, V. Randall-Selitto Paw Pressure Test. In *Encyclopedia of Pain*; Gebhart, G.F., Schmidt, R.F., Eds.; Springer: Berlin/Heidelberg, Germany, 2013. [CrossRef]
60. ARRP Guideline 20: Guidelines for the Housing of Rats in Scientific Institutions. Available online: http://www.animalethics.org.au (accessed on 1 August 2021).

61. Solinas, M.; Justinova, Z.; Goldberg, S.R.; Tanda, G. Anandamide administration alone and after inhibition of fatty acid amide hydrolase (FAAH) increases dopamine levels in the nucleus accumbens shell in rats. *J. Neurochem.* **2006**, *98*, 408–419. [CrossRef]
62. da Veiga, M.A.L.C.; Fonseca Bloise, F.; Costa-e-Sousa, R.H.; Souza, L.L.; Almeida, N.A.d.S.; Oliveira, K.J.; Pazos-Moura, C.C. Acute effects of endocannabinoid anandamide and CB1 receptor antagonist, AM251 in the regulation of thyrotropin secretion. *J. Endocrinol.* **2008**, *199*, 235–242. [CrossRef]
63. Randall, L.O.; Selitto, J.J. A method for measurement of analgesic activity on inflamed tissue. *Arch. Int. Pharmacodyn. Ther.* **1957**, *111*, 409–419. [PubMed]
64. Pääkkönen, T.; Leppäluoto, J. Cold exposure, and hormonal secretion: A review. *Int. J. Circumpolar Health* **2002**, *61*, 265–276. [CrossRef] [PubMed]
65. Lichtman, A.H.; Cook, S.A.; Martin, B.R. Investigation of brain sites mediating cannabinoid induced antinociception in rats: Evidence supporting periaqueductal gray involvement. *J. Pharmacol. Exp. Ther.* **1996**, *276*, 585–593. [PubMed]
66. Martin, W.J.; Patrick, S.L.; Coffin, P.O.; Tsou, K.; Walker, J. An examination of the central sites of action of cannabinoid-induced antinociception in the rat. *Life Sci.* **1995**, *56*, 2103–2109. [CrossRef] [PubMed]
67. Martin, W.J.; Hohmann, A.G.; Walker, J.M. Suppression of Noxious Stimulus-Evoked Activity in the Ventral Posterolateral Nucleus of the Thalamus by a Cannabinoid Agonist: Correlation between Electrophysiological and Antinociceptive Effects. *J. Neurosci.* **1996**, *16*, 6601–6611. [CrossRef] [PubMed]
68. Martin, W.J.; Tsou, K.; Walker, J.M. Cannabinoid receptor-mediated inhibition of the rat tail-flick reflex after microinjection into the rostral ventromedial medulla. *Neurosci. Lett.* **1998**, *242*, 33–36. [CrossRef] [PubMed]
69. Meng, I.D.; Manning, B.H.; Martin, W.J.; Fields, H.L. An analgesia circuit activated by cannabinoids. *Nature* **1998**, *395*, 381–383. [CrossRef] [PubMed]
70. Martin, W.J.; Coffin, P.O.; Attias, E.; Balinsky, M.; Tsou, K.; Walker, J. Anatomical basis for cannabinoid-induced antinociception as revealed by intracerebral microinjections. *Brain Res.* **1999**, *822*, 237–242. [CrossRef] [PubMed]
71. Guindon, J.; Hohmann, A.G. The Endocannabinoid System and Pain. *CNS Neurol. Disord. Drug Targets* **2009**, *8*, 403–421. [CrossRef]
72. Smith, P.B.; Martin, B.R. Spinal mechanisms of delta9-tetrahydrocannabinol-induced analgesia. *Brain Res.* **1992**, *578*, 8–12. [CrossRef]
73. Yaksh, T.L. The Antinociceptive Effects of Intrathecally Administered Levonantradol and Desacetyllevonantradol in the Rat. *J. Clin. Pharmacol.* **1981**, *21*, 334S–340S. [CrossRef]
74. Hohmann, A.G.; Tsou, K.; Walker, J.M. Cannabinoid modulation of wide dynamic range neurons in the lumbar dorsal horn of the rat by spinally administered WIN55,212-2. *Neurosci. Lett.* **1998**, *257*, 119–122. [CrossRef]
75. Johanek, L.M.; Simone, D.A. Cannabinoid Agonist, CP 55,940, Prevents Capsaicin-Induced Sensitization of Spinal Cord Dorsal Horn Neurons. *J. Neurophysiol.* **2005**, *93*, 989–997. [CrossRef] [PubMed]
76. Sokal, D.M.; Elmes, S.J.R.; Kendall, D.A.; Chapman, V. Intraplantar injection of anandamide inhibits mechanically evoked responses of spinal neurones via activation of CB2 receptors in anaesthetised rats. *Neuropharmacology* **2003**, *45*, 404–411. [CrossRef] [PubMed]
77. Hohmann, A.G.; Tsou, K.; Walker, J.M. Intrathecal cannabinoid administration suppresses noxious stimulus-evoked Fos protein-like immunoreactivity in rat spinal cord: Comparison with morphine. *Acta Pharmacol. Sin.* **1999**, *20*, 1132–1136.
78. Richardson, J.D.; Aanonsen, L.; Hargreaves, K.M. Hypoactivity of the Spinal Cannabinoid System Results in NMDA-Dependent Hyperalgesia. *J. Neurosci.* **1998**, *18*, 451–457. [CrossRef] [PubMed]
79. Hohmann, A.G. Spinal and peripheral mechanisms of cannabinoid antinociception: Behavioral, neurophysio-logical, and neu-roanatomical perspectives. *Chem. Phys. Lipids* **2002**, *121*, 173–190. [CrossRef] [PubMed]
80. Guindon, J.; Hohmann, A.G. Cannabinoid CB2 receptors: A therapeutic target for the treatment of inflamma-tory and neuro-pathic pain. *Br. J. Pharmacol.* **2008**, *153*, 319–334. [CrossRef] [PubMed]
81. Rice, A.S.C.; Farquhar-Smith, W.P.; Nagy, I. Endocannabinoids and pain: Spinal and peripheral analgesia in inflammation and neuropathy. *Prostaglandins Leukot. Essent. Fat. Acids* **2002**, *66*, 243–256. [CrossRef]
82. Patel, S.; Roelke, C.T.; Rademacher, D.J.; Cullinan, W.E.; Hillard, C.J. Endocannabinoid Signaling Negatively Modulates Stress-Induced Activation of the Hypothalamic-Pituitary-Adrenal Axis. *Endocrinology* **2004**, *145*, 5431–5438. [CrossRef]
83. Mariotti, A. The effects of chronic stress on health: New insights into the molecular mechanisms of brain-body communication. *Future Sci. OA* **2015**, *1*, FSO23. [CrossRef]
84. Harris, R.B.S. Chronic and acute effects of stress on energy balance: Are there appropriate animal models? *Am. J. Physiol. Regul. Integr. Comp. Physiol.* **2015**, *308*, R250–R265. [CrossRef] [PubMed]
85. James, K.A.; Stromin, J.I.; Steenkamp, N.; Combrinck, M.I. Understanding the relationships between physiological and psychosocial stress, cortisol and cognition. *Front. Endocrinol.* **2023**, *14*, 1085950. [CrossRef] [PubMed]
86. Stuart, K.E.; Padgett, C. A systematic review of the association between psychological stress and dementia risk in humans. *J. Alzheimer's Dis.* **2020**, *78*, 335–352. [CrossRef] [PubMed]
87. Han, B.; Wang, J.-H.; Geng, Y.; Shen, L.; Wang, H.-L.; Wang, Y.-Y.; Wang, M.-W. Chronic stress contributes to cognitive dysfunction and hippocampal metabolic abnormalities in app/ps1 mice. *Cell Physiol. Biochem.* **2017**, *41*, 1766–1776. [CrossRef] [PubMed]
88. Kvetnansky, R.; McCarty, R. Immobilization Stress. In *Encyclopedia of Stress*, 2nd ed.; Fink, G., Ed.; Academic Press: Cambridge, MA, USA, 2007; pp. 445–449, ISBN 9780123739476. [CrossRef]

89. Becker, M.; Pinhasov, A.; Ornoy, A. Animal models of depression: What can they teach us about the human disease? *Diagnostics* **2021**, *11*, 123. [CrossRef] [PubMed]
90. Cao, G.; Meng, G.; Zhu, L.; Zhu, J.; Dong, N.; Zhou, X.; Zhang, S.; Zhang, Y. Susceptibility to chronic immobilization stress-induced depressive-like behaviour in middle-aged female mice and accompanying changes in dopamine D1 and GABAA receptors in related brain regions. *Behav. Brain Funct.* **2021**, *17*, 2. [CrossRef] [PubMed]
91. Stasiulewicz, A.; Znajdek, K.; Grudzień, M.; Pawiński, T.; Sulkowska, A.J.I. A Guide to Targeting the Endocannabinoid System in Drug Design. *Int. J. Mol. Sci.* **2020**, *21*, 2778. [CrossRef] [PubMed]
92. Godfrey, L.; Bailey, I.; Toms, N.J.; Clarke, G.D.; Kitchen, I.; Hourani, S.M. Paracetamol inhibits nitric oxide synthesis in murine spinal cord slices. *Eur. J. Pharmacol.* **2007**, *562*, 68–71. [CrossRef]
93. Ottani, A.; Leone, S.; Sandrini, M.; Ferrari, A.; Bertolini, A. The analgesic activity of paracetamol is prevented by the blockade of cannabinoid CB1 receptors. *Eur. J. Pharmacol.* **2006**, *531*, 280–281. [CrossRef]
94. Pickering, G.; Loriot, M.A.; Libert, F.; Eschalier, A.; Beaune, P.; Dubray, C. Analgesic effect of acetaminophen in humans: First, evidence of a central serotonergic mechanism. *Clin. Pharmacol. Ther.* **2006**, *79*, 371–378. [CrossRef]
95. Baldo, B.A.; Rose, M.A. The anaesthetist, opioid analgesic drugs, and serotonin toxicity: A mechanistic and clinical review. *Br. J. Anaesth.* **2020**, *124*, 44–62. [CrossRef]
96. Gillman, P.K. Extracting value from case reports: Lessons from serotonin toxicity. *Biol. Psychiatr.* **2006**, *61*, 419–422. [CrossRef]
97. Bouaboula, M.; Perrachon, S.; Milligan, L.; Canat, X.; Rinaldi-Carmona, M., Portier, M.; Barth, F.; Calandra, B.; Pecceu, F.; Lupker, J. A Selective Inverse Agonist for Central Cannabinoid Receptor Inhibits Mitogen-activated Protein Kinase Activation Stimulated by Insulin or Insulin-like Growth Factor 1. Evidence for a new model of receptor/ligand interactions. *J. Biol. Chem.* **1997**, *272*, 22330–22339. [CrossRef]
98. Console-Bram, L.; Marcu, J.; Abood, M.E. Cannabinoid receptors: Nomenclature and pharmacological principles. Prog. *Neuro-Psychopharmacol. Biol. Psychiatry* **2012**, *38*, 4–15. [CrossRef]
99. Ibsen, M.S.; Connor, M.; Glass, M. Cannabinoid CB1 and CB2 receptor signaling and bias. *Cannabis Cannabinoid Res.* **2017**, *2*, 48–60. [CrossRef]
100. Kalant, H. Adverse effects of cannabis on health: An update of the literature since 1996. *Prog. Neuropsychopharmacol. Biol. Psychiatry* **2004**, *28*, 849–863. [CrossRef] [PubMed]
101. Whiting, P.F.; Wolff, R.F.; Deshpande, S.; Di Nisio, M.; Duffy, S.; Hernandez, A.V.; Keurentjes, J.C.; Lang, S.; Misso, K.; Ryder, S.; et al. Cannabinoids for medical use: A systematic review and meta-analysis. *J. Am. Med. Assoc.* **2015**, *313*, 2456–2473. [CrossRef] [PubMed]
102. Todaro, B. Cannabinoids in the treatment of chemotherapy-induced nausea and vomiting. *J. Natl. Compr. Cancer Netw.* **2012**, *10*, 487–492. [CrossRef]
103. Lutge, E.E.; Gray, A.; Siegfried, N. The medical use of cannabis for reducing morbidity and mortality in patients with HIV/AIDS. *Cochrane Database Syst. Rev.* **2013**, *4*, CD005175. [CrossRef] [PubMed]
104. Marx, W.; McGuinness, A.J.; Rocks, T.; Ruusunen, A.; Cleminson, J.; Walker, A.J.; Gomes-da-Costa, S.; Lane, M.; Sanches, M.; Diaz, A.P.; et al. The kynurenine pathway in major depressive disorder, bipolar disorder, and schizophrenia: A meta-analysis of 101 studies. *Mol. Psychiatry* **2021**, *26*, 4158–4178. [CrossRef] [PubMed]
105. Savitz, J. The kynurenine pathway: A finger in every pie. *Mol. Psychiatry* **2020**, *25*, 131–147. [CrossRef]

biomedicines

MDPI

Article

Beyond the Brain: Perinatal Exposure of Rats to Serotonin Enhancers Induces Long-Term Changes in the Jejunum and Liver

Romana Gračan [1], Sofia Ana Blažević [2,*], Matea Brižić [2] and Dubravka Hranilovic [2]

[1] Division of Zoology, Department of Biology, Faculty of Science, University of Zagreb, 10000 Zagreb, Croatia; romana.gracan@biol.pmf.unizg.hr

[2] Division of Animal Physiology, Department of Biology, Faculty of Science, University of Zagreb, 10000 Zagreb, Croatia; matea305@gmail.com (M.B.); dubravka.hranilovic@biol.pmf.unizg.hr (D.H.)

* Correspondence: sofia.ana.blazevic@biol.pmf.unizg.hr

Abstract: Serotonin (5-hydroxytryptamine, 5HT) homeostasis is essential for many physiological processes in the central nervous system and peripheral tissues. Hyperserotonemia, a measurable sign of 5HT homeostasis disruption, can be caused by 5HT-directed treatment of psychiatric and gastrointestinal diseases. Its impact on the long-term balance and function of 5HT in the peripheral compartment remains unresolved and requires further research due to possible effects on human health. We explored the effects of perinatal 5HT imbalance on the peripheral organs responsible for serotonin metabolism—the jejunum, a synthesis site, and the liver, a catabolism site—in adult rats. Hyperserotonemia was induced by subchronic treatment with serotonin precursor 5-hydroxytryptophan (5HTP) or serotonin degradation inhibitor tranylcypromine (TCP). The jejunum and liver were collected on postnatal day 70 and analyzed histomorphometrically. Relative mRNA levels of 5HT-regulating proteins were determined using qRT-PCR. Compared to controls, 5HTP- and TCP-treated rats had a reduced number of 5HT-producing cells and expression of the 5HT-synthesising enzyme in the jejunum, and an increased expression of 5HT-transporter accompanied by karyomegaly in hepatocytes, with these differences being more pronounced in the TCP-treated animals. Here, we report that perinatal 5HT disbalance induced long-term cellular and molecular changes in organs regulating 5HT-metabolism, which may have a negative impact on 5HT availability and function in the periphery. Our rat model demonstrates a link between the developmental abnormalities of serotonin homeostasis and 5HT-related changes in adult life and may be suitable for exploring the neurobiological substrates of vulnerability to behavioral and metabolic disorders, as well as for modeling the adverse effects of the prenatal exposure to 5HT enhancers in the human population.

Keywords: serotonin; 5-hydroxytryptophan; tranylcypromine; monoamine oxidase; liver; jejunum; histological techniques; qRT-PCR; enterochromaffin cells; rat

1. Introduction

Serotonin (5-hydroxytryptamine, 5HT) is a biologically active amine present in the central nervous system (CNS) and the peripheral tissues of mammals. In the "central 5HT compartment", it is best known as a neurotransmitter that modulates neural activity and a range of neuropsychological processes including mood, perception, reward, anger, aggression, appetite, memory, cognition, pain sensitivity, thermoregulation, sleep, sexual behavior, and circadian rhythm [1,2]. The cell bodies of 5HT-synthesizing neurons are located in the raphe nuclei of the brain stem and project their axons throughout the cortical and subcortical regions of the brain. The first step in serotonin biosynthesis, the conversion of L-tryptophan to 5-hydroxytryptophan (5HTP), is catalyzed by the enzyme tryptophan hydroxylase (TPH2 isoform), which is followed by the reduction to 5HT via aromatic L-amino acid decarboxylase and active transport into synaptic vesicles by vesicular monoamine transporter (VMAT2 isoform). 5HT synaptic action is terminated through its reuptake by 5HT transporter (5HTt) and degradation to 5-hydroxyindoleacetic acid by the enzyme monoamine oxidase (MAO), preferentially the MAOA isoform [3].

Nonetheless, most serotonin is found outside the CNS, in the "peripheral compartment". 5HT is primarily produced in the gut enterochromaffin (EC) cells of the mucosa [4] by the TPH1 isoform and packed into dense granules by the VMAT1 isoform [5]. Upon its release into circulation, platelets accumulate the majority of peripheral serotonin, while small amounts of 5HT remaining in platelet-free plasma can activate more than seventeen 5HT receptors located in various peripheral tissues [6] before 5HT is taken up by 5HTt and catabolized by MAOA in the endothelial cells of the lungs and liver [7]. Peripheral 5HT regulates numerous biological processes in cardiovascular, pulmonary, gastrointestinal (GI), and genitourinary systems [1]. 5HT from the circulatory system governs hemodynamics, modifies blood pressure, and changes body temperature through cutaneous vasodilation [4,7]. Previous studies have suggested that EC cells are pressure sensors that secrete serotonin into the wall of the GI tract, initiate peristaltic and secretory reflexes, and activate sensory nerves [8]. However, recent studies imply that 5HT from the neurons of the enteric system is more important for constitutive gastrointestinal transit than is enteric serotonin from EC cells. Neuronal 5HT also promotes the growth/maintenance of the mucosa and neurogenesis, while enteric serotonin induces a GI inflammatory response [9]. Enteric serotonin enters the liver through the portal vein and affects several key processes: gluconeogenesis [6], hepatic lipid metabolism via a gut–liver endocrine axis, hepatic blood flow (portal and sinusoidal), regeneration, innervation, and wound healing [10,11].

The central and the peripheral serotonergic systems are functionally separated by a blood–brain barrier and regulated independently. However, during the fetal and early postnatal development of the brain, the blood–brain barrier is not fully formed, and the two systems can freely communicate [12]. Considering the role of 5-HT in neurodevelopment [13] and prenatal programming [14], genetic or environmental disruption of optimal serotonin concentrations can affect serotonin homeostasis in both compartments, leading to an increased vulnerability to behavioral and/or metabolic disorders [15,16]. One of the measurable signs of 5HT homeostasis disruption is hyperserotonemia—a state of elevated blood 5HT levels. It has been identified in some developmental disorders such as those of autism spectrum but can also be caused by the use of serotonergic medications developed for medical treatments of psychiatric, neurological, and some gastrointestinal disorders [17–19]. In addition to the "classical" 5HT-targeting drugs, such as MAO inhibitors, selective serotonin reuptake inhibitors (SSRIs), or agents targeting specific serotonin receptors, the immediate 5HT precursor 5-HTP has been widely offered for alleviating depressive symptoms, binge eating, headache, or insomnia [20]. Although the effects of serotonergic drugs have been examined in detail and are fully understood in the CNS and partially in the digestive tract [21], some side effects (e.g., diabetes, metabolic syndrome, and valvular heart disease [8,22]) reveal that the physiological role of the peripheral serotonergic system is still unclear and needs to be studied further. This especially holds true for 5HTP, whose safety of use has hardly been studied in the human population or in animal models [23].

To identify the consequences of developmentally disturbed serotonin homeostasis, we pharmacologically induced elevated blood 5HT levels by the perinatal treatment of rats with serotonin precursor 5-hydroxytryptophan (5HTP) or MAO inhibitor tranylcypromine (TCP) during the most intensive development of 5HT neurons. The aim was to induce perinatal hyperserotonemia through endogenous serotonin, i.e., not through an analog but through the inhibition of catabolism or the stimulation of synthesis at two levels. First, primarily at the peripheral level, the administration of 5-hydorxytryptophan, the immediate precursor of 5HT, allowed us to bypass the rate-limiting step in the synthesis of 5HT and significantly increase peripheral serotonin (treatment explained in more detail in [24]). Second, both at the central and peripheral levels, TCP inhibited both monoamine oxidase isoforms inducing long-term hyperserotonemia (explained in more detail in [25]). In our previous studies, we showed the immediate effects of the treatments and their long-lasting impact on the central

5HT compartment at the molecular, neurochemical, and behavioral level. While treatment with 5HTP significantly raised peripheral but not central 5HT concentrations, treatment with TCP induced significant 5HT elevations in both "compartments" [26]. Still, both treatments increased pup mortality, reduced weight gain, compromised thermoregulation, and altered affiliative behavior [24,25,27]. At adult age, 5HTP-treated rats displayed a modest but significant decrease in 5HT concentration [26] and an increase in *MaoA* and *MaoB* mRNA abundance [28] in the frontal cortex, accompanied by increased exploratory activity [29]. More prominent long-lasting effects were observed in TCP-treated rats. Disturbed peripheral 5HT homeostasis was reflected in hyperserotonemia, altered bone remodeling, and hematopoiesis [30]. Disturbed central 5HT homeostasis was reflected in a significant increase in mRNA abundance for both *Mao* genes [28] and, consequently, increased brain 5HT metabolism and drastically decreased 5HT concentrations in the frontal cortex and raphe nuclei [26], accompanied by highly anxiolytic behavior [29].

In this study, we further explored the structural and molecular backgrounds of the disturbed peripheral homeostasis by focusing on the peripheral organs responsible for serotonin metabolism—the digestive tract, where enteric 5HT is synthesized, and the liver, where enteric 5HT is primarily metabolized. Our aim was to analyze the long-lasting histomorphological and 5HT-regulating gene expression changes in the jejunum and liver tissue after 5HTP-induced and TCP-induced perinatal hyperserotonemia. Jejunum and liver samples were collected from 13 5HTP-treated, 13 TCP-treated, and 11 saline-treated rats of both sexes on postnatal day (P) 70; the samples were analyzed histomorphometrically; and the relative expression of the genes coding for TPH1 and VMAT1 in the jejunum and 5HTt and MAOA in the liver was compared among the three groups.

2. Materials and Methods

We performed a two-step chronic treatment of animals with either of the two 5HT-enhancers—5-hydorxytryptophan (5HTP) and tranylcypromine (TCP)—or with saline. In the first step, we treated pregnant females (3 with each of the 5HT enhancers and 2 with saline) from gestational day 12 until parturition. In the second step, we treated pups (13 with TCP, 13 with 5HTP, and 11 with saline) from postnatal day (PND) 1 until PND21. At PND70, blood, jejunum, and liver samples were collected from all experimental and control rats. Serum 5HT concentrations were measured with ELISA, jejunum and liver tissue was examined histomorphologically, and the relative expression of the genes of the serotonin pathway proteins, including tryptophan hydroxylase 1 (*Tph1*) and vesicular monoamine transporter 1 (*Vmat1*)—responsible for serotonin synthesis and storage in the jejunum—and serotonin transporter (*5HTt*) and monoamine oxidase A (*MaoA*)—responsible for 5HT elimination in liver—were determined via quantitative PCR.

2.1. Housing and Breeding of Animals

The experiment was performed on eight nulliparous Wistar females acquired from the animal facility of the Croatian Institute for Brain Research (University of Zagreb, Zagreb, Croatia), weighing 220–250 g, which were randomly assigned to a saline, 5-hydroxytryptophan (5HTP), or tranylcypromine (TCP) group and mated with males of the same strain and age in a 3:1 or 2:1 ratio in order to synchronize paring and parturition [31] and reduce the number of male progenitors in accordance with the 3R's principle [32]. Nulliparous females were used in order to eliminate the effect of previous pregnancies and lactation on the dam's affiliative behavior influenced by serotonin [33] through the HPA axis [34] and to allow for the same conditions for all pups being reared. After gravidity was confirmed in all females, the male was removed from the cage. Females remained together until 2 days before parturition when they were separated and remained singly housed until weaning of the pups. After weaning, animals were kept 3–4 per cage in polycarbonate cages under 12 h light:12 h dark conditions at a temperature of 22 ± 2 °C, with free access to rat chow and tap water. Animals were kept at the Animal facility of the Division of Animal

Physiology, Department of Biology, Faculty of Science, University of Zagreb (Facility reg. num. HR-POK-027).

The animals' health status was monitored throughout the experiments by a health surveillance program according to Federation of European Laboratory Animal Science Associations (FELASA) guidelines. The rats were free of all viral, bacterial, and parasitic pathogens listed in the FELASA recommendations. All efforts were made to reduce the number of animals used and to minimize animal suffering. The study was approved by the ethics committee of the University of Zagreb (251-58-508-10-19) and was conducted in accordance with the Directive of The European Parliament and of the Council (2010/63/EU) and the Croatian Animal Protection Law (NN, 102/2017, NN 32/2019) as well as the directive on animal protection in scientific research (NN 55/2013, NN, 116/2019).

2.2. Pharmacological Treatments

Rats were treated with serotonin synthesis precursor, 5-hydroxytryptophan (5HTP), or with the nonselective MAO inhibitor, tranylcypromine (TCP), in order to increase the level of serotonin and induce hyperserotonemia. The treatment started prenatally from the 12th until the 21st gestation day by treating pregnant females—three with 2 mg/kg of TCP (Sigma–Aldrich, St. Louis, MO, USA), three with 25 mg/kg of 5HTP (Sigma–Aldrich), and two with saline. The experiment continued with postnatal treatment of pups from P1 to P21—13 rats with TCP, 13 rats with 5HTP, and 11 rats with saline (control group). Young adult rats of both sexes were used to check for the potential differences in vulnerability to disbalance in 5HT homeostasis and avoid a sex-biased interpretation of the results [35]. Solutions were delivered in volumes of 1.51 mL per kg of body mass to dams, in volumes of 3.3 mL per kg of body mass to pups until they reached 15 g, and in volumes of 5 mL per kg of body mass until the end of treatment. The control group was treated with saline in the same manner. All subcutaneous injections were performed between 2 and 3 pm. 5HTP was dissolved in acidified saline, neutralized with NaOH, and warmed to body temperature, while TCP was dissolved in ethanol and saline, neutralized with HCl, and again warmed to body temperature.

2.3. Collection and Processing of Tissue Samples

On P 70 $\pm$ 1, all 37 rats were decapitated under isofluorane anesthesia (C3H2ClF5O; Mr = 184.49 g/mol; Baxter, Deerfield, IL, USA). Blood samples were collected as reported in Blazevic et al. [30] and analyzed as reported in our previous study. Tissue samples were collected for histological and gene expression analysis from the second part of the small intestine (jejunum) and from the left liver lobe. For mRNA expression analysis, approximately 85 mg of the liver and 65 mg of jejunum tissue were immediately cut with a scalpel, washed in cold saline, placed in microtubes, and frozen in liquid nitrogen. Samples for histological processing were fixed in 10% neutral formalin for 24 h, dehydrated through graded alcohol series (70–100%), cleared in xylene, and embedded in Paraplast embedding media (Sherwood Medical, Norfolk, NE, USA). Cross sections were cut on a rotating microtome (Shandon Finesse 325, Thermo Fisher Scientific, Waltham, MA, USA) at 5–7 μm in thickness, stained with hematoxylin–eosin (HE), and processed for general histology examination and analysis. Additionally, small intestine sections were stained with the histochemical Masson–Fontana method to identify neuroendocrine argentaffin cells, while liver sections were stained with periodic acid–Schiff (PAS) to highlight basement membranes and enable precise morphometry. The tissue samples from all of the groups were coded and studied independently in a blinded fashion, with 1–2 sections being selected at random for each rat.

2.4. qRT-PCR

Samples were disrupted and homogenized with an ultrasonic homogenizer (Bandelin electronic, Mecklenburg-Vorpommern, Germany) in 500 μL of guanidinium thiocyanate solution and frozen at −80 °C until further processing. RNA isolation was performed utilizing the phenol-free RNAqueous-4PCR kit (Ambion Inc., Austin, TX, USA), following the manufacturer's guidelines. Subsequently, genomic DNA was eliminated as per the provided instructions. RNA quality and concentrations were assessed through agarose gel (1.5%) electrophoresis and measured in a spectrophotometer (Biochrome). Samples with degraded RNA or 260/280 nm ratios outside the 1.7–2.1 range were excluded from further processing (Supplementary Materials). Following the manufacturer's instructions, mRNA was reversely transcribed from 1 μg of total RNA using MuLV reverse transcriptase (Applied Biosystems, Foster City, CA, USA) and oligo dT primers (Applied Biosystems, Foster City, CA, USA). The efficacy of reverse transcription was assessed through end-point PCR with the primers provided in the kit. Until further analysis, cDNA was stored at −20 °C.

Relative expression was assessed through qPCR using the TaqMan gene expression master mix (Applied Biosystems, Foster City, CA, USA) according to the manufacturer's instructions for the following genes of interest (all primer probe sets predesigned and acquired from Applied Biosystems): tryptophan hydroxylase (*Tph1*, Rn01476869_m1), monoamine oxidase A (*MaoA*, Rn01430961_m1), vesicle-monoamine transporter (*Vmat*, Rn00564688_m1), and serotonin transporter (*5HTt*, Rn00564737_m1). Serial dilutions were employed to validate primers, duplex reactions, and ascertain the initial concentrations of cDNA. All reactions were performed in a duplex setup with primer limited rat β-actin (ACTB, VIC labelled, 4352340E, Applied Biosystems) or glyceraldehyde 3-phosphate dehydrogenase (GAPDH, VIC labelled, 4352338E, Applied Biosystems) as endogenous control reference genes (REF) and completed in duplicate. GOIs were amplified in duplex with each REF gene separately. Pipetting errors were minimized and efficiency maximized using duplexing, reducing the need for multiple technical replicates, especially with limited samples.

The qPCR setup on the AB 7300 real-time PCR System involved a two-minute incubation at 50 °C, followed by 10 min at 95 °C, and then 40 cycles of 95 °C for 15 s and 60 °C for 60 s. Amplification results were analyzed using 7300 System SDS v1.4. software (Applied Biosystems, Foster City, CA, USA). Relative gene expression was calculated according to the Pfaffl method with efficiency (E) correction [36] according to the following equation: (EGOI)ΔCt GOI/Geometric Mean [(EREF)ΔCt REF]. Experiments were conducted following the Minimum Information for Publication of Quantitative Real-Time PCR Experiments (MIQE) guidelines [37]. *Tph1* and *MaoA* gene expression was analyzed and partially reported (for saline and TCP) in our previous study [25], in which we applied a different method for calculating relative gene expression.

2.5. Quantitative Histomorphometric Analysis

To determine whether experimentally caused hyperserotonemia increased the number of argentaffin cells which produce serotonin in the mucosal epithelial layer, we counted the number of positive cells stained with the specific Masson–Fontana method. The whole digestive tract surface (without lumen) was measured, and cells were counted on 1 cross section of the jejunum in the surface epithelial and crypt epithelial area separately. These values were expressed as the average number of argentaffin cells on 1 mm of referent space. In some cases, there was a positive reaction in lymphocytes, erythrocytes, and Paneth cells, which were all excluded from counting.

To determine the quantity of argentaffin granules in positive cells, we examined each cell with 1000× magnification, assigned the values from 1 (low intensity of stain) to 3 (high intensity of stain), and averaged these results for each animal (Figure 1A–C). We also measured the thickness of the tunica mucosa, the height of the mucosal epithelial cells, and the thickness of the outer muscle wall (tunica muscularis) at 5 randomly chosen test fields at magnification of 100× for each animal.

To investigate whether altered serotonin homeostasis affected structures in the liver, we morphometrically analyzed 10 randomly chosen test fields (at a magnification of 200×) per animal and digitally captured the pericentral zone around the central vein in hepatic lobules from 34 liver samples stained with PAS. In each field, we measured the following:

the minimum and maximum width of 10 hepatocytes, the width of 10 hepatocyte nuclei, the diameter of 10 sinusoids, and the minimum and maximum diameter of a central vein (Figure 1D,E). All morphometric measures were performed with a computerized image analysis system comprised of a light microscope (Nikon Eclipse E600), a digital camera (AxioCamErc 5s, Zeiss), and ZENlite 2.1 software (Carl Zeiss Microscopy, GmbH, Jena, Germany).

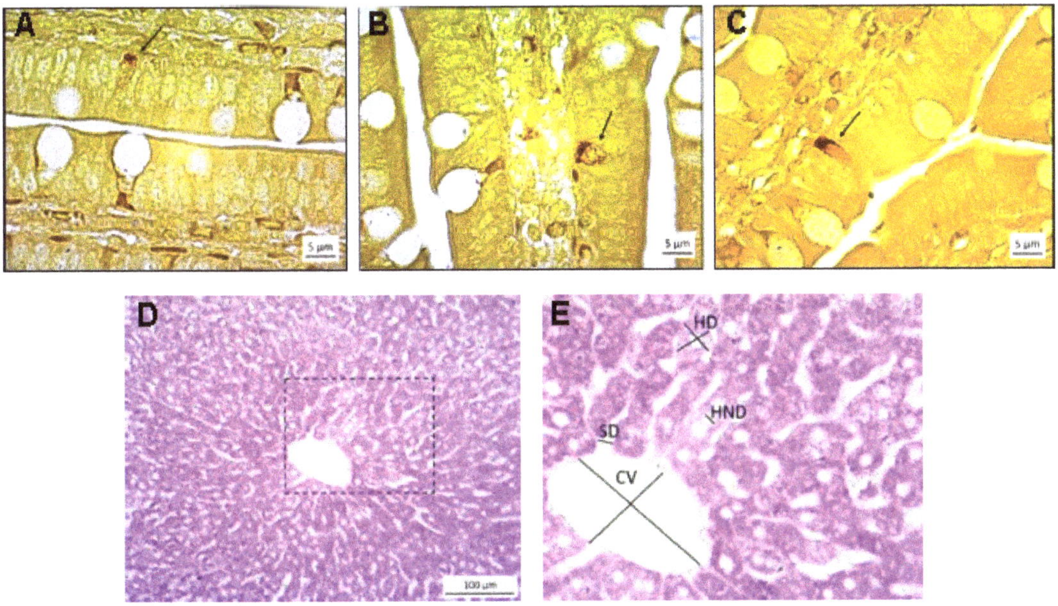

Figure 1. Histological sections of the jejunum with three representative argentaffin (serotonin-producing) cells (arrow) of different staining intensity: (**A**) low staining intensity, (**B**) medium staining intensity, and (**C**) high staining intensity (Masson–Fontana technique, magnification: 1000×). Normal histological structure of the (**D**) hepatic lobule in the rat liver with a rectangular area enlarged at (**E**) showing analyzed histomorphometric parameters. CV—central vein; HND—hepatocyte nuclei diameter; HD—hepatocyte diameter; SD—sinusoid diameter. PAS stain, magnification: 100×.

2.6. Statistical Analysis

Data were processed with GraphPad Prism 9.1.2 software (GraphPad Software, Inc., La Jolla, CA, USA). The normality of distribution was checked with Kolmogorov–Smirnov test. Original or transformed values of all parameters were analyzed with two-way ANOVA with treatment and sex as the main effects. Tukey's multiple comparison test was used for post hoc analyses. Correlation was analyzed with Pearson r correlation factor on all measured parameters. Values are presented as the median with interquartile range. The level of significance was set to 0.05 (two-tail p value). Some samples were lost during processing, and a female TCP-treated rat was excluded from all analyses, as the results were consistently outliers. The final number of samples on which the statistical analyses were performed is given in Table 1.

Table 1. 5-hydorxytryptophan and tranylcypromine induced changes in peripheral organs.

		Saline				5-Hydroxytryptophan				Tranilcypromine			
	5HT Conc.	Female Median (Q1,Q3)	N	Male Median (Q1,Q3)	N	Female Median (Q1,Q3)	N	Male Median (Q1,Q3)	N	Female Median (Q1,Q3)	N	Male Median (Q1,Q3)	N
	(ng 5-HT/mL PRP)	349 (1069,176)	5	711 (1005,242)	5	827 (1277,600)	5	484 (794,188)	5	927 (1478,558)	4	959 (1238,718)	6
	Gene expression (arbitrary units)												
Jejunum	TPH1	1.00 (1.27,0.72)	5	1.06 (1.56,0.80)	4	0.80 (0.93,0.67)	5	0.85 (1.15,0.60)	3	0.64 (0.80,0.59)	5	0.81 (1.00,0.63)	5
	VMAT	0.82 (1.33,0.67)		1.17 (1.34,0.95)		0.67 (0.73,0.65)		0.89 (1.11,0.81)	4	0.64 (1.11,0.57)		0.87 (1.26,0.79)	
Liver	5HTt	1.06 (1.13,0.74)	3	1.13 (1.53,0.67)	4	1.56 (1.75,1.10)	5	0.98 (1.22,0.93)	5	1.73 (1.85,1.50)	5	1.41 (1.76,0.97)	5
	MAOA	1.42 (1.90,1.15)		0.75 (0.93,0.63)		1.50 (1.81,0.97)		0.77 (0.97,0.64)		1.35 (1.62,1.11)		0.64 (0.66,0.60)	
	Histology												
Jejunum	Mucosal layer width (μm)	685.9 (741.5,644.3)	5	688.8 (706.8,566.4)	6	756.6 (766.5,725.4)	5	653.4 (776.0,589.6)	7	624.2 (697.8,525.3)	6	739.3 (779.4,637.9)	6
	Muscle layer width (μm)	67.5 (111.4,60.0)		82.6 (96.3,70.8)		71.0 (82.0,67.2)		90.9 (95.2,74,4)		71.9 (104.7,66.9)		92.8 (105.8,67.7)	
	Epithelial layer width (μm)	33.1 (36.0,31.6)		31.1 (35.0,28.4)		34.3 (36.0,32.7)		33.7 (38.4,31.6)		31.8 (33.7,29.5)		31.2 (34.7,28.6)	
	Total number of argentaffin-positive cells/mm^2	11.2 (12.2,8.9)		12.1 (14.6,7.0)		8.8 (10.9,7.0)		8.9 (10.4,8.0)		6.3 (6.9,5.0)		5.8 (6.7,4.5)	
	Number of cells in villi/1 mm^2	5.66 (8.37,4.84)		7.63 (9.17,4.86)		5.38 (6.41,4.76)		5.70 (7.03,4.99)		4.38 (5.07,3.39)		3.70 (4.21,2.95)	
	Number of cells in the crypts/1 mm^2	3.40 (6.24,2.79)		4.47 (5.20,2.31)		3.47 (4.41,2.19)		3.05 (3.22,2.42)		1.91 (2.15,1.62)		2.10 (2.53,1.58)	
	Argentaffin cell intensity	1.80 (2.20,1.30)		2.10 (2.40,1.75)		1.80 (1.85,1.60)		1.60 (2.00,1.40)		2.20 (2.60,1.95)		1.00 (1.20,1.00)	
Liver	Central vein diameter (μm)	109.6 (121.6,99.9)	5	98.7 (115.3,84.4)	3	145.4 (164.5,112.5)	5	114.7 (154.0,97.0)	6	81.4 (116.2,62.5)	6	109.1 (147.9,59.7)	6
	Hepatocyte nuclei diameter (μm)	6.30 (6.60,6.27)		6.55 (6.79,6.50)		6.72 (7.07,6.14)		7.09 (7.32,6.69)		6.79 (7.67,6.56)		7.26 (7.68,7.02)	
	Hepatocyte diameter (μm)	20.0 (20.9,19.6)		21.2 (21.3,20.7)		20.0 (21.0,19.0)		21.5 (22.3,19.9)		18.9 (20.1,17.8)		21.1 (21.7,20.4)	
	Sinusoid diameter (μm)	4.44 (5.36,3.81)		4.30 (5.87,4.05)		4.15 (4.63,4.00)		5.03 (5.27,4.48)		5.31 (6.08,4.93)		4.93 (6.72,4.22)	

3. Results

3.1. Blood 5HT Concentrations

Although blood 5HT concentrations were analyzed and partially reported (for saline and TCP) in our previous study [30], it is important to re-examine them in the context of the current study. As shown in Figure 2, there was a tendency of increase in blood 5HT concentrations after TCP treatment (males 959 (1238, 718) ng/mL, females 927 (1478, 558) ng/mL) in comparison to saline (males 711 (1005, 242) ng/mL, females 349 (1069, 176) ng/mL) and 5HTP (males 484 (794, 188) ng/mL, females 827 (1277, 600) ng/mL) treatment. However, two-way ANOVA did not show significant effects of treatment ($F(2,24) = 2.396$; $p = 0.1125$), sex ($F(1,24) = 0.7624$; $p = 0.3912$), or treatment × sex interaction ($F(2,24) = 1.156$; $p = 0.3318$) on 5HT concentrations in the blood of adult animals.

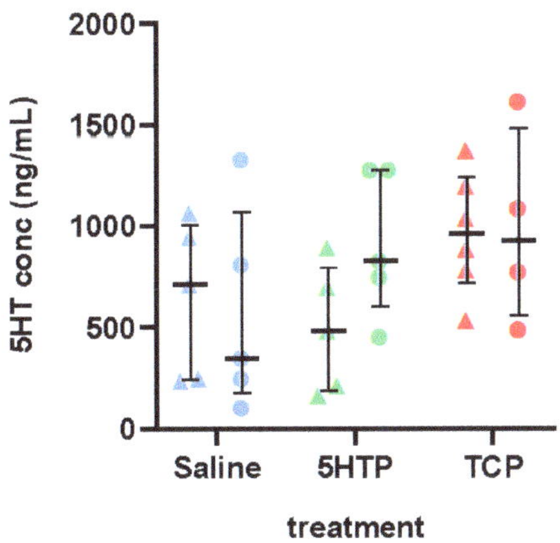

Figure 2. Effects of chronic treatment with 25 mg/kg 5-hydroxytryptophan (5HTP) or 2 mg/kg tranylcypromine (TCP) on 5HT concentrations in whole blood expressed as ng 5HT per mL of blood. Results are shown as the median with interquartile range; males are depicted as triangles and females as circles.

3.2. Histomorphological and Gene Expression Changes in Jejunum

Histological sections of the jejunum viewed under a light microscope showed normal architecture in all layers of the digestive tract. All examined samples from the three experimental groups exhibited intact epithelial lining of the mucosa, well-preserved cellular integrity, and no evidence of distortion or crypt atrophy in the mucosa or signs of inflammation. Consequently, histomorphometric characteristics of digestive tract layers showed similar mean values for the measured parameters in all three groups (Table 1). Indeed, as analyzed by two-way ANOVA, treatment, sex, and treatment × sex interaction did not have a significant effect on either the epithelial layer width ($F(2,30) = 2.08$, $p = 0.14$; $F(1,30) = 0.47$, $p = 0.4978$ and $F(2,30) = 0.33$, $p = 0.7181$, respectively) or the muscle layer width ($F(2,30) = 0.14$, $p = 0.8732$; $F(1,30) = 1.00$, $p = 0.3242$ and $F(2,30) = 0.39$, $p = 0.6775$, respectively). The mucosal layer width was significantly affected by treatment × sex interaction ($F(2,30) = 4.01$, $p = 0.0274$), but no effect of treatment or sex ($F(2,30) = 1.0$, $p = 0.3682$ and $F(1,30) = 0.029$, $p = 0.8653$, respectively) was observed.

An extremely significant effect of treatment was observed on the total number of argentaffin-positive cells ($F(2,30) = 17.53$, $p < 0.0001$), with no effects of sex ($F(1,30) = 0.11$, $p = 0.7388$) or treatment × sex interaction ($F(21,30) = 0.15$, $p = 0.8621$). As can be seen in Figure 3A, post hoc analysis revealed significantly lower values in the TCP-treated group in comparison to controls, with intermediate values of 5HTP-treated animals. Interestingly, the total number of argentaffin-positive cells significantly negatively correlated with blood 5HT concentration ($r = -0.465$, $p = 0.01$). The argentaffin-positive cells were stained brownish to black, with varying intensity depending on the number of granules within cells. The staining intensity of argentaffin cells was not significantly affected by treatment (F(2,30) = 1.98, $p = 0.1558$), although a significant effect was observed for both sex (F(1,30) = 5.864, $p = 0.0217$) and sex x treatment interaction (F(2,30) = 11.92, $p = 0.0002$). Post hoc analysis showed that this significance was due to males from the TCP treatment group having a significantly lower staining intensity than that of animals from the other subgroups (Figure 3B).

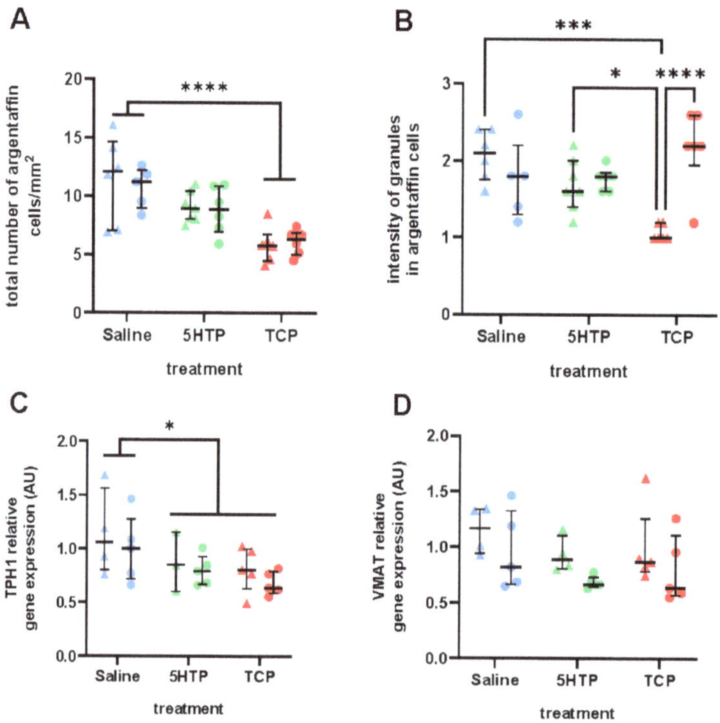

Figure 3. Effects of chronic treatment with serotonin enhancers 5-hydroxytryptophan (5HTP, 25 mg/kg) and tranylcypromine (TCP, 2 mg/kg) or saline on the small intestine (jejunum). (**A**) Number of argentaffin-positive cells, which produce serotonin, per mm^2 of surface in the epithelial layer of the jejunum. Two-way ANOVA revealed a significant effect of treatment. (**B**) Staining intensity corresponding to the number of granules in argentaffin cells. Cells were rated subjectively from 1 (low intensity) to 3 (high intensity), and averages of 5 measurements per animal are shown. Two-way ANOVA revealed the significant effect of treatment × sex interaction. (**C**) Relative expression of tryptophan hydroxylase (TPH1) mRNA. Two-way ANOVA revealed the significant effect of treatment. (**D**) Relative expression of vesicular monoamine transporter (VMAT) mRNA. Results are shown as the median with interquartile range; males are depicted as triangles, and females as circles. * $p < 0.05$, *** $p < 0.001$, **** $p < 0.0001$, Tukey's multiple comparison test for post hoc analyses.

Treatment (F(2,21) = 4.013, $p = 0.0334$), but not sex (F(1,21) = 1.362, $p = 0.2562$) or treatment × sex interaction (F(2,21) = 0.05219, $p = 0.9493$), had a significant effect on the relative gene expression for TPH1. Post hoc analysis showed significantly lower mean levels of mRNA for TPH1 in both the treatment groups compared to the controls (Figure 3C). Although treatment (F(2,22) = 1.908, $p = 0.1722$, Figure 3D), as well as sex and treatment × sex interaction (F(1,22) = 4.192, $p = 0.0527$; and F(2,22) = 0.03419, $p = 0.9664$, respectively), did not significantly affect mRNA levels for *Vmat*, relative expression of this gene significantly positively correlated with the expression of the *Tph1* gene (r = 0.440, $p = 0.022$).

3.3. Histomorphological and Gene Expression Changes in Liver

Microscopically, liver sections from all three groups appeared normal, with no heavy pathological findings such as inflammation, fat deposits, fibrosis, or necrosis. The hepatic parenchyma was organized into polygonal lobules with hepatocytes, normal portal tracts, and a regular pattern of the central veins. However, quantitative morphometric parameters revealed some changes in the treated groups. According to two-way ANOVA, treatment had a significant (F(2,26) = 6.259, p = 0.006) effect on hepatocyte nuclei diameter, with the values of TCP-treated group being significantly higher and the values of the 5HTP group being intermediate as compared to the values of the control group (Figure 4A). Sex had a marginally significant effect (F(1,26) = 4.399, p = 0.0458), and sex × treatment interaction had no effect (F(2,27) = 0.1107, p = 0.8956). Interestingly, the effect of treatment on nuclear enlargement (karyomegaly) was not followed by enlargement of hepatocytes (hepatocellular hypertrophy). Two-way ANOVA revealed only a significant effect of sex (F(1,27) = 9.252, p = 0.0052) but not of treatment or sex × treatment interaction on hepatocyte diameter (F(2,27) = 1.556, p = 0.2292 and F(2,27) = 1.031, p = 0.3703, respectively).

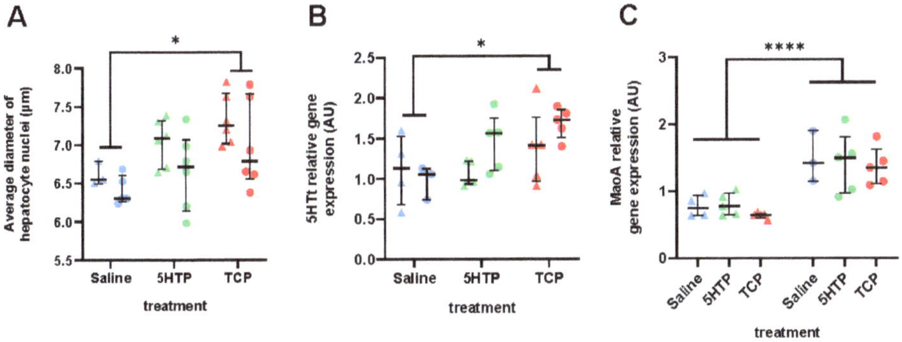

Figure 4. Effects of chronic treatment with serotonin enhancers 5-hydroxytryptophan (5HTP, 25 mg/kg) and tranylcypromine (TCP, 2 mg/kg) or saline on the liver. (**A**) Average diameter of hepatocyte nuclei. Each measure represents the average of the measured width of 100 hepatocyte nuclei. Two-way ANOVA revealed a significant effect of treatment. (**B**) Relative gene expression for 5HT transporter (5HTt) mRNA. Two-way ANOVA revealed a significant effect of treatment. (**C**) Relative gene expression for monoamine oxidase A (MAOA) mRNA. Two-way ANOVA revealed a significant effect of sex. Results are shown as the median with interquartile range; males are depicted as triangles and females as circles. * $p < 0.05$, **** $p < 0.0001$, Tukey's multiple comparison test.

Although some early signs of connective tissue deposition around the central veins (perivenular fibrosis) were visible in females treated with 5HTP, no significant differences between the treated groups were detected with two-way ANOVA for structural dilatation of the sinusoid diameter or central veins.

Treatment had a significant effect on the gene expression for 5HTt (F(2,21) = 4.636, p = 0.0215) due to a significantly higher expression in the TCP-treated group, with the values of the 5HTP-treated group again being in between (Figure 4B). No effect of sex (F(1,21) = 2.149, p = 0.1575) or sex × treatment interaction (F(2,21) = 1.453, p = 0.2565) was observed. A strong effect of sex was noticed for MAOA mRNA expression (F(1,21) = 38.69, p < 0.0001), with no effect of treatment or treatment × sex interaction (F(2,21) = 0.5400, p = 0.5906 and F(2,22) = 2.599, p = 0.0970; respectively).

We studied the long-lasting effects of perinatal exposure to excessive 5HT concentrations on the organs responsible for the maintenance of peripheral 5HT homeostasis. Animals treated perinatally with 5HT enhancers displayed decreased number and function of serotonin-producing cells in the jejunum, enlarged nuclei of the liver cells, and an increase in 5HTt mRNA expression. In comparison to TCP, 5HTP had smaller yet visible effects on the measured parameters.

4. Discussion

We showed earlier that blood serotonin levels were significantly increased in both treatment groups during treatment, while TCP, unlike 5HTP, also caused a significant increase in brain 5HT concentrations [26]. TCP seemed to have induced a more prominent disbalance in 5HT homeostasis, which affected both 5HT compartments, and we therefore expected to see more serious effects in TCP-treated animals than in 5HTP-treated animals. At adult age, differences in blood 5HT levels of the TCP- and 5HTP-treated animals were not significantly different from those in saline-treated rats, but a tendency of gradual saline-5HTP-TCP increase was still observed. The fact that 5HT levels did not fully return to normal seven weeks after the end of treatment indicates that peripheral 5HT homeostasis was not fully reestablished in spite of the compensatory mechanisms. Indeed, we observed specific, 5HT-related changes, which is in accordance with the reported findings that high levels of neurotransmitters during development induce permanent changes at the histological and cellular level [38,39].

As expected, perinatal treatment with 5HT enhancers did not have a gross effect on the enteric tissue, as the thickness of tunica mucosa, height of the mucosal epithelial cells, and thickness of the outer muscle wall remained unchanged. Argentaffin-positive cells from our study were pyramidal or triangular in shape (Figure 1A–C), similar to the description by Gustafsson et al. [40], and clearly showed the presence of secretory granules in the basal portion of the cells, which can activate vagal afferent fibers inducing intestinal motility and modulating brain–gut axis signaling, or they can be released into the cardiovascular system and stimulate glucose and lipid metabolism [41]. The TCP-treated group from our study showed a significantly lower number of argentaffin-positive cells and a lower presence of 5HT in the granules in these cells (significant only for males), which was reflected in the lower level of gene expression for TPH1 (significantly so in both the TCP- and 5HTP-treated groups). Although mRNA levels for VMAT1 significantly positively correlated with mRNA levels for TPH1, as it would be expected that less synthesis leads to less need for storage, the expression of this gene was not significantly lowered in the treated groups. Takahashi and colleagues [42] found that heterozygous *Vmat2* knock-out mice had reduced neuronal 5HT concentrations probably due to the lack of storage and, therefore, easier availability for degradation. A more stable concentration of VMAT than of TPH1 might be explained by an attempt to compensate for the decrease in the number of cells and synthesis rate and to protect the remaining 5HT from degradation. We assume that the reduction in number of 5HT-producing cells and down-regulation of *Tph1* expression, long after a washout-period, are the results of the extensive compensatory mechanism that occurred during the increased availability of the immediate 5HT precursor (in the case of 5HTP treatment) or the lack of degradation of 5HT during MAO inhibition (in the case of TCP treatment). In contrast with these results, a high-tryptophan diet during fetal and early postnatal development, caused, besides hyperserotonemia, an increase in the number of serotonin-producing cells [43]. The discrepancy between these results could be explained by the type of administered 5HT enhancer—5HT precursor tryptophan requires TPH1 as the rate-limiting enzyme crucial for the first step of serotonin synthesis, which might have caused an increase in both *Tph1* gene expression and the number of TPH1-expressing cells. In our experiment, there was no need for increased TPH1 activity, allowing for the compensatory reduction of serotonin-producing cells and enzymes.

As in the jejunum, changes at the tissue level were also absent in the liver—both sinusoid and central vein diameters showed no difference between the groups. At the cellular level, the hepatocyte nuclei diameter showed an increase in the treated groups paralleled by an increase in *5HTt* gene expression. The increase in both parameters was significant in the TCP-treated group with intermediate values in the 5HTP-treated group. A highly significant difference in *MaoA* expression between the sexes, with females having double the expression than males, was expected due to the location of this gene on the X chromosome. Interestingly, our earlier study demonstrated a marked, long-lasting compensatory increase in mRNA expression for MAOA and 5HTt in the brains of TCP-treated animals [28], yet no changes were observed in the liver *MaoA* gene expression after 5HT enhancement. Although we cannot rule out an increased *MaoA* expression in the lungs (another site of 5HT degradation), it seems that in the liver, serotonin enhancement specifically upregulates *5HTt* expression. Serotonin promotes liver regeneration [44] yet may cause hepatotoxicity due to the generation of reactive oxygen species (ROS) during degradation by MAOA [45]. This might be the reason why we did not see an increase in the peripheral expression of *MaoA* after chronic inhibition since the compensatory mechanism of increasing *MaoA* expression might have a deleterious effect on liver cells due to excess ROS. Instead, 5HT uptake into hepatocytes increased (as demonstrated by increased *5HTt* expression), after which the excess of 5HT might have been converted to melatonin, as hepatocytes were shown to express serotonin N-acetyltransferase and hydroxyindole-O-methyl transferase [46]. Alternatively, hepatocyte 5HT content might have remained increased, potentially inducing karyomegaly, as serotonin was reported to mediate the induction of DNA synthesis in primary cultures of rat hepatocytes [47] and stimulate liver regeneration after hepatectomy in humans [48].

Taken all together, our current results indicate that in the periphery, a reduction in 5HT synthesis (lower number of 5HT-producing cells and decreased *Tph1* expression) coupled with an enhanced removal of 5HT from blood plasma (increased *5HTt* expression) are the main means of compensation for excessive blood 5HT levels. The resulting alteration in 5HT production might have induced dysregulation of 5HT signaling and caused impairments in 5HT-regulated peripheral functions, such as bone maintenance and leukocyte development and/or the sustainment previously observed in adult TCP-treated rats [30]. Future investigation of the gene expression of proinflammatory molecules and the expression of serotonin receptors in both tissues should provide a deeper understanding of the physiological changes in the digestive tract as a consequence of perinatal 5HT enhancement.

In humans, inadequate 5HT production leads to various disorders such as inflammatory bowel diseases (IBDs), celiac disease, and neuroendocrine disorders [41]. Studies on 5HT signaling in IBD show that the number of EC cells and the presence of 5HT in secretory granules can be either increased or decreased both in animal and human models [49–52]. These differences may arise from different model organisms of induced diseases and from the severity and location of the disease [52]. Serotonin's role in gut inflammation is well known [49,53–57]. In studies, inflammation in the intestine was present in *Tph1* or *5HTt* KO models fully lacking the ability of 5HT synthesis or removal, respectively. The administration of 5HTP to $Tph1^{-/-}$ mice increased the number of 5HT-expressing cells and intestinal histologic damage [58], while gastrointestinal inflammation was induced with 2,4,6-trinitrobenzene sulfonic acid (TNBS) in a *5HTt* KO model [59]. The lack of inflammation in the intestines of the 5HTP- and TCP-treated rats 2 months after the end of treatment might be the result of the compensatory decrease in intestine *Tph1* expression and a parallel increase in liver *5HTt* expression. Still, both 5HTP- and TCP-treated rats had previously shown a slower rate of increase in body mass compared to the saline-treated rats [24,25], pointing to a possible inadequacy in nutrient absorption and storage and/or consumption and rendering them a potential model for studying gastrointestinal and metabolic disorders.

The fact that the period of 5HTP and TCP treatment used in our study corresponds to the second and third trimester of human pregnancy [13] provides another point of potential clinical relevance to our model. Selective serotonin reuptake inhibitors (SSRIs) are commonly used 5HT enhancers during pregnancy [60], and the consequences of developmental exposure to SSRIs have been thoroughly studied in both animal models and human populations [61,62]. On the other hand, the use of MAO inhibitors is restricted to SSRI-nonresponsive patients; hence, reports on the prenatal exposure to MAO inhibitors are limited. Even less is known about the prenatal exposure to 5HTP, which is often offered as a natural alternative to antidepressant drugs, and the versatility of the potential therapeutic effects, easy availability, and convenience of unsupervised use increase the probability of prenatal exposure [20]. Effects analogous to those observed in our model, such as impeded growth and potential behavioral and/or metabolic alterations, might occur in exposed humans, suggesting that systematic studies on the prenatal impact of these 5HT enhancers in the human population are needed.

Our study has several advantages. First, by employing the inhibition of catabolism or the stimulation of synthesis, we were able to study the consequences of 5HT metabolic alterations, which complemented previously reported studies focused on 5HT synaptic action, i.e., treatment with SSRI's [63] and 5HT receptor agonists [64,65]. Second, parallel use of the two compounds, one altering 5HT homeostasis only in the peripheral 5HT compartment and the other altering 5HT homeostasis both peripherally and centrally, enabled us to study the relationship between the two compartments and to examine the contribution of central 5HT disbalance to the alterations in the peripheral compartment. Third, the use of 5HTP instead of tryptophan (Trp) as a 5HT precursor allowed us to avoid the rate-limiting step in the synthesis of serotonin and to mimic the effect of increased serotonin synthesis through the chosen 5HTP dose. As opposed to Trp, which is an essential amino acid with many functions in the body (more than 90% of Trp enters the kynurenine metabolic pathway, about 5% is metabolized through the indole pathway by the gut microbiota, and only the remaining Trp is used in the serotonin synthesis [66,67]), 5HTP is only found in the serotonin synthesis pathway and is quantitatively converted to 5HT [20]. Fourth, experimenting on both male and female animals enabled us to check for the potential sex differences in the vulnerability to disbalance in 5HT homeostasis and to avoid a sex-biased interpretation of the results. Finally, the low chronic doses used in this study ae similar to those taken by humans, enhancing the translatability of the obtained results.

We also have to mention several limitations of our study, which could affect the reliability and interpretation of the results. The major limitation of the study lies in the relatively small number of animals, which could have caused some false-negative results due to insufficient sample power. The number of females included in the experiment was determined from our previous experience and according to the 3R principle [32], but rather small litter sizes and the loss of several samples resulted in a suboptimal sample number, rendering our findings only as preliminary and requiring further confirmation. We should note that TCP, as a nonselective MAO inhibitor, also affects catecholamine metabolism, allowing for the possibility that other monoamines influenced our results. Still, unlike 5HT, catecholamines can enter an alternative degradation pathway through catechol-O-methyltransferase, which is present in the brain and peripheral tissues and increases its activity when MAO is blocked [68]. Accordingly, we showed earlier that TCP treatment raised central dopamine and noradrenaline concentrations to a considerably lower extent than did that of 5HT, while it did not affect peripheral catecholamine levels [27]. Finally, our study did not include analysis at the protein level, which would have enabled us to establish a link between gene expression and structural changes and provide a clearer view of the mild yet significant effects of the 5HT enhancers.

5. Conclusions

We have shown that the perinatal exposure to the increased 5HT concentrations induces long-lasting cellular and molecular changes in the two organs responsible for serotonin metabolism, which may have a negative impact on 5HT availability and, consequently, on the 5HT-regulated peripheral functions. Our current and previous results demonstrate a link between developmental abnormalities of serotonin homeostasis and 5HT-related molecular, neurochemical, structural, and functional changes in adult life, suggesting our rat model to be suitable for exploring the neurobiological substrates of vulnerability to behavioral and metabolic disorders, as well as for modeling the adverse effects of the prenatal exposure to 5HT enhancers in the human population. Future studies

biomedicines

MDPI

Review

The Orexin/Hypocretin System, the Peptidergic Regulator of Vigilance, Orchestrates Adaptation to Stress

Miklós Jászberényi [1], Balázs Thurzó [1,2], Zsolt Bagosi [1], László Vécsei [3,4] and Masaru Tanaka [4,*]

1. Department of Pathophysiology, University of Szeged, H-6701 Szeged, Hungary; miklos.jaszberenyi@med.u-szeged.hu (M.J.); bazska82@gmail.com (B.T.); bagosi.zsolt@med.u-szeged.hu (Z.B.)
2. Emergency Patient Care Unit, Albert Szent-Györgyi Health Centre, University of Szeged, H-6725 Szeged, Hungary
3. Department of Neurology, Albert Szent-Györgyi Medical School, University of Szeged, H-6725 Szeged, Hungary; vecsei.laszlo@med.u-szeged.hu
4. HUN-REN-SZTE Neuroscience Research Group, Hungarian Research Network, University of Szeged (HUN-REN-SZTE), Danube Neuroscience Research Laboratory, Tisza Lajos krt. 113, H-6725 Szeged, Hungary

* Correspondence: tanaka.masaru.1@med.u-szeged.hu

Abstract: The orexin/hypocretin neuropeptide family has emerged as a focal point of neuroscientific research following the discovery that this family plays a crucial role in a variety of physiological and behavioral processes. These neuropeptides serve as powerful neuromodulators, intricately shaping autonomic, endocrine, and behavioral responses across species. Notably, they serve as master regulators of vigilance and stress responses; however, their roles in food intake, metabolism, and thermoregulation appear complementary and warrant further investigation. This narrative review provides a journey through the evolution of our understanding of the orexin system, from its initial discovery to the promising progress made in developing orexin derivatives. It goes beyond conventional boundaries, striving to synthesize the multifaceted activities of orexins. Special emphasis is placed on domains such as stress response, fear, anxiety, and learning, in which the authors have contributed to the literature with original publications. This paper also overviews the advancement of orexin pharmacology, which has already yielded some promising successes, particularly in the treatment of sleep disorders.

Keywords: orexins; neuropeptides; neurotransmitters; stress; feeding; temperature regulation; fear; anxiety; learning; sleep–wake disorders

1. Introduction: Neuropeptides as the Modulators of the Connectome

In Sections 1 and 2, a general overview of the orexin system is given, and Sections 3 and 4 will be devoted to those fields in which the authors have considerably contributed to the literature. Neuropeptide research started more than a hundred years ago with the discovery of the effects of vasopressin [1] and oxytocin [2] and tissue extraction of the first classical neuropeptide: substance P [3]. Since then, more and more distinct features of neuropeptides have been identified that clearly separate them from classical neurotransmitters [4–6]. First, some obvious biochemical features justify the differentiation. They are much larger molecules than classical neurotransmitters; therefore, the energy requirements for their synthesis and transport well exceed those of these neurotransmitters. Functionally, their release is not confined to the synapses, although some portions of their pool are also frequently co-secreted together with classic neurotransmitters. In contrast, they can be released from the dense core vesicles of practically any portion of the neurons [4–6]. Unlike classic neurotransmitters, neuropeptides are not taken back economically by a reuptake system but are metabolized by peptidases. Nonetheless, this process frequently yields biologically active compounds [6]. Further, due to their prolonged half-life, neuropeptides can diffuse to long distances; therefore, they act not only post- and pre-synaptically (i.e., in a paracrine and autocrine fashion) but also in an endocrine manner [6] through the operation of G-protein-coupled receptors (GPCRs) [6]. Due to these characteristics, their effects develop slowly but are usually longer lasting. Their impact, compared to that of classic small molecular and even gaseous neurotransmitters, is almost always less robust, which strongly resembles the activity of hormones [7]. That is why in the literature some members are still referred to as neurohormones and their activity has been formulated as "neuromodulation" [4–6], which represents a "mild" or "functionally buffered" form of signal transduction [4–6]. A unique feature of neuromodulation is that it is realized using a much broader arsenal of receptors than that of neurotransmitters [5]. Also, the ligands themselves show immense structural versatility because, in some families, almost infinite splice variants can be produced from several copies of an ancestral gene [5]. Therefore, it is not surprising that neuroscience has struggled to formulate a rigid functional definition of neuromodulation, in contrast with that of neurotransmission and neurotransmitters [8].

Accordingly, neuropeptides appear to represent an individual and separate form of transfer of biological information, somewhere in between that of the classical neurotransmitters and peripheral hormones. The secretion of these modulators gives rise to less acute but, in the long run, more profound changes in the neural connectome, the operative framework of neurophysiology [9]. The multi-faceted activity and redundancy of these signaling molecules provide an indispensable component of the plasticity and resilience of the central nervous system (CNS). This is further augmented by the bewildering diversity and extremely broad distribution of several neuropeptide families. Certain groups and their receptors are expressed at every level of neuroendocrine control [4–6].

It is apparent that the challenges to which the CNS is exposed ultimately will give rise to changes in translational processes. These will manifest themselves in the modification of receptor and enzyme expression, synaptic plasticity, and the dendritic pattern and structure and finally the complete wiring of the connectome [9,10]. Neuropeptides represent an essential but so-far overlooked element of the translational machinery, bridging the gap between volatile functional alterations and permanent structural changes. As peptides, they represent one of the earliest steps (along with neurotransmission-evoked peptide and protein synthesis) in the translational processes of information signaling in the CNS. Their modulatory action via extremely versatile ligands, the corresponding receptors, and a multitude of stimulated signaling cascades make them the most flexible line of neuroendocrine plasticity and adaptation [4–6].

The experiments carried out on the orexin/hypocretin system especially support this view: its cooperation with other neuropeptides appears to harmonize the autonomic, behavioral, and endocrine response to arousal [11–20]. Hence, firstly, the present paper gives a general overview of the general biochemical, anatomical–histological, physiological, and pathophysiological features of the orexin/hypocretin system. This review focuses on those specific fields (stress response, thermoregulation, fear, anxiety, and learning) in which the authors have also contributed to the literature.

2. The Hypocretin/Orexin Peptide and Receptor Family

The hypocretin/orexin system represents an extremely complex neuropeptide network in the CNS [21,22]. The seminal papers [23–25] that dealt with the discovery of these ligands and their receptors also demonstrated the hyperphagic [23] and neuroexcitatory activity [24] of orexins and the unique distribution pattern of the system. The orexin/hypocretin system, similarly to melanin-concentrating hormone (MCH)-positive neurons [26], has a well-circumscribed expression in the hypothalamus (Figure 1) [24,27]. Its cell bodies are restricted to the lateral, dorsal, dorsomedial, and perifornical areas, and the whole population does not exceed 50,000–80,000 cells in the hypothalamus. However, its axon terminals reach distant regions, and its receptors are scattered throughout the whole CNS [25].

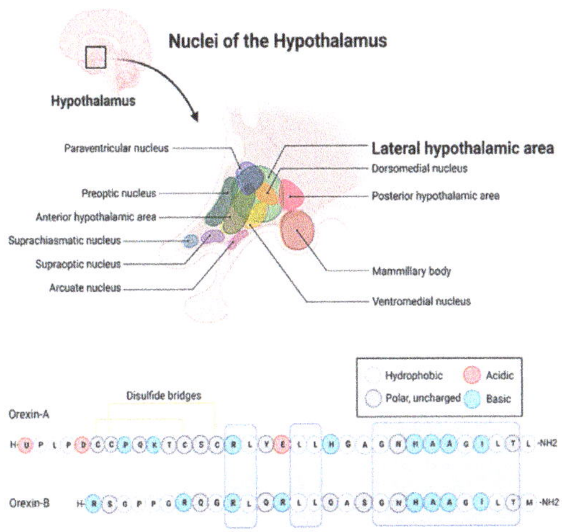

Figure 1. The localization of the lateral hypothalamic area and the amino acid sequences of the orexin/hypocretin family peptides. The letters stand for the one letter code of amino acids. A: Alanine, C: Cysteine, D: Aspartic acid, E: Glutamic acid, G: Glycine, H: Histidine, I: Isoleucine, K: Lysine, L: Leucine, M: Methionine, N: Asparagine, P: Proline, Q: Glutamine, R: Arginine, S: Serine, T: Threonine, U: Pyroglutamic acid, Y: Tyrosine.

At the cellular level, so far, two ligands (orexin-A, orexin-B) and two receptors (OX1R and OX2R) of the system have been described (Figure 1) [23,24]. The peptides biochemically belong to the incretin family, but they bear weak structural resemblance only to a few members of the group [23,24]. Even orexin-A and orexin-B differ by 50% of their primary structure. Both peptides are cleft from pre-pro-orexin (PPO) and are amidated C-terminally, but orexin-A is larger, comprising 33 amino acids, while orexin-B consists of only 28 residues [28]. Orexin-A is also less prone to proteolytic degradation because it comprises an N-terminal pyroglutamate residue and two disulfide bonds. Additionally, orexin-A is more hydrophobic, and therefore it can bypass more efficiently the blood–brain barrier (BBB) [29]. These orexins also exhibit significantly different receptor affinities [23,24,30], which is definitely attributed to the fact that the orexin receptors (OXRs) share only 64% amino acid identity [28,31]. The two receptor subtypes create diversity within the cellular signaling pathways [28,31–34]. Both OX1R and OX2R activity is mediated by Gq_{11}, which, in turn, leads to the activation of phospholipase C (PLC), phospholipase A (PLA), and phospholipase D, ultimately resulting in an increase in cytosolic Ca^{2+} and the activation of protein kinase C (PKC). In addition, OX1R can elevate the intracellular Ca^{2+} level by activating non-selective cation channels (NSCCs) [31]. On the other hand, OX2R can also inhibit adenyl cyclase (AC) and protein kinase A (PKA) through the G-protein-coupled pathway. The potential dimerization of the OXRs and the structural overlap between OXRs and some other GPCRs lend further diversity to the signal transduction of the system [31]. For example, certain neuropeptide receptors, such as the type-2 neuropeptide-Y (NPY) receptor, the thyrotropin-releasing hormone (TRH) receptor, the cholecystokinin (CCK) type-A receptor, and the NK2 neurokinin receptor, show some similarities (26%, 25%, 23%, and 20% identity, respectively) to the orexin receptors [23]. The highest structural similarity is exhibited by the neuropeptide FF (NPFF) receptor of the RF-amide peptide family, which is 37% identical to OX1R and 35% identical to OX2R, respectively [35,36].

Neither the distribution of the immunoreactivity of the two orexins [37,38] nor the expression of OX1R [30,39–41] and OX2R [30,40–42] completely overlaps. This, together with the aforementioned distinct features of the pharmacokinetics of orexin peptides and the differences in the signal transduction of OX1R and OX2R [32–34], must be responsible for some divergence in the physiologic and pathophysiologic actions of orexin-A and orexin-B [38].

3. The Orexin System, as an Indispensable Regulator of Arousal, Cooperates with the Central Oscillator to Control Circadian Activities

At the systemic level, the function of target areas of the orexin neurons has suggested numerous clues on the feasible actions of orexins [25] (Table 1). Although, at first, orexins were proved to play an important role in hedonic feeding [23,43], later publications unveiled that the most important aspect of their functional spectrum could be the regulation of arousal [44]. Later studies also verified that the orexin network receives important input from the neurons of the circadian system [45,46], the most important center of which is the suprachiasmatic nucleus (SCN). These results substantiated the way circadian rhythms and arousal are synchronized in the mammalian brain. The mammalian circadian clock itself is hierarchically organized [47–50]. Its main components are the input signaling pathways, the main pacemaker, and the output signaling pathways [47–50]. The most important inputs to the SCN are photic stimuli, which arrive from the retina through the retinohypothalamic pathway [47,48,51]. The SCN serves as the "master clock" for the brain and the body and controls the activity of "local clocks". In the CNS, its outputs reach several autonomic centers in the hypothalamus, such as the ventrolateral preoptic nucleus (VLPO), the arcuate nucleus (ARC), the organum vasculosum laminae terminalis (OVLT), the median preoptic area (MnPO), the lateral hypothalamus, the medial preoptic area (MPO), and the paraventricular nucleus (PVN) [48]. Therefore, the central oscillator determines the circadian, diurnal, or mensual characteristics of the sleep–wake cycle, food and fluid intake, core temperature, vigilance, and several endocrine activities, such as the estrous cycle and the activity of the hypothalamic–pituitary–adrenal cortex (HPA). The SCN also targets several extrahypothalamic centers from the brainstem, through the pineal gland to the hippocampus [47]. This way, it also provides temporal clues on the entrainment of arousal, autonomic control, pain sensation, and even higher cortical activities such as mood, affection, and learning. The connection between the SCN and the orexin neurons has two-way bidirectional components, as described in recent publications [48]. However, a strong endocrine connection has also been verified between the two centers, through the melatonin secretion of the pineal gland [51]. Ultimately, indirect communication is established between the central oscillator and the orexin neurons at the level of the ascending reticular activation system (ARAS). First, the ARAS is undoubtedly the most important output of the lateral hypothalamus since orexinergic cells target several important centers of the ARAS, such as the pedunculopontine tegmental (PPT) and lateral dorsal tegmental (LDT) nuclei in the mesopontine tegmentum (MT), the nucleus raphe (NR), the locus coeruleus (LC), and the periaqueductal gray (PG) [25,52]. Second, these nuclei also provide the most important non-photic inputs to the central oscillator [48].

The nuclei of the ARAS operate with the classical neurotransmitters (acetylcholine, serotonin, norepinephrine, and dopamine, respectively) and foster the inputs to the dualistic centers of sleep–wakefulness regulation: the tuberomammillary nucleus (TMN) and the VLPO of the hypothalamus. The histaminergic TMN and the galanin- and γ-amino-butyric-acid (GABA)-positive VLPO control sleep onset according to a flip-flop mechanism [53–55]. It seems that the orexin-positive cells facilitate arousal through indirect disinhibition: they block the GABAergic output of the VLPO through the stimulation of the above-mentioned cholinergic and monoaminergic nuclei of the ARAS [25,56–61]. In this activity, OX2R mediation appears to play a predominant role. OX2R antagonism is sufficient to induce sleep, while OX1R blockade even attenuates this phenomenon [62–64]. This way, the orexin system could be easily categorized not only as the master regulator of arousal [65] but also as a significant modulator of the sleep–wake cycle and other circadian rhythms [44,53,66,67]. The indispensable role of the orexin system in the maintenance of vigilance is strongly supported by the finding that narcolepsy and cataplexy observed in dogs [68] and mice [69] can be solely attributed to the deficiency of the orexin/hypocretin system. Moreover, by now, it has been supported by several observations that human cases of narcolepsy with cataplexy [70–72] can also be attributed to either the abnormal development [73] or acquired immunological destruction [74] of the orexin–hypocretin system. Narcolepsy is characterized by REM intrusion into wakefulness, and REM sleep depends on the cholinergic activity of the ARAS, which is gated by the histaminergic neurons of the system [60,61,64]. These antagonistic centers both receive orexinergic input [25]. However, it appears that it is the selective deficiency of histaminergic gating that is responsible for the disease. This can be attributed to the absence of OX2R in the histaminergic neurons [60,61,64]. These observations offer great therapeutic opportunities not only for sleep disorders but also for abnormalities of these physiological functions, which are influenced by the orexin/hypocretin network. The most important physiological processes the circadian control of which the orexin system modulates are food and fluid intake [75–77], metabolism and thermoregulation [78], the activity of the HPA axis [11,13,65,79–82], and reproduction [83,84]. As mentioned above, the anatomical connections, which provide the foundation of these physiological actions, have also been verified: the orexinergic axons target the ARC, the PVN, and the preoptic and supraoptic nuclei (PON and SON, respectively) of the hypothalamus [10,53].

Even the initial publications suggested that orexins increase body weight and acutely stimulate food intake [23,85]. Due to the hyperphagic activity and specific localization of the orexin neurons, at least a group of their population can certainly be identified with some portion of the classic glucose-sensitive feeding center of the ventrolateral hypothalamus [86–90]. The orexin-positive neurons are bidirectionally connected to the ARC and the PVN, which operate in a well-known dualistic manner in food intake regulation. The most important stimulatory neuropeptides are NPY and agouti-related peptide (AgRP) in the ARC and TRH in the PVN. The inhibitory neurohormones are cocaine- and amphetamine-regulated transcript (CART) and melanocortins (MCs) in the ARC and CRH in the PVN [91,92]. According to the literature, orexin-A evokes the activation [93] of the OX1Rs [77] in the ARC, and the PVN mediates the hyperphagic effect of the system. However, the role of orexins is more complex since, in the long run, it is their deficiency that is associated with weight gain [94], which is attributed to their two-pronged action in thermoregulation. The anatomical substrate of this activity is the connection of the orexin system to the PON and the dorsomedial hypothalamus (DMH) [25]. The orexins concurrently activate heat loss and thermogenesis. That is why they can either decrease or increase the core temperature depending on the experimental settings [12,95–97]. In summary, they stimulate heat dissipation [12,97] through sympathetic vasodilation [95], which is mediated by OX1R. However, it is accompanied by the modulation of metabolism in the brown adipose tissue (BAT) [98]. In the sympathetic nervous system, OX1Rs apparently activate [96,99] while OX2Rs inhibit [100] non-shivering thermogenesis in the BAT. Obviously, concomitant increases in heat generation and heat dissipation prevent the excessive accumulation of fat.

Orexins also modulate the activity of the reproductive axis [83,84,101,102]. This action is bidirectional and brain-region- and, in females, estrous-cycle-dependent. Further, both orexin-A and orexin-B and both OXR1 and OXR2 take part in the control of the hypothalamic–pituitary–gonadal (HPG) axis [103]. The orexin system may supply period-dependent inputs to the HPG axis. Moreover, it can provide the link between self-preservation and species preservation since a well-fed but not overweight subject can optimally guarantee the survival of its offspring. It appears, that in the regulation of the HPG axis, the interaction between the orexigenic and anorexigenic (such as leptin) peptides plays a pivotal role [104,105]. As far as self-preservation is concerned, orexins have also been proved to be one of the most important orchestrators of the stress response [80,81]. Further, they modulate all threat-related adaptive behavioral processes [106–108], even fear-related learning [109–112].

Table 1. An outline of the orexin/hypocretin connectome in physiologic regulation [113].

Input Region	Core Region	Target Region	Receptor	Function
Thalamus, TMN, SCN	PFA, LHA	Thalamus, LC, DR, VTA, TMN	OX2R	Circadian regulation, arousal, wakefulness [44,53,65–67]
Peripheral signals, ARC, PVN, SCN	LHA, DMH	VMH, ARC, PVN, NAc	OX1R	Food intake [23,43,85]
Peripheral receptors, brainstem, septum	LHA, PFA	PAG, NST, PON, PVN, RVLM, RVMM, VTA	OX1R, OX2R	Autonomic regulation: thermoregulation [12,95–97], cardiovascular responses [114,115]
Thalamus, hippocampus, PVN, BNST	PFA, DMH	CeA, LA, LC, PPT, PVT, BNST and MTL	OX1R	Emotions (anxiety, fear, mood) [109,110,116]
Thalamus, hippocampus, SCN	LHA, DMH	VTA, NAc, DR, IC, and PFC	OX1R, OX2R	Cognition, reward, and addiction [117,118]
Pituitary, adrenal gland, thalamus, brainstem, SCN	LHA, DMH	PVN, PON	OX1R, OX2R	GAS [11,65,119] and fight-or-flight response [80,81]
Pituitary, ovary, brainstem, SCN	LHA, DMH	ARC	OX1R, OX2R	Gonadal functions [83,103]

ARC: arcuate nucleus, CeA: central amygdala, DMH: dorsomedial hypothalamus, BNST: bed nucleus of stria terminals, DR: dorsal raphe, IC: insular cortex, LA: lateral amygdala, LC: locus coeruleus, LHA: lateral hypothalamic area, MTL: medial temporal lobe, NAc: nucleus accumbens, NST: nucleus of the solitary tract, OX1R: orexin-1 receptor, OX2R: orexin-2 receptor, PAG: periaqueductal gray material, PFA: perifornical area, PFC: prefrontal cortex, PON: preoptic nucleus, PVN: paraventricular nucleus, PPT: pedunculopontine tegmental nucleus, RVLM: rostral ventrolateral medulla, RVMM: rostral ventromedial medulla, TMN: tuberomammillary nucleus, VMH: ventromedial hypothalamus, VTA: ventral tegmental area.

However, the orexin system has been proven to act as an important regulator even in physiological and pathophysiological processes which possess less obvious temporal characteristics: to mention a few of them, pain sensation [120,121], anxiety, mood, reward processes, and addiction [21,79,106,122,123]. The orexin system represents the poster child of neuropeptide regulation: its perikarya are confined to a small region, but it signals diverse evolutionarily conserved functions to distant targets. In summary, we can say that its principal role must be the temporal gating of brainstem functions [10,53].

4. The Role of Orexins in the Regulation of the Stress Response

The reaction of our neuroendocrine regulation to adverse challenges is provided by the interaction between the sympathoadrenal (SA) system and the HPA axis [124]. Although they represent two distinct pathways, the line between them is frequently blurred, even in scientific literature. Perhaps this is due to their interwoven functions, as they complement each other's activity while trying to maintain the homeostatic balance of challenged individuals. However, the SA response described by Cannon [125] is carried out according to the cooperation of the autonomic nervous system and the adrenal medulla, while the stress response, discovered by Selye [126], relies on the reaction of the HPA system, one of the central neuroendocrine axes later described by Schally, Guillemin [127], and Vale [128]. Unfortunately, by now, the terminology has been oversimplified, and stress response (though it has several stages) is frequently used as an umbrella term for both responses. Only in meticulous descriptions are these two neuroendocrine reactions clearly separated. To avoid confusion, for the HPA response, the most suitable term is the synonym (general adaptation syndrome: GAS) coined later by Selye [129]. Nonetheless, the distinction between the two pathways is of crucial importance because it helps clarify many contradictions in the literature. Some conflicting responses to certain stress paradigms could be easily resolved by clear discrimination between the two potential targets of adverse stimuli, that is, the SA system and the HPA axis.

It is well known that many neuropeptides modulate the activity of the HPA axis. For instance, NPY, neurotensin (NT), ghrelin, apelin, and endomorphins activate [14,17,20,130–133] while oxytocin and natriuretic peptides inhibit the system [134–137]. The output of the HPA axis is quite uniform: it begins with the pituitary translation and cleavage of proopiomelanocortin (POMC), yielding adrenocorticotropic hormone (ACTH), which, upon secretion, stimulates glucocorticoid release from the adrenal cortex [126,129]. However, in sharp contrast with the output, the input of the HPA axis is extremely diverse and involves a multitude of neuropeptides in signal transduction [131]. Therefore, it is not surprising that the modality (systemic or neurogenic) and schedule (acute, repeated, or chronic) of the stressors strongly influence the extent of the HPA response [138]. Systemic challenges (e.g. osmotic, immune, etc.) perturb the homeostatic balance of the organism, which is directly projected to the brainstem, while neurogenic paradigms (fear, pain) are processed by the cerebral centers [124]. The responses to these two types of challenges are signaled in a dichotomized manner in the brain. The corticotrope-releasing hormone (CRH)-positive neurons of the PVN are responsible for the acute and processed stimuli, while parvocellular arginine vasopressin (AVP) cells in the PVN and the SON maintain responsiveness to chronic, repeated, and homeostatic challenges [139]. It is also worth noting that neuropeptide modulation perfectly complements the built-in brakes of the GAS: the stepwise ultrashort, short, and long loop feedback mechanisms provided by CRH, ACTH, and the glucocorticoids, as well as the potent anti-inflammatory action of the glucocorticoids [124]. These mechanisms are called stress coping or stress resilience, and they harness the severe inflammatory response (SIRS), which otherwise could consume the organism [124,140,141].

As far as the effect of orexins on the HPA axis and the SA system is concerned, the two responses work hand in hand. Namely, in both responses, orexins play a predominantly stimulatory role [80,81]. However, according to the data from the literature, they are stimulated separately. It seems that the SA system is uniformly activated by orexin-A, which stimulates the OX1Rs expressed in the neurons of the nucleus of the solitary tract (NST), the LC, and the sympathetic neurons [53,65,75,80,142–144]. Ultimately, it is not a far-fetched idea to state that the perifornical, dorsal, dorsomedial, and lateral hypothalamic foci of orexin-positive neurons can be identified with those in the caudal hypothalamic region, which were demonstrated to be essential for an intact "fight or flight" and "sham rage" response by Philip Bard and Walter Hess [8,106].

However, as for the HPA axis, the picture is more complex. Soon after the discovery of the dense orexinergic innervation of the hypothalamic centers (PVN and SON) of the GAS, the scientific rivalry surrounding this highly coveted topic begot several important papers, which established that orexin neurons can activate the HPA axis predominantly at the hypothalamic level [11,65,119]. The main targets of the orexin neurons are the OX2Rs [145] expressed in the CRH-positive perikarya of the PVN [25,119]. Nonetheless, later publications showed that the connection between the orexin- and CRH-positive neuron population is bidirectional since abundant CRH-positive fibers land in the orexinergic perikarya of the hypothalamus [146–148]. Apparently, orexin-evoked HPA activation also involves the release of noradrenaline and NPY [13,149–151], which can significantly diversify its processing [140,141].

As far as the input of the HPA axis is concerned, the activity of orexins appears to be stressor- and schedule-specific [80,81]. In an acute setting, the challenges processed with heightened arousal (aversive odors, novelty, and contextual fear) give rise to more conspicuous activation of the orexin neurons (verified according to *c-fos* expression) than systemic challenges (e.g., cold exposure) or long-lasting procedures (e.g., restraint and immobilization) [80,81,108,152]. Nevertheless, while acute stress mostly activates the orexin neurons, experiments with chronic or repeated stressors returned mixed results [80,81], the findings of which may reflect an adaptation to unavoidable and permanent challenges. Further studies have revealed that the involvement of the orexins in the GAS depends on not only the modalities and schedule of the applied stressor but also the species and gender of the investigated subjects. Females and strains with better stress resilience phenotypes release less orexin in response to adverse stimuli [80,81].

Regarding the output of the HPA axis, orexins have been proven to stimulate the HPA axis not only at the hypothalamic but also at the pituitary and adrenal levels [80,81]. This finding is of crucial importance as peripheral activation stabilizes the HPA response to prolonged stimuli. It nurtures sufficient basal activity but also prevents an exaggerated hypothalamic response by maintaining negative feedback through the release of ACTH and glucocorticoids. Apparently, the orexin/hypocretin system also plays a crucial role in the cooperation and seamless integration of the GAS and the "fight or flight" response. Even the earliest publications which dealt with the orexin system demonstrated the dense innervation of the BNST, a limbic center, which harmonizes the activity of the SA system and the GAS [25]. Therefore, it is not unrealistic at all to conceive of orexins as the coordinators of the stress response to challenges with heightened arousal [80,81].

5. The Role of the Orexins in the Regulation of Anxiety and Reward-Related Learning Processes

There is a consensus in the scientific community that the orexin system is the most important peptidergic mediator of the ARAS [44,53,65] and thus arousal processes. Its indispensable role in the regulation of vigilance was ultimately confirmed by the observation that its deficit leads to irreversible functional consequences both in congenital and acquired disorders of arousal and sleep: narcolepsy and cataplexy [68,70–73]. However, over time, it became obvious that not only the maintenance of wakefulness but also the fine-tuning of arousal-related behavior belongs to the functional repertoire of the orexin system [109]. This concept is supported by the experimental data, which have demonstrated that orexins stimulate attention, rearing, and locomotion as well as such anxiety-related stereotyped behaviors as grooming and freezing [44,53,65,153–156]. Further experiments are needed to verify its role in such ancient behavioral patterns as thanatosis [157,158].

It is well known that threats are the strongest activators of vigilance. They evoke alertness and attention and then provoke an emotional response, that is, fear. And fear has a huge impact on all aspects of behavior, which manifests itself in anxiety and alterations in mood and cognition, among other things [159]. This strong association considered, it is not surprising that the appropriate behavioral responses to both transient and permanent threats are accompanied by the stimulation of the orexin system, one of the key components of arousal regulation [160]. It seems that in the central processing of threats, first, the robust stimulation of the ARAS involves activation of the orexinergic network [44,53,65]. In turn, its hypothalamic foci fine-tune the neurotransmitter release [107,111,112,116,160,161] of those brainstem and limbic centers which are responsible for the regulation of emotions, affections, mood, and learning processes [80,160,162]. The neuroanatomical substrate of fear- and reward-related learning consists of three components: first, the sensory center, the thalamus, and second, the primary modulator, the amygdala. However, the third, the output, is modality-dependent. Reward-related learning is controlled by the ventral striatum and the ventral tegmental area (VTA), while it is the medial temporal lobe (MTL) that synchronizes fear-related learning [159,163]. Both the central (CeA) and the extended amygdala (e.g., BNST) take part in the facilitation of fear-related memory engraving. Then, contextual memory consolidation is achieved through the activity of such components of the MTL as the hippocampus and the entorhinal, perirhinal, and parahippocampal cortices [163]. On the other hand, reward-related memory is processed by the basolateral amygdala, and the output reaches the prefrontal cortex (PFC). This connection, however, is permanently fine-tuned by such mesolimbic reward centers as the VTA and the nucleus accumbens (NAc) [164]. The orexin-induced activation, similarly to the neuroendocrine parallels, is bidirectional, as inputs from the limbic structures (the septum, BNST, basal forebrain, central amygdala, and hippocampus) account for most of the telencephalic inputs to the orexin neurons [165]. The activity of this connection was demonstrated in a multitude of experiments, which revealed that anxiogenic stimuli, such as exposure to cat odor or novelty [106–108,166], gave rise to the activation of the orexin network. In this way, it is not surprising that orexin treatment enhances the startle response [167] and passive avoidance [112]. Later studies specified that the function of the amygdala, which monitors emotional learning and arousal-driven memory consolidation [168], is controlled by the orexin network indirectly and directly. The amygdala receives direct orexinergic projections [25], but the indirect pathway (through the LC) is more important: it carries rich noradrenergic projections to the lateral amygdala [160]. These studies ultimately revealed that orexins play an especially important role in cue-dependent fear memory formation, mainly indirectly through the release of noradrenaline in the LC [109–111]. Both this indirect pathway and the direct pathway utilize OX1Rs. The LC expresses exclusively OX1Rs [169], and the direct pathway targets the OX1Rs in the lateral nucleus of the amygdala and hippocampus [160,170]. This hypothesis was confirmed by the finding that orexin-A, which prefers OX1R, proved to promote emotional learning, memory consolidation, and retrieval processes in a passive avoidance paradigm and in social learning [112,171]. Hence, facilitation of learning ensures the avoidance of potentially harmful events, which ultimately is preventive and therefore the most effective technique in stress coping.

Recently, more and more attention has been paid to specific aspects of orexin-mediated behavioral responses: reward and addiction [117]. Functionally, orexins are prime examples of hedonistic neuropeptides [172]. In the past two decades, orexins have been proven to take part in the control of such strong natural rewards as food and fluid intake [23,43,75–77] and reproduction [83,102]. They especially stimulate binge eating of palatable food [85,173]. These physiological data have already been substantiated by the histological findings, as well. The cells of the two principal dopaminergic pathways (mesolimbic and mesocortical tracts) of the reward system [8] bear orexin-positive boutons [25]. The beginning (the VTA) of the pathways, the relay centers (the BNST, the CeA, and the hippocampus), and the endings (the NAc, the target of the mesolimbic tract, and the PFC, the target of the mesocortical fibers) receive rich orexinergic inputs [25]. Perhaps the orexinergic inputs can fine-tune the SCN-independent circadian activity of the reward system [118]. However, this hypothesis requires experimental verification.

In addition to these primary hedonistic features, orexins appear to control stress resilience, especially in chronic and repeated experimental conditions [80,81]. This concept was reinforced by the histological data when the interaction between the orexin network and another hedonistic peptide, ghrelin, was verified [89,174,175]. It was suggested that they should augment each other's activity in stress coping, which could dampen the detrimental psychological consequences of adverse stimuli. Therefore, it was postulated early on that they could take part in the mediation and modulation of behavioral responses evoked by not only natural but also pharmacological rewards. Since then, numerous publications have revealed that the orexin connectomics shows significant alterations not only in obesity [89,174,175] but also in drug dependence [176]. This way, several pathophysiological responses in addiction, such as reinforcement, drug-seeking, and self-administration, were attributed to its modified activity [177]. The orexin network is unambiguously upregulated in cocaine [178–180] and opiate abuse [181–183], while in the case of other substances, the reaction is more complex [177]. Acute alcohol consumption increased while chronic alcohol, Δ^{19}-tetrahydrocannabinol, and nicotine abuse decreased the orexin expression in the hypothalamus [177,184–186]. Acute changes must be related to the direct effect of the addictive substance. However, chronic changes may reflect the response to a specific stress paradigm: drug withdrawal. Ultimately, these schedule-dependent bimodal changes also appear to reflect adaptation, a form of stress coping.

6. The Cooperation between Orexinergic and Other Peptidergic Neuronal Networks

As has been discussed, the somas of the orexin/hypocretin neurons are restricted to the caudal portion of the hypothalamus [23] but their axon terminals reach distant regions, and their receptors are scattered throughout the whole CNS [25]. This spatial concentration of the cell bodies is not unique in the CNS since it can be observed among other neuropeptides such as MCH [187], ghrelin [188,189], and neuromedin-S [190]. As is the case with other neuropeptides, the feasible interaction of the orexin system and other networks greatly broadens the regulatory repertoire of the orexin/hypocretin neurons. The potential partners are MCH- [191], NPY- [192], apelin- [14,193–195], ghrelin- [15–17,196], and neuromedin-positive [20,197] networks, which show a marked functional overlap with orexins in the regulation of food intake, the sleep–wake cycle, stress response, and behavior. These networks may cooperate with each other, but the intact function of the orexin system is required for normal processing of arousal-related processes [68–72].

So far, besides releasing hormones of the hypothalamic–pituitary–target organ axis, only the orexin system has proven to be an essential neuropeptide in the regulation of the CNS. However, the interpolations of other neuropeptides and neurotransmitters in the signal transduction of the orexin neurons lend immense diversity and flexibility to the orexin-regulated responses [83]. This is because the neuropeptide ligand and receptor families typically consist of several members, which may have numerous splice variants, can also be modified by peptidases after secretion, and can act on an arsenal of receptors [4–6,131,140,198]. With the different binding affinities and activities taken into consideration, the number of potential interactions between this abundance of ligands and receptors is infinite and may span from full agonism to complete antagonism [4,5,7,198].

Cooperation both in the afferent and efferent pathways of the orexin system has been verified. In the input, monoamines [25], NPY [199,200], and ghrelin [89,174,175] seem to play the most important role, while in the output, NPY [12,13,151,199,201], POMC [202], and also monoamines [25,107,112,161,203] have been identified. Unambiguously, the pathways between the LC and the lateral hypothalamus are the most important connections of the orexin network in the regulation of arousal-related behavioral and endocrine responses [24,25]. Also, circulating peripheral or centrally released ghrelin significantly contributes to the hyperphagic activity of the orexins [89]. In efferentation, the orexin connectomics cooperates with the corticotrope-releasing hormone (CRH)–urocortin system [11], the network of NPY-positive [12,13] and monoaminergic [203] cells in the orchestration of the neuroendocrine responses to processed and homeostatic challenges [11,13]. Such interactions were established in other functions such as thermoregulation, mood, anxiety, learning [12,107,112,148,161,204,205], and reproduction [151]. Regarding arousal, one of the most important connections between the orexinergic system of the organism and the environment is established through the SCN [46]. The neuromedin-S released from the SCN of the hypothalamus might interpret these photic stimulations, which arrive at the SCN through the retinohypothalamic pathway [190]. Nevertheless, this aspect of hypocretin physiology must be further scrutinized and confirmed using experimental data.

During the investigation of pathophysiological alterations in the hypocretin/orexin network, some unique features of the system were unveiled. It is a well-known phenomenon in neuropeptide pathophysiology that the deficiency of a given neuropeptide or its secretory neurons usually does not bring about significant functional disturbances in the affected organism. This is due to the functional overlap between and redundancy of different neuropeptides or neuropeptide families. Typically, in congenital cases, during embryonic and fetal development, other neuropeptides can functionally compensate for the deficiency of the affected transcript even in knockout animals. Obviously, acquired abnormalities are less prone to correction due to the much more limited adaptation of the adult brain. Therefore, neuropeptide deficiencies do not cause such dramatic pathophysiological and clinical changes as is the case in congenital or acquired disorders of neurotransmission such as dopamine (phenylketonuria, Parkinson's disease, and Sydenham's chorea minor), GABA (Huntington's disease and some forms of congenital epilepsies), or acetylcholine (myasthenia gravis, Lambert–Eaton myasthenic syndrome, and Alzheimer's disease) metabolism disorders. However, the orexin/hypocretin system is different in this respect. Not only acquired but also congenital deficiency inevitably leads to severe pathophysiological changes, as exemplified in narcolepsy [70,71] or the blunted stress response exhibited by OX2R-deficient knockout mice [145]. This might be attributed to the fact that the orexin-positive neuron population does not exceed 50,000–80,000 cells in the hypothalamus [72], which makes it peculiarly sensitive to injuries. Furthermore, orexins bear weak structural resemblance only to a few members of the incretin family [23,24]. Even orexin-A and orexin-B differ in 50% of their primary structure, and they exhibit significantly different receptor affinities [23,24]. Therefore, it is not surprising that hardly any other neuronal network can take over the function of the orexinergic system. Some functional overlap might be provided by other GPCRs since certain neuropeptide receptors, such as the type-2 NPY receptor, the TRH receptor, the CCK type-A receptor, and the NK2 neurokinin receptor show some similarities (26%, 25%, 23%, and 20% identity, respectively) to the orexin receptors (OX1R and OX2R) [23]. However, their binding affinity to orexins is negligible [206]. The highest structural similarity is exhibited by the NPFF receptor of the RF-amide peptide family, which is 37% identical to OX1R and 35% identical to OX2R, respectively, and shows significant affinity to the orexins [35,36].

7. Aspects of Human Pathophysiology: The Present and Future Therapeutic Potential of Orexin Receptor Ligands

Even the first results of experiments carried out on the orexin/hypocretin system suggested that several human pathophysiological conditions could be explained by alterations in the orexin neurons [207]. Dysfunctions of the ARAS and sleep disorders, such as obstructive sleep apnea–hypopnea syndrome, were the first and somewhat obvious culprits, which were thoroughly and successfully investigated. Since then, both in narcolepsy with cataplexy [70–73,208] and in obstructive sleep apnea–hypopnea syndrome [209–211], the dysfunction of the orexin system has been established. Moreover, the acquired form of narcolepsy proved to be a classic example of a neuroinflammatory disorder. It seems to be evoked by H1N1 influenza virus infection or vaccination, which gives rise to an autoimmune reaction against the hypocretin neurons [74,212,213].

Increased tone of the orexinergic system, especially in cooperation with the ghrelin network, has also been suspected in disorders of the reward system. It appears that their synergistic hyperactivity is accountable for a rare form of monogenic obesity, Prader–Willi syndrome (PWS) [214]. However, the picture is more complex, as the orexin system is a double-edged sword; it increases feeding and energy expenditure simultaneously depending on the environmental cues. Accordingly, it has been implicated in both weight gain and weight loss [85], as well as in such disorders of food consumption as binge eating [215], bulimia, and anorexia nervosa [216]. Furthermore, in Kleine–Levin syndrome [217,218], the alternation of the alert and hyperphagic stages of hypersomnia has been connected to fluctuations in the orexin levels in the cerebrospinal fluid (CSF). It seems that, like the HPA response, the actual eating disorder is determined by the schedule and the modality of the psychological stressor [219], and it can manifest itself in seemingly opposite conditions.

Regarding reproductive processes, hypoactivity of the orexin system was observed in mothers suffering from gestational diabetes [220] and in patients diagnosed with polycystic ovary syndrome (PCOS) [221,222]. This might be related to the concomitant increase in the body weight and leptin levels of the patients, which downregulates orexin expression [223]. As for the pharmacological rewards, it is substance withdrawal that represents the common mechanism of orexin upregulation in different forms of drug addictions. Apparently, withdrawal symptoms are managed by individuals as stress stimuli, and they increase arousal, attention, and drug-seeking behavior [172,224,225].

In humans, the dysfunction of the orexin system in the regulation of the ARAS may also bring about the development of such diseases as attention deficit hyperactivity disorder (ADHD), anxiety, epilepsy, panic, and phobias [106,160,162,172,226]. As far as hyperactivity is concerned, the role of the orexin system has also been verified since the exaggerated startle response in anxious patients could be effectively reduced with an orexin receptor antagonist [227]. These conditions accompany the pathophysiological regulation of neuronal excitation and show clear circadian fluctuation, which reinforces the view that alteration in the orexin/hypocretin system plays a causative role in their development. Long periods of overexcitation have a detrimental impact on the neurons. In the burnt-out phase, these diseases give way to such chronic conditions as major depression, post-traumatic stress disorder (PTSD), psychosomatic problems like hypertension [228–231], and even neurodegenerative disorders [232]. Some further conditions such as cognitive disorders [233] and abnormal pain sensation [234–236] may also be related to alterations in alertness and the gating mechanism and therefore can be connected to the orexin/hypocretin system. However, it is important to emphasize that orexin receptors show some structural similarities to those of RF-amides [233]. Accordingly, their direct action may be mediated by not only their own receptors, expressed on the crucial gating elements (LC and PAG) of pain signaling, but also can be reinforced indirectly via the RF-amide receptors, which are expressed in both the ascending and descending pathways of pain sensation [237]. Abnormalities in orexin physiology have already been identified in chronic pain disorders, such as fibromyalgia [238], and especially in primary headaches such as migraine and cluster headaches [120,121,198]. The latter condition deserves special attention since these attacks show a clear diurnal pattern, and in its pathogenesis, the role of the SCN has already been verified [121]. According to the data from the literature, this analgesic action of the orexin network is mediated by orexin-A and OX1Rs [239].

The previously mentioned conformational overlap between the RF-amide and orexin receptors may also account for the reproductive and antineoplastic activities of orexins [28,240,241]. This is because RF-amides play a well-known role in the inhibition of metastasis formation [242], and in the past few years, they have emerged as metabolic regulators of the gonadal axis [243]. Since the activity of the RF-amide system shows clear periodicity, it is quite reasonable to imply that the orexin system may modulate its function either directly or indirectly [240].

Finally, it must be mentioned that the dysfunction of the orexin system was demonstrated in common neuropsychiatric, neuroinflammatory, and neurodegenerative disorders such as schizophrenia, Parkinson's disease, Alzheimer's disease, Huntington's disease, multiple sclerosis (MS), and amyotrophic lateral sclerosis (ALS) [232,244–247]. Nevertheless, in these pathologic conditions, the dysfunction of the orexin system is not specific but can be attributed to the widespread devastation of the connectome. In these conditions, ultimately, all neural networks will be affected, but the orexin system is specifically frail and sensitive to focal injuries since it has a limited number of neurons, which are confined to a relatively small region. Therefore, it is among the first centers that succumb to the detrimental effects of misfolded protein aggregation and neuroinflammation. That is why some shared, conspicuous symptoms of the above-mentioned fatal disorders were identified as resulting from the failure of the orexin network. Cataplexy and dysfunction of the postural reflexes can be observed in Parkinson's, Huntington's, and prion diseases. Alterations in sleep patterns and vigilance are common findings in Alzheimer's, MS, and prion diseases. Rapid fluctuations in mood, unwarranted anxiety, irrational fears, and extreme irritability are the common behavioral symptoms [248,249] in the above-mentioned diseases. Later, in all these symptom categories, either hyperactivity or hypoactivity of the orexin system has been suspected or already verified [232,244].

8. Promising Results in Translational Pharmacology

It is a well-known hindrance in neuropeptide pharmacology that often those compounds which possess the most promising biochemical features (affinity, activity, half-life, etc.) cannot bypass the blood–brain barrier (BBB) [7]. In several instances, only circumscribed areas (the lamina cribrosa or the circumventricular organs) provide access to the cerebrospinal fluid (CSF) to native ligands [7], or sophisticated nanocarriers (liposomes, nanoparticles, etc.) are required to surmount this pharmacokinetic obstacle [250]. However, in the case of the previously discussed feed-promoting neuropeptides such as ghrelin and the orexin system, both natural ligands and their chemically designed analogs can freely bypass the BBB [7,251,252]. Derivatives of orexins are especially successful in this regard because some of these antagonists have already been approved by the Food and Drug Administration (FDA) in the treatment of insomnia [113] (Table 2). Other antagonists, which are suggested for the treatment of panic, major depressive disorder, anxiety, and binge eating, are under investigation [113]. Studies on antagonists which are recommended for the treatment of narcolepsy are also in the clinical phase of pharmacological trials [113].

Table 2. Orexin analogs under clinical investigation [113,253].

Classes	Indications	Stage
OX2R agonists	Narcolepsy	Phase II. [254,255]
OX2R antagonists	Major depressive disorder (MDD)	Phase III. [256]
Dual antagonists	Insomnia	approved (e.g., Suvorexant [257,258], Lemborexant [259])
OX1R antagonists	Binge eating disorder Panic disorder, MDD, anxiety	Phase II. [260] Phase II. [261]

At present, the most coveted aim in neuroendocrine research is to engineer orexin derivatives which could relieve the abnormalities of the sleep–wake cycle in neurodegenerative disorders. They would be game-changers in palliative therapy, as traditional hypnotics are strong depressants and further deteriorate the function of the otherwise failing CNS. Therefore, present and future orexin derivatives are among the most pioneering and successful compounds in neuropeptide pharmacology and have huge potential in pharmaceutical development [113].

Additionally, emerging research explores the potential of non-invasive brain stimulation techniques (NIBS), such as transcranial magnetic stimulation (TMS) and transcranial direct current stimulation (tDCS). These NIBS techniques seem to be promising therapeutic alternatives as the orexin system occupies a well-circumscribed region in the CNS. Therefore, the symptoms of conditions like narcolepsy, cluster headaches, and affective and cognitive disorders that are associated with the dysfunction of the orexin system could be mitigated by them [262–264].

9. Discussion

Orexin/hypocretin neuropeptides are pivotal players in regulating various physiological processes, such as food intake, metabolism, the HPA axis, reproduction, and behavior [10,21,23,43,82,83,85,109,136,265,266]. They were primarily described to orchestrate such parameters of homeostatic balance as feeding, thermogenesis, and heat dissipation [12,23,43,85,97]. Later research shed light on their intricate involvement in the mediation and modulation of such behavioral paradigms as arousal, anxiety, fear, and the stress response [11,44,65,82,106,111,116,160]. The orexin system is also implicated in the regulation of pain sensation and the behavioral changes evoked by natural and pharmacological rewards such as addiction [79,106,117,120,181,198,224,267,268]. This way, dysfunctions in the orexin system have been associated with various human pathophysiological conditions, such as obesity, addictive disorders, narcolepsy, obstructive sleep apnea–hypopnea syndrome, anxiety, cognitive disorders, and abnormal mood fluctuations [10,109,122,215,227,230,269]. This review tries to seamlessly integrate the diverse activities of orexins and provides a more in-depth understanding of those fields such as stress response, fear, anxiety, and learning in which the authors have significantly contributed to the literature [11–13,107,112,161].

Regarding the limits of this article, it is important to note that the review is based on the existing literature and does not present any new experimental data. As a result, the caliber and scope of the studies included in the analysis limit the conclusions drawn from this review. Additionally, the review focuses on preclinical research on the orexin/hypocretin system, and the translation of these findings into clinical practice may be challenging. However, the review has several merits, including its interdisciplinary approach to understanding the orexin/hypocretin system, synthesizing information from various fields, including neuroscience, endocrinology, and pharmacology [10,21,83,85,109,113,270,271]. It could provide "food for thought" to researchers and clinicians interested in the orexin/hypocretin system, and it could inspire future research by identifying the knowledge gaps and areas that require further investigation.

The ultimate goal of the research on the orexin/hypocretin system is to develop effective therapeutic interventions for various disorders, such as sleep disorders, obesity, addiction, and anxiety [23,53,66,68,69,85,106,108,116,160,162,217,272–275]. However, this goal presents several challenges, including the need to understand the complex and multifaceted role of orexins in physiology and behavior, as well as the need to develop safe and effective drugs that target the orexin system. To achieve this goal, researchers need to have a deep understanding of the orexin/hypocretin system, including its molecular and cellular mechanisms, as well as its interactions with other systems in the body. They also need to develop advanced technologies for studying the orexin system, such as optogenetics, chemogenetics, and advanced imaging techniques. In addition, researchers need to develop safe and effective drugs that target selectively the orexin system, which requires a thorough understanding of the pharmacokinetics and pharmacodynamics of orexin derivatives. Overall, this line of research has the potential to improve the lives of millions of people worldwide, making it a crucial area of investigation, as is their potential therapeutic applications. Nevertheless, since several derivatives of orexins with high affinity and activity to their receptors can bypass the blood–brain barrier, some antagonists have already been approved by the FDA for the treatment of insomnia, and other antagonists and agonists are under investigation for the treatment of various disorders of food intake and behavior [113,271,276].

10. Conclusions

The interdisciplinary approach of this review has enhanced our understanding of the orexin/hypocretin neuropeptide family and its potential therapeutic applications. However, there are still several theoretical and methodological avenues that require refinement, such as the need for more precise and selective orexin receptor agonists and antagonists. Future research directions could focus on developing innovative drug delivery systems that can effectively target the orexin system while minimizing the off-target effects. Additionally, further research is needed to understand the complex interactions between the orexin system and other physiological and behavioral processes, such as the immune system and circadian rhythms. Overall, the orexin/hypocretin system is a fascinating area of research with significant theoretical and translational implications. By understanding the complex and multifaceted role of the orexin system, researchers can identify new drug targets and develop innovative drug delivery systems that can effectively treat various disorders. We hope that this review serves as a valuable resource for researchers and clinicians interested in the orexin/hypocretin system and the development of agents targeting this system.

Author Contributions: Conceptualization, M.J.; writing—original draft preparation, M.J.; writing—review and editing, M.J., M.T., L.V., B.T. and Z.B.; visualization, M.T.; supervision, M.J., L.V. and M.T.; project administration, M.T.; funding acquisition, M.T. All authors have read and agreed to the published version of the manuscript.

Funding: This work was supported by the National Research, Development, and Innovation Office—NKFIH K138125, SZTE SZAOK-KKA No:2022/5S729, and the HUN-REN Hungarian Research Network.

Institutional Review Board Statement: Not applicable.

Informed Consent Statement: Not applicable.

Data Availability Statement: Data sharing is not applicable to this article.

Acknowledgments: The figures were created using BioRender.com.

Conflicts of Interest: The authors declare no conflicts of interest.

Abbreviations

ACTH	adrenocorticotropic hormone
ALS	amyotrophic lateral sclerosis
ARAS	ascending reticular activation system
ARC	arcuate nucleus
BAT	brown adipose tissue
BBB	blood–brain barrier
BNST	bed nucleus of stria terminalis
CeA	central amygdala
CCK	cholecystokinin
CNS	central nervous system
CSF	cerebrospinal fluid
CRH	corticotrope-releasing hormone
DMH	dorsomedial hypothalamus
DR	dorsal raphe
FDA	the Food and Drug Administration
GABA	γ-amino-butyric-acid
GAS	general adaptation syndrome
GPCRs	G-protein-coupled receptors
HPA	hypothalamic–pituitary–adrenal cortex
HPG	hypothalamic–pituitary–gonadal axis
IC	insular cortex
LA	lateral amygdala
LC	locus coeruleus
LDT	lateral dorsal tegmental nuclei
LHA	lateral hypothalamic area
MCH	melanin-concentrating hormone
MDD	major depressive disorder
MnPO	median preoptic nucleus
MPO	medial preoptic nucleus
MS	multiple sclerosis
MT	mesopontine tegmentum
MTL	medial temporal lobe
NAc	nucleus accumbens
NIBS	non-invasive brain stimulation techniques
NK	neurokinin
NM	neuromedin
NMS	neuromedin S
NPY	neuropeptide Y
NST	nucleus of the solitary tract
NT	neurotensin
OVLT	organum vasculosum laminae terminalis
OX1R	orexin-1 receptor
OX2R	orexin-2 receptor
OXR	orexin receptor
PAG	periaqueductal gray
PCOS	polycystic ovary syndrome
PFA	perifornical area
PFC	prefrontal cortex
POMC	pro-opiomelanocortin
PON	preoptic nucleus
PPT	pedunculopontine tegmental nucleus
PVN	paraventricular nuclei
RVLM	rostral ventrolateral medulla
RVMM	rostral ventromedial medulla
SA	sympathoadrenal

SCN	suprachiasmatic nucleus
SON	supraoptic nucleus
tDCS	transcranial direct current stimulation
TMs	transcranial magnetic stimulation
TMN	tuberomammillary nucleus
VMH	ventromedial hypothalamus
VTA	ventral tegmental area
VLPO	ventrolateral preoptic nucleus

References

1. Oliver, G.; Schafer, E.A. On the Physiological Action of Extracts of Pituitary Body and certain other Glandular Organs: Preliminary Communication. *J. Physiol.* **1895**, *18*, 277–279. [CrossRef]
2. Dale, H.H. On some physiological actions of ergot. *J. Physiol.* **1906**, *34*, 163–206. [CrossRef] [PubMed]
3. US, V.E.; Gaddum, J.H. An unidentified depressor substance in certain tissue extracts. *J. Physiol.* **1931**, *72*, 74–87. [CrossRef]
4. van den Pol, A.N. Neuropeptide transmission in brain circuits. *Neuron* **2012**, *76*, 98–115. [CrossRef] [PubMed]
5. Elphick, M.R.; Mirabeau, O.; Larhammar, D. Evolution of neuropeptide signalling systems. *J. Exp. Biol.* **2018**, *221*, jeb151092. [CrossRef] [PubMed]
6. Marvar, P.J.; Andero, R.; Hurlemann, R.; Lago, T.R.; Zelikowsky, M.; Dabrowska, J. Limbic Neuropeptidergic Modulators of Emotion and Their Therapeutic Potential for Anxiety and Post-Traumatic Stress Disorder. *J. Neurosci.* **2021**, *41*, 901–910. [CrossRef] [PubMed]
7. Hokfelt, T.; Bartfai, T.; Bloom, F. Neuropeptides: Opportunities for drug discovery. *Lancet Neurol.* **2003**, *2*, 463–472. [CrossRef] [PubMed]
8. Purves, D. *Neuroscience*, 6th ed.; Oxford University Press: New York, NY, USA, 2018.
9. Seguin, C.; Sporns, O.; Zalesky, A. Brain network communication: Concepts, models and applications. *Nat. Rev. Neurosci.* **2023**, *24*, 557–574. [CrossRef] [PubMed]
10. Sakurai, T.; Mieda, M. Connectomics of orexin-producing neurons: Interface of systems of emotion, energy homeostasis and arousal. *Trends Pharmacol. Sci.* **2011**, *32*, 451–462. [CrossRef]
11. Jaszberenyi, M.; Bujdoso, E.; Pataki, I.; Telegdy, G. Effects of orexins on the hypothalamic-pituitary-adrenal system. *J. Neuroendocrinol.* **2000**, *12*, 1174–1178. [CrossRef]
12. Jaszberenyi, M.; Bujdoso, E.; Kiss, E.; Pataki, I.; Telegdy, G. The role of NPY in the mediation of orexin-induced hypothermia. *Regul. Pept.* **2002**, *104*, 55–59. [CrossRef]
13. Jaszberenyi, M.; Bujdoso, E.; Telegdy, G. The role of neuropeptide Y in orexin-induced hypothalamic-pituitary-adrenal activation. *J. Neuroendocrinol.* **2001**, *13*, 438–441. [CrossRef]
14. Jaszberenyi, M.; Bujdoso, E.; Telegdy, G. Behavioral, neuroendocrine and thermoregulatory actions of apelin-13. *Neuroscience* **2004**, *129*, 811–816. [CrossRef] [PubMed]
15. Palotai, M.; Bagosi, Z.; Jaszberenyi, M.; Csabafi, K.; Dochnal, R.; Manczinger, M.; Telegdy, G.; Szabo, G. Ghrelin and nicotine stimulate equally the dopamine release in the rat amygdala. *Neurochem. Res.* **2013**, *38*, 1989–1995. [CrossRef] [PubMed]
16. Palotai, M.; Bagosi, Z.; Jaszberenyi, M.; Csabafi, K.; Dochnal, R.; Manczinger, M.; Telegdy, G.; Szabo, G. Ghrelin amplifies the nicotine-induced dopamine release in the rat striatum. *Neurochem. Int.* **2013**, *63*, 239–243. [CrossRef]
17. Jaszberenyi, M.; Bujdoso, E.; Bagosi, Z.; Telegdy, G. Mediation of the behavioral, endocrine and thermoregulatory actions of ghrelin. *Horm. Behav.* **2006**, *50*, 266–273. [CrossRef]
18. Tanaka, M.; Telegdy, G. Neurotransmissions of antidepressant-like effects of neuromedin U-23 in mice. *Behav. Brain Res.* **2014**, *259*, 196–199. [CrossRef]
19. Telegdy, G.; Adamik, A. Anxiolytic action of neuromedin-U and neurotransmitters involved in mice. *Regul. Pept.* **2013**, *186*, 137–140. [CrossRef]
20. Jaszberenyi, M.; Bagosi, Z.; Thurzo, B.; Foldesi, I.; Telegdy, G. Endocrine and behavioral effects of neuromedin S. *Horm. Behav.* **2007**, *52*, 631–639. [CrossRef] [PubMed]
21. Xia, L.; Liu, H.Y.; Wang, B.Y.; Lin, H.N.; Wang, M.C.; Ren, J.X. A review of physiological functions of orexin: From instinctive responses to subjective cognition. *Medicine* **2023**, *102*, e34206. [CrossRef]
22. Soya, S.; Sakurai, T. Evolution of Orexin Neuropeptide System: Structure and Function. *Front. Neurosci.* **2020**, *14*, 691. [CrossRef] [PubMed]
23. Sakurai, T.; Amemiya, A.; Ishii, M.; Matsuzaki, I.; Chemelli, R.M.; Tanaka, H.; Williams, S.C.; Richardson, J.A.; Kozlowski, G.P.; Wilson, S.; et al. Orexins and orexin receptors: A family of hypothalamic neuropeptides and G protein-coupled receptors that regulate feeding behavior. *Cell* **1998**, *92*, 573–585. [CrossRef] [PubMed]
24. de Lecea, L.; Kilduff, T.S.; Peyron, C.; Gao, X.; Foye, P.E.; Danielson, P.E.; Fukuhara, C.; Battenberg, E.L.; Gautvik, V.T.; Bartlett, F.S., 2nd; et al. The hypocretins: Hypothalamus-specific peptides with neuroexcitatory activity. *Proc. Natl. Acad. Sci. USA* **1998**, *95*, 322–327. [CrossRef]
25. Peyron, C.; Tighe, D.K.; van den Pol, A.N.; de Lecea, L.; Heller, H.C.; Sutcliffe, J.G.; Kilduff, T.S. Neurons containing hypocretin (orexin) project to multiple neuronal systems. *J. Neurosci.* **1998**, *18*, 9996–10015. [CrossRef] [PubMed]

26. Bittencourt, J.C.; Presse, F.; Arias, C.; Peto, C.; Vaughan, J.; Nahon, J.L.; Vale, W.; Sawchenko, P.E. The melanin-concentrating hormone system of the rat brain: An immuno- and hybridization histochemical characterization. *J. Comp. Neurol.* **1992**, *319*, 218–245. [CrossRef]
27. Lopez-Lopez, C.; Dietrich, M.O.; Metzger, F.; Loetscher, H.; Torres-Aleman, I. Disturbed cross talk between insulin-like growth factor I and AMP-activated protein kinase as a possible cause of vascular dysfunction in the amyloid precursor protein/presenilin 2 mouse model of Alzheimer's disease. *J. Neurosci.* **2007**, *27*, 824–831. [CrossRef]
28. Couvineau, A.; Nicole, P.; Gratio, V.; Voisin, T. The Orexin receptors: Structural and anti-tumoral properties. *Front. Endocrinol.* **2022**, *13*, 931970. [CrossRef]
29. Kastin, A.J.; Akerstrom, V. Orexin A but not orexin B rapidly enters brain from blood by simple diffusion. *J. Pharmacol. Exp. Ther.* **1999**, *289*, 219–223.
30. Sutcliffe, J.G.; de Lecea, L. The hypocretins: Excitatory neuromodulatory peptides for multiple homeostatic systems, including sleep and feeding. *J. Neurosci. Res.* **2000**, *62*, 161–168. [CrossRef]
31. Wang, C.; Wang, Q.; Ji, B.; Pan, Y.; Xu, C.; Cheng, B.; Bai, B.; Chen, J. The Orexin/Receptor System: Molecular Mechanism and Therapeutic Potential for Neurological Diseases. *Front. Mol. Neurosci.* **2018**, *11*, 220. [CrossRef]
32. Kukkonen, J.P. G-protein-dependency of orexin/hypocretin receptor signalling in recombinant Chinese hamster ovary cells. *Biochem. Biophys. Res. Commun.* **2016**, *476*, 379–385. [CrossRef] [PubMed]
33. Kukkonen, J.P. OX2 orexin/hypocretin receptor signal transduction in recombinant Chinese hamster ovary cells. *Cell. Signal.* **2016**, *28*, 51–60. [CrossRef] [PubMed]
34. Kukkonen, J.P. Orexin/Hypocretin Signaling. *Curr. Top. Behav. Neurosci.* **2017**, *33*, 17–50. [CrossRef] [PubMed]
35. Bonini, J.A.; Jones, K.A.; Adham, N.; Forray, C.; Artymyshyn, R.; Durkin, M.M.; Smith, K.E.; Tamm, J.A.; Boteju, L.W.; Lakhlani, P.P.; et al. Identification and characterization of two G protein-coupled receptors for neuropeptide FF. *J. Biol. Chem.* **2000**, *275*, 39324–39331. [CrossRef] [PubMed]
36. Laemmle, B.; Schindler, M.; Beilmann, M.; Hamilton, B.S.; Doods, H.N.; Wieland, H.A. Characterization of the NPGP receptor and identification of a novel short mRNA isoform in human hypothalamus. *Regul. Pept.* **2003**, *111*, 21–29. [CrossRef]
37. Cutler, D.J.; Morris, R.; Sheridhar, V.; Wattam, T.A.; Holmes, S.; Patel, S.; Arch, J.R.; Wilson, S.; Buckingham, R.E.; Evans, M.L.; et al. Differential distribution of orexin-A and orexin-B immunoreactivity in the rat brain and spinal cord. *Peptides* **1999**, *20*, 1455–1470. [CrossRef]
38. Smart, D.; Jerman, J. The physiology and pharmacology of the orexins. *Pharmacol. Ther.* **2002**, *94*, 51–61. [CrossRef]
39. Hervieu, G.J.; Cluderay, J.E.; Harrison, D.C.; Roberts, J.C.; Leslie, R.A. Gene expression and protein distribution of the orexin-1 receptor in the rat brain and spinal cord. *Neuroscience* **2001**, *103*, 777–797. [CrossRef]
40. Trivedi, P.; Yu, H.; MacNeil, D.J.; Van der Ploeg, L.H.; Guan, X.M. Distribution of orexin receptor mRNA in the rat brain. *FEBS Lett.* **1998**, *438*, 71–75. [CrossRef] [PubMed]
41. Lu, X.Y.; Bagnol, D.; Burke, S.; Akil, H.; Watson, S.J. Differential distribution and regulation of OX1 and OX2 orexin/hypocretin receptor messenger RNA in the brain upon fasting. *Horm. Behav.* **2000**, *37*, 335–344. [CrossRef] [PubMed]
42. Mitsukawa, K.; Kimura, H. Orexin 2 receptor (OX2R) protein distribution measured by autoradiography using radiolabeled OX2R-selective antagonist EMPA in rodent brain and peripheral tissues. *Sci. Rep.* **2022**, *12*, 8473. [CrossRef] [PubMed]
43. Saper, C.B.; Chou, T.C.; Elmquist, J.K. The need to feed: Homeostatic and hedonic control of eating. *Neuron* **2002**, *36*, 199–211. [CrossRef] [PubMed]
44. Burlet, S.; Tyler, C.J.; Leonard, C.S. Direct and indirect excitation of laterodorsal tegmental neurons by Hypocretin/Orexin peptides: Implications for wakefulness and narcolepsy. *J. Neurosci.* **2002**, *22*, 2862–2872. [CrossRef] [PubMed]
45. Smale, L.; Lee, T.; Nunez, A.A. Mammalian diurnality: Some facts and gaps. *J. Biol. Rhythms* **2003**, *18*, 356–366. [CrossRef]
46. Chen, H.; Huang, H.; Chen, X.; Deng, S.; Zhu, C.; Huang, H.; Li, G. Structural and functional characterization of neuromedin S in the teleost fish, zebrafish (Danio rerio). *Comp. Biochem. Physiol. B Biochem. Mol. Biol.* **2016**, *191*, 76–83. [CrossRef] [PubMed]
47. Hastings, M.H.; Maywood, E.S.; Brancaccio, M. Generation of circadian rhythms in the suprachiasmatic nucleus. *Nat. Rev. Neurosci.* **2018**, *19*, 453–469. [CrossRef]
48. Starnes, A.N.; Jones, J.R. Inputs and Outputs of the Mammalian Circadian Clock. *Biology* **2023**, *12*, 508. [CrossRef]
49. Fuhr, L.; Abreu, M.; Pett, P.; Relogio, A. Circadian systems biology: When time matters. *Comput. Struct. Biotechnol. J.* **2015**, *13*, 417–426. [CrossRef]
50. Lehmann, R.; Childs, L.; Thomas, P.; Abreu, M.; Fuhr, L.; Herzel, H.; Leser, U.; Relogio, A. Assembly of a comprehensive regulatory network for the mammalian circadian clock: A bioinformatics approach. *PLoS ONE* **2015**, *10*, e0126283. [CrossRef] [PubMed]
51. Ruan, W.; Yuan, X.; Eltzschig, H.K. Circadian rhythm as a therapeutic target. *Nat. Rev. Drug Discov.* **2021**, *20*, 287–307. [CrossRef] [PubMed]
52. Shiromani, P.J.; Kilduff, T.S.; Bloom, F.E.; McCarley, R.W. Cholinergically induced REM sleep triggers Fos-like immunoreactivity in dorsolateral pontine regions associated with REM sleep. *Brain Res.* **1992**, *580*, 351–357. [CrossRef] [PubMed]
53. Saper, C.B.; Scammell, T.E.; Lu, J. Hypothalamic regulation of sleep and circadian rhythms. *Nature* **2005**, *437*, 1257–1263. [CrossRef] [PubMed]

54. Cheng, J.; Wu, F.; Zhang, M.; Ding, D.; Fan, S.; Chen, G.; Zhang, J.; Wang, L. The Interaction Between the Ventrolateral Preoptic Nucleus and the Tuberomammillary Nucleus in Regulating the Sleep-Wakefulness Cycle. *Front. Neurosci.* **2020**, *14*, 615854. [CrossRef] [PubMed]
55. Arrigoni, E.; Fuller, P.M. The Sleep-Promoting Ventrolateral Preoptic Nucleus: What Have We Learned over the Past 25 Years? *Int. J. Mol. Sci.* **2022**, *23*, 2905. [CrossRef] [PubMed]
56. Barcomb, K.; Olah, S.S.; Kennedy, M.J.; Ford, C.P. Properties and modulation of excitatory inputs to the locus coeruleus. *J. Physiol.* **2022**, *600*, 4897–4916. [CrossRef]
57. Chou, T.C.; Bjorkum, A.A.; Gaus, S.E.; Lu, J.; Scammell, T.E.; Saper, C.B. Afferents to the ventrolateral preoptic nucleus. *J. Neurosci.* **2002**, *22*, 977–990. [CrossRef]
58. Hasegawa, E.; Yanagisawa, M.; Sakurai, T.; Mieda, M. Orexin neurons suppress narcolepsy via 2 distinct efferent pathways. *J. Clin. Investig.* **2014**, *124*, 604–616. [CrossRef]
59. Kim, J.; Nakajima, K.; Oomura, Y.; Wayner, M.J.; Sasaki, K. Orexin-A and ghrelin depolarize the same pedunculopontine tegmental neurons in rats: An in vitro study. *Peptides* **2009**, *30*, 1328–1335. [CrossRef]
60. Feng, H.; Wen, S.Y.; Qiao, Q.C.; Pang, Y.J.; Wang, S.Y.; Li, H.Y.; Cai, J.; Zhang, K.X.; Chen, J.; Hu, Z.A.; et al. Publisher Correction: Orexin signaling modulates synchronized excitation in the sublaterodorsal tegmental nucleus to stabilize REM sleep. *Nat. Commun.* **2020**, *11*, 4910. [CrossRef]
61. Feng, H.; Wen, S.Y.; Qiao, Q.C.; Pang, Y.J.; Wang, S.Y.; Li, H.Y.; Cai, J.; Zhang, K.X.; Chen, J.; Hu, Z.A.; et al. Orexin signaling modulates synchronized excitation in the sublaterodorsal tegmental nucleus to stabilize REM sleep. *Nat. Commun.* **2020**, *11*, 3661. [CrossRef]
62. Gotter, A.L.; Forman, M.S.; Harrell, C.M.; Stevens, J.; Svetnik, V.; Yee, K.L.; Li, X.; Roecker, A.J.; Fox, S.V.; Tannenbaum, P.L.; et al. Orexin 2 Receptor Antagonism is Sufficient to Promote NREM and REM Sleep from Mouse to Man. *Sci. Rep.* **2016**, *6*, 27147. [CrossRef]
63. Dugovic, C.; Shelton, J.E.; Aluisio, L.E.; Fraser, I.C.; Jiang, X.; Sutton, S.W.; Bonaventure, P.; Yun, S.; Li, X.; Lord, B.; et al. Blockade of orexin-1 receptors attenuates orexin-2 receptor antagonism-induced sleep promotion in the rat. *J. Pharmacol. Exp. Ther.* **2009**, *330*, 142–151. [CrossRef]
64. Willie, J.T.; Chemelli, R.M.; Sinton, C.M.; Tokita, S.; Williams, S.C.; Kisanuki, Y.Y.; Marcus, J.N.; Lee, C.; Elmquist, J.K.; Kohlmeier, K.A.; et al. Distinct narcolepsy syndromes in Orexin receptor-2 and Orexin null mice: Molecular genetic dissection of Non-REM and REM sleep regulatory processes. *Neuron* **2003**, *38*, 715–730. [CrossRef]
65. Hagan, J.J.; Leslie, R.A.; Patel, S.; Evans, M.L.; Wattam, T.A.; Holmes, S.; Benham, C.D.; Taylor, S.G.; Routledge, C.; Hemmati, P.; et al. Orexin A activates locus coeruleus cell firing and increases arousal in the rat. *Proc. Natl. Acad. Sci. USA* **1999**, *96*, 10911–10916. [CrossRef]
66. Hung, C.; Yamanaka, A. The role of orexin neuron activity in sleep/wakefulness regulation. *Peptides* **2023**, *165*, 171007. [CrossRef] [PubMed]
67. Jones, B.E. Arousal and sleep circuits. *Neuropsychopharmacology* **2020**, *45*, 6–20. [CrossRef] [PubMed]
68. Lin, L.; Faraco, J.; Li, R.; Kadotani, H.; Rogers, W.; Lin, X.; Qiu, X.; de Jong, P.J.; Nishino, S.; Mignot, E. The sleep disorder canine narcolepsy is caused by a mutation in the hypocretin (orexin) receptor 2 gene. *Cell* **1999**, *98*, 365–376. [CrossRef] [PubMed]
69. Chemelli, R.M.; Willie, J.T.; Sinton, C.M.; Elmquist, J.K.; Scammell, T.; Lee, C.; Richardson, J.A.; Williams, S.C.; Xiong, Y.; Kisanuki, Y.; et al. Narcolepsy in orexin knockout mice: Molecular genetics of sleep regulation. *Cell* **1999**, *98*, 437–451. [CrossRef]
70. Scammell, T.E. Narcolepsy. *N. Engl. J. Med.* **2015**, *373*, 2654–2662. [CrossRef] [PubMed]
71. Mahoney, C.E.; Cogswell, A.; Koralnik, I.J.; Scammell, T.E. The neurobiological basis of narcolepsy. *Nat. Rev. Neurosci.* **2019**, *20*, 83–93. [CrossRef]
72. Thannickal, T.C.; Moore, R.Y.; Nienhuis, R.; Ramanathan, L.; Gulyani, S.; Aldrich, M.; Cornford, M.; Siegel, J.M. Reduced number of hypocretin neurons in human narcolepsy. *Neuron* **2000**, *27*, 469–474. [CrossRef]
73. Peyron, C.; Faraco, J.; Rogers, W.; Ripley, B.; Overeem, S.; Charnay, Y.; Nevsimalova, S.; Aldrich, M.; Reynolds, D.; Albin, R.; et al. A mutation in a case of early onset narcolepsy and a generalized absence of hypocretin peptides in human narcoleptic brains. *Nat. Med.* **2000**, *6*, 991–997. [CrossRef] [PubMed]
74. Liblau, R.S.; Vassalli, A.; Seifinejad, A.; Tafti, M. Hypocretin (orexin) biology and the pathophysiology of narcolepsy with cataplexy. *Lancet Neurol.* **2015**, *14*, 318–328. [CrossRef]
75. Zheng, H.; Patterson, L.M.; Berthoud, H.R. Orexin-A projections to the caudal medulla and orexin-induced c-Fos expression, food intake, and autonomic function. *J. Comp. Neurol.* **2005**, *485*, 127–142. [CrossRef]
76. Hurley, S.W.; Arseth, H.A.; Johnson, A.K. Orexin neurons couple neural systems mediating fluid balance with motivation-related circuits. *Behav. Neurosci.* **2018**, *132*, 284–292. [CrossRef] [PubMed]
77. Backberg, M.; Hervieu, G.; Wilson, S.; Meister, B. Orexin receptor-1 (OX-R1) immunoreactivity in chemically identified neurons of the hypothalamus: Focus on orexin targets involved in control of food and water intake. *Eur. J. Neurosci.* **2002**, *15*, 315–328. [CrossRef]
78. Plazzi, G.; Moghadam, K.K.; Maggi, L.S.; Donadio, V.; Vetrugno, R.; Liguori, R.; Zoccoli, G.; Poli, F.; Pizza, F.; Pagotto, U.; et al. Autonomic disturbances in narcolepsy. *Sleep Med. Rev.* **2011**, *15*, 187–196. [CrossRef]
79. Peleg-Raibstein, D.; Burdakov, D. Do orexin/hypocretin neurons signal stress or reward? *Peptides* **2021**, *145*, 170629. [CrossRef] [PubMed]

80. Grafe, L.A.; Bhatnagar, S. Orexins and stress. *Front. Neuroendocrinol.* **2018**, *51*, 132–145. [CrossRef]
81. Sargin, D. The role of the orexin system in stress response. *Neuropharmacology* **2019**, *154*, 68–78. [CrossRef]
82. Spinazzi, R.; Andreis, P.G.; Rossi, G.P.; Nussdorfer, G.G. Orexins in the regulation of the hypothalamic-pituitary-adrenal axis. *Pharmacol. Rev.* **2006**, *58*, 46–57. [CrossRef]
83. Lopez, M.; Tena-Sempere, M., Dieguez, C. Cross-talk between orexins (hypocretins) and the neuroendocrine axes (hypothalamic-pituitary axes). *Front. Neuroendocrinol.* **2010**, *31*, 113–127. [CrossRef]
84. Kohsaka, A.; Watanobe, H.; Kakizaki, Y.; Suda, T.; Schioth, H.B. A significant participation of orexin-A, a potent orexigenic peptide, in the preovulatory luteinizing hormone and prolactin surges in the rat. *Brain Res.* **2001**, *898*, 166–170. [CrossRef]
85. Sakurai, T. Roles of orexins in the regulation of body weight homeostasis. *Obes. Res. Clin. Pract.* **2014**, *8*, e414–e420. [CrossRef]
86. Hetherington, A.W.; Ranson, S.W. Hypothalamic lesions and adiposity in the rat. *Anat. Rec.* **1940**, *78*, 149–172. [CrossRef]
87. Anand, B.K.; Brobeck, J.R. Hypothalamic control of food intake in rats and cats. *Yale J. Biol. Med.* **1951**, *24*, 123–140.
88. Oomura, Y.; Ono, T.; Ooyama, H.; Wayner, M.J. Glucose and osmosensitive neurones of the rat hypothalamus. *Nature* **1969**, *222*, 282–284. [CrossRef]
89. Funahashi, H.; Takenoya, F.; Guan, J.L.; Kageyama, H.; Yada, T.; Shioda, S. Hypothalamic neuronal networks and feeding-related peptides involved in the regulation of feeding. *Anat. Sci. Int.* **2003**, *78*, 123–138. [CrossRef]
90. Elmquist, J.K.; Elias, C.F.; Saper, C.B. From lesions to leptin: Hypothalamic control of food intake and body weight. *Neuron* **1999**, *22*, 221–232. [CrossRef]
91. Valassi, E.; Scacchi, M.; Cavagnini, F. Neuroendocrine control of food intake. *Nutr. Metab. Cardiovasc. Dis.* **2008**, *18*, 158–168. [CrossRef]
92. Barsh, G.S.; Schwartz, M.W. Genetic approaches to studying energy balance: Perception and integration. *Nat. Rev. Genet.* **2002**, *3*, 589–600. [CrossRef]
93. Wang, C.; Han, X.; Guo, F.; Sun, X.; Luan, X.; Xu, L. Orexin-A signaling in the paraventricular nucleus modulates spontaneous firing of glucose-sensitive neurons and promotes food intake via the NPY pathway in rats. *Biochem. Biophys. Res. Commun.* **2018**, *505*, 162–167. [CrossRef]
94. Schuld, A.; Hebebrand, J.; Geller, F.; Pollmacher, T. Increased body-mass index in patients with narcolepsy. *Lancet* **2000**, *355*, 1274–1275. [CrossRef]
95. Federici, L.M.; Caliman, I.F.; Molosh, A.I.; Fitz, S.D.; Truitt, W.A.; Bonaventure, P.; Carpenter, J.S.; Shekhar, A.; Johnson, P.L. Hypothalamic orexin's role in exacerbated cutaneous vasodilation responses to an anxiogenic stimulus in a surgical menopause model. *Psychoneuroendocrinology* **2016**, *65*, 127–137. [CrossRef]
96. Madden, C.J.; Tupone, D.; Morrison, S.F. Orexin modulates brown adipose tissue thermogenesis. *Biomol. Concepts* **2012**, *3*, 381–386. [CrossRef]
97. Szekely, M.; Petervari, E.; Balasko, M. Thermoregulation, energy balance, regulatory peptides: Recent developments. *Front. Biosci.* **2010**, *2*, 1009–1046. [CrossRef]
98. Folgueira, C.; Beiroa, D.; Porteiro, B.; Duquenne, M.; Puighermanal, E.; Fondevila, M.F.; Barja-Fernandez, S.; Gallego, R.; Hernandez-Bautista, R.; Castelao, C.; et al. Hypothalamic dopamine signaling regulates brown fat thermogenesis. *Nat. Metab.* **2019**, *1*, 811–829. [CrossRef]
99. Murakami, M.; Ohba, T.; Kushikata, T.; Niwa, H.; Kurose, A.; Imaizumi, T.; Watanabe, H.; Yanagisawa, T.; Nakaji, S.; Ono, K.; et al. Involvement of the orexin system in sympathetic nerve regulation. *Biochem. Biophys. Res. Commun.* **2015**, *460*, 1076–1081. [CrossRef]
100. Jia, M.Q.; Wang, Y.J.; Fu, K.; Jiao, H.; Sun, J.; Gao, Y. Orexin receptor type 2 agonism inhibits thermogenesis in brown adipose tissue by attenuating afferent innervation. *J. Biomed. Res.* **2022**, *36*, 195–207. [CrossRef]
101. Sasson, R.; Dearth, R.K.; White, R.S.; Chappell, P.E.; Mellon, P.L. Orexin A induces GnRH gene expression and secretion from GT1-7 hypothalamic GnRH neurons. *Neuroendocrinology* **2006**, *84*, 353–363. [CrossRef]
102. Di Sebastiano, A.R.; Wilson-Perez, H.E.; Lehman, M.N.; Coolen, L.M. Lesions of orexin neurons block conditioned place preference for sexual behavior in male rats. *Horm. Behav.* **2011**, *59*, 1–8. [CrossRef]
103. Kim, H.J.J.; Dickie, S.A.; Laprairie, R.B. Estradiol-dependent hypocretinergic/orexinergic behaviors throughout the estrous cycle. *Psychopharmacology* **2023**, *240*, 15–25. [CrossRef]
104. Iwasa, T.; Noguchi, H.; Aoki, H.; Tamura, K.; Maeda, T.; Takeda, A.; Uchishiba, M.; Arakaki, R.; Minato, S.; Kamada, S.; et al. Effects of undernutrition and low energy availability on reproductive functions and their underlying neuroendocrine mechanisms. *Endocr. J.* **2022**, *69*, 1363–1372. [CrossRef]
105. Iwasa, T.; Yamamoto, Y.; Noguchi, H.; Takeda, A.; Minato, S.; Kamada, S.; Imaizumi, J.; Kagawa, T.; Yoshida, A.; Kawakita, T.; et al. Neuroendocrine mechanisms of reproductive dysfunctions in undernourished condition. *J. Obstet. Gynaecol. Res.* **2022**, *48*, 568–575. [CrossRef]
106. Johnson, P.L.; Molosh, A.; Fitz, S.D.; Truitt, W.A.; Shekhar, A. Orexin, stress, and anxiety/panic states. *Prog. Brain Res.* **2012**, *198*, 133–161. [CrossRef]
107. Palotai, M.; Telegdy, G.; Jaszberenyi, M. Orexin A-induced anxiety-like behavior is mediated through GABA-ergic, alpha- and beta-adrenergic neurotransmissions in mice. *Peptides* **2014**, *57*, 129–134. [CrossRef]
108. Vanderhaven, M.W.; Cornish, J.L.; Staples, L.G. The orexin-1 receptor antagonist SB-334867 decreases anxiety-like behavior and c-Fos expression in the hypothalamus of rats exposed to cat odor. *Behav. Brain Res.* **2015**, *278*, 563–568. [CrossRef]

109. Sakurai, T. The role of orexin in motivated behaviours. *Nat. Rev. Neurosci.* **2014**, *15*, 719–731. [CrossRef]
110. Sears, R.M.; Fink, A.E.; Wigestrand, M.B.; Farb, C.R.; de Lecea, L.; Ledoux, J.E. Orexin/hypocretin system modulates amygdala-dependent threat learning through the locus coeruleus. *Proc. Natl. Acad. Sci. USA* **2013**, *110*, 20260–20265. [CrossRef]
111. Soya, S.; Shoji, H.; Hasegawa, E.; Hondo, M.; Miyakawa, T.; Yanagisawa, M.; Mieda, M.; Sakurai, T. Orexin receptor-1 in the locus coeruleus plays an important role in cue-dependent fear memory consolidation. *J. Neurosci.* **2013**, *33*, 14549–14557. [CrossRef]
112. Telegdy, G.; Adamik, A. The action of orexin A on passive avoidance learning. Involvement of transmitters. *Regul. Pept.* **2002**, *104*, 105–110. [CrossRef]
113. Jacobson, L.H.; Hoyer, D.; de Lecea, L. Hypocretins (orexins): The ultimate translational neuropeptides. *J. Intern. Med.* **2022**, *291*, 533–556. [CrossRef]
114. Carrive, P.; Kuwaki, T. Orexin and Central Modulation of Cardiovascular and Respiratory Function. *Curr. Top. Behav. Neurosci.* **2017**, *33*, 157–196. [CrossRef]
115. Carrive, P. Orexin, orexin receptor antagonists and central cardiovascular control. *Front. Neurosci.* **2013**, *7*, 257. [CrossRef] [PubMed]
116. Soya, S.; Takahashi, T.M.; McHugh, T.J.; Maejima, T.; Herlitze, S.; Abe, M.; Sakimura, K.; Sakurai, T. Orexin modulates behavioral fear expression through the locus coeruleus. *Nat. Commun.* **2017**, *8*, 1606. [CrossRef]
117. Baimel, C.; Bartlett, S.E.; Chiou, L.C.; Lawrence, A.J.; Muschamp, J.W.; Patkar, O.; Tung, L.W.; Borgland, S.L. Orexin/hypocretin role in reward: Implications for opioid and other addictions. *Br. J. Pharmacol.* **2015**, *172*, 334–348. [CrossRef]
118. Becker-Krail, D.D.; Walker, W.H., 2nd; Nelson, R.J. The Ventral Tegmental Area and Nucleus Accumbens as Circadian Oscillators: Implications for Drug Abuse and Substance Use Disorders. *Front. Physiol.* **2022**, *13*, 886704. [CrossRef] [PubMed]
119. Samson, W.K.; Taylor, M.M.; Follwell, M.; Ferguson, A.V. Orexin actions in hypothalamic paraventricular nucleus: Physiological consequences and cellular correlates. *Regul. Pept.* **2002**, *104*, 97–103. [CrossRef] [PubMed]
120. Holland, P.; Goadsby, P.J. The hypothalamic orexinergic system: Pain and primary headaches. *Headache* **2007**, *47*, 951–962. [CrossRef]
121. Hoffmann, J.; May, A. Diagnosis, pathophysiology, and management of cluster headache. *Lancet Neurol.* **2018**, *17*, 75–83. [CrossRef]
122. Villano, I.; La Marra, M.; Di Maio, G.; Monda, V.; Chieffi, S.; Guatteo, E.; Messina, G.; Moscatelli, F.; Monda, M.; Messina, A. Physiological Role of Orexinergic System for Health. *Int. J. Environ. Res. Public. Health* **2022**, *19*, 8353. [CrossRef]
123. Vaseghi, S.; Zarrabian, S.; Haghparast, A. Reviewing the role of the orexinergic system and stressors in modulating mood and reward-related behaviors. *Neurosci. Biobehav. Rev.* **2022**, *133*, 104516. [CrossRef] [PubMed]
124. Melmed, S.; Auchus, R.J.; Goldfine, A.B.; Koenig, R.J.; Rosen, C.J. *Williams Textbook of Endocrinology*, 14th ed.; Elsevier: Philadelphia, PA, USA, 2020.
125. Cannon, W.B. The emergency function of the adrenal medulla in pain and the major emotions. *Am. J. Physiol.-Leg. Content* **1914**, *33*, 356–372. [CrossRef]
126. Selye, H. A Syndrome produced by Diverse Nocuous Agents. *Nature* **1936**, *138*, 32. [CrossRef]
127. Wade, N. Guillemin and schally: A race spurred by rivalry. *Science* **1978**, *200*, 510–513. [CrossRef] [PubMed]
128. Vale, W.; Spiess, J.; Rivier, C.; Rivier, J. Characterization of a 41-residue ovine hypothalamic peptide that stimulates secretion of corticotropin and beta-endorphin. *Science* **1981**, *213*, 1394–1397. [CrossRef] [PubMed]
129. Selye, H. The general adaptation syndrome and the diseases of adaptation. *J. Allergy* **1946**, *17*, 231. [CrossRef] [PubMed]
130. Bujdoso, E.; Jaszberenyi, M.; Tomboly, C.; Toth, G.; Telegdy, G. Behavioral and neuroendocrine actions of endomorphin-2. *Peptides* **2001**, *22*, 1459–1463. [CrossRef]
131. Aguilera, G. Regulation of the hypothalamic-pituitary-adrenal axis by neuropeptides. *Horm. Mol. Biol. Clin. Investig.* **2011**, *7*, 327–336. [CrossRef]
132. Bujdoso, E.; Jaszberenyi, M.; Tomboly, C.; Toth, G.; Telegdy, G. Effects of endomorphin-1 on open-field behavior and on the hypothalamic-pituitary-adrenal system. *Endocrine* **2001**, *14*, 221–224. [CrossRef]
133. Rostene, W.H.; Alexander, M.J. Neurotensin and neuroendocrine regulation. *Front. Neuroendocrinol.* **1997**, *18*, 115–173. [CrossRef]
134. Perras, B.; Schultes, B.; Behn, B.; Dodt, C.; Born, J.; Fehm, H.L. Intranasal atrial natriuretic peptide acts as central nervous inhibitor of the hypothalamo-pituitary-adrenal stress system in humans. *J. Clin. Endocrinol. Metab.* **2004**, *89*, 4642–4648. [CrossRef]
135. Kuppusamy, T.; Ramaswamy, P.; Perumal, M.; Silambanan, S.; Prabu Kumar, A. A short note on oxytocin and stress attenuation. *Bioinformation* **2021**, *17*, 921–923. [CrossRef]
136. Jaszberenyi, M.; Bujdoso, E.; Telegdy, G. Effects of C-type natriuretic peptide on pituitary-adrenal activation in rats. *Neuroreport* **1998**, *9*, 2601–2603. [CrossRef] [PubMed]
137. Jaszberenyi, M.; Bujdoso, E.; Telegdy, G. Effects of brain natriuretic peptide on pituitary-adrenal activation in rats. *Life Sci.* **2000**, *66*, 1655–1661. [CrossRef] [PubMed]
138. Kronenberg, H.; Williams, R.H. *Williams Textbook of Endocrinology*, 11th ed.; Saunders/Elsevier: Philadelphia, PA, USA, 2008.
139. Carrasco, G.A.; Van de Kar, L.D. Neuroendocrine pharmacology of stress. *Eur. J. Pharmacol.* **2003**, *463*, 235–272. [CrossRef]
140. Pan, W.; Kastin, A.J. Urocortin and the brain. *Prog. Neurobiol.* **2008**, *84*, 148–156. [CrossRef]
141. Henckens, M.J.; Deussing, J.M.; Chen, A. Region-specific roles of the corticotropin-releasing factor-urocortin system in stress. *Nat. Rev. Neurosci.* **2016**, *17*, 636–651. [CrossRef] [PubMed]

142. de Oliveira, C.V.; Rosas-Arellano, M.P.; Solano-Flores, L.P.; Ciriello, J. Cardiovascular effects of hypocretin-1 in nucleus of the solitary tract. *Am. J. Physiol. Heart Circ. Physiol.* **2003**, *284*, H1369–H1377. [CrossRef]
143. Yamashita, A.; Moriya, S.; Nishi, R.; Kaminosono, J.; Yamanaka, A.; Kuwaki, T. Aversive emotion rapidly activates orexin neurons and increases heart rate in freely moving mice. *Mol. Brain* **2021**, *14*, 104. [CrossRef] [PubMed]
144. Kuwaki, T. Orexin (hypocretin) participates in central autonomic regulation during fight-or-flight response. *Peptides* **2021**, *139*, 170530. [CrossRef] [PubMed]
145. Yun, S.; Wennerholm, M.; Shelton, J.E.; Bonaventure, P.; Letavic, M.A.; Shireman, B.T.; Lovenberg, T.W.; Dugovic, C. Selective Inhibition of Orexin-2 Receptors Prevents Stress-Induced ACTH Release in Mice. *Front. Behav. Neurosci.* **2017**, *11*, 83. [CrossRef] [PubMed]
146. Winsky-Sommerer, R.; Yamanaka, A.; Diano, S.; Borok, E.; Roberts, A.J.; Sakurai, T.; Kilduff, T.S.; Horvath, T.L.; de Lecea, L. Interaction between the corticotropin-releasing factor system and hypocretins (orexins): A novel circuit mediating stress response. *J. Neurosci.* **2004**, *24*, 11439–11448. [CrossRef]
147. Sakamoto, F.; Yamada, S.; Ueta, Y. Centrally administered orexin-A activates corticotropin-releasing factor-containing neurons in the hypothalamic paraventricular nucleus and central amygdaloid nucleus of rats: Possible involvement of central orexins on stress-activated central CRF neurons. *Regul. Pept.* **2004**, *118*, 183–191. [CrossRef]
148. Blasiak, A.; Gundlach, A.L.; Hess, G.; Lewandowski, M.H. Interactions of Circadian Rhythmicity, Stress and Orexigenic Neuropeptide Systems: Implications for Food Intake Control. *Front. Neurosci.* **2017**, *11*, 127. [CrossRef]
149. Hirota, K.; Kushikata, T.; Kudo, M.; Kudo, T.; Lambert, D.G.; Matsuki, A. Orexin A and B evoke noradrenaline release from rat cerebrocortical slices. *Br. J. Pharmacol.* **2001**, *134*, 1461–1466. [CrossRef] [PubMed]
150. Brunton, P.J.; Bales, J.; Russell, J.A. Neuroendocrine stress but not feeding responses to centrally administered neuropeptide Y are suppressed in pregnant rats. *Endocrinology* **2006**, *147*, 3737–3745. [CrossRef] [PubMed]
151. Russell, S.H.; Small, C.J.; Dakin, C.L.; Abbott, C.R.; Morgan, D.G.; Ghatei, M.A.; Bloom, S.R. The central effects of orexin-A in the hypothalamic-pituitary-adrenal axis in vivo and in vitro in male rats. *J. Neuroendocrinol.* **2001**, *13*, 561–566. [CrossRef]
152. Furlong, T.M.; Vianna, D.M.; Liu, L.; Carrive, P. Hypocretin/orexin contributes to the expression of some but not all forms of stress and arousal. *Eur. J. Neurosci.* **2009**, *30*, 1603–1614. [CrossRef]
153. Kotz, C.M.; Wang, C.; Teske, J.A.; Thorpe, A.J.; Novak, C.M.; Kiwaki, K.; Levine, J.A. Orexin A mediation of time spent moving in rats: Neural mechanisms. *Neuroscience* **2006**, *142*, 29–36. [CrossRef]
154. Kotz, C.M. Integration of feeding and spontaneous physical activity: Role for orexin. *Physiol. Behav.* **2006**, *88*, 294–301. [CrossRef] [PubMed]
155. Villano, I.; Messina, A.; Valenzano, A.; Moscatelli, F.; Esposito, T.; Monda, V.; Esposito, M.; Precenzano, F.; Carotenuto, M.; Viggiano, A.; et al. Basal Forebrain Cholinergic System and Orexin Neurons: Effects on Attention. *Front. Behav. Neurosci.* **2017**, *11*, 10. [CrossRef] [PubMed]
156. Li, Y.; Li, S.; Wei, C.; Wang, H.; Sui, N.; Kirouac, G.J. Changes in emotional behavior produced by orexin microinjections in the paraventricular nucleus of the thalamus. *Pharmacol. Biochem. Behav.* **2010**, *95*, 121–128. [CrossRef] [PubMed]
157. Humphreys, R.K.; Ruxton, G.D. A review of thanatosis (death feigning) as an anti-predator behaviour. *Behav. Ecol. Sociobiol.* **2018**, *72*, 22. [CrossRef] [PubMed]
158. Peinkhofer, C.; Martial, C.; Cassol, H.; Laureys, S.; Kondziella, D. The evolutionary origin of near-death experiences: A systematic investigation. *Brain Commun.* **2021**, *3*, fcab132. [CrossRef] [PubMed]
159. Steimer, T. The biology of fear- and anxiety-related behaviors. *Dialogues Clin. Neurosci.* **2002**, *4*, 231–249. [CrossRef] [PubMed]
160. Soya, S.; Sakurai, T. Orexin as a modulator of fear-related behavior: Hypothalamic control of noradrenaline circuit. *Brain Res.* **2020**, *1731*, 146037. [CrossRef]
161. Palotai, M.; Telegdy, G.; Ekwerike, A.; Jaszberenyi, M. The action of orexin B on passive avoidance learning. Involvement of neurotransmitters. *Behav. Brain Res.* **2014**, *272*, 1–7. [CrossRef]
162. Flores, A.; Saravia, R.; Maldonado, R.; Berrendero, F. Orexins and fear: Implications for the treatment of anxiety disorders. *Trends Neurosci.* **2015**, *38*, 550–559. [CrossRef]
163. LaBar, K.S.; Cabeza, R. Cognitive neuroscience of emotional memory. *Nat. Rev. Neurosci.* **2006**, *7*, 54–64. [CrossRef]
164. Rosen, L.G.; Sun, N.; Rushlow, W.; Laviolette, S.R. Molecular and neuronal plasticity mechanisms in the amygdala-prefrontal cortical circuit: Implications for opiate addiction memory formation. *Front. Neurosci.* **2015**, *9*, 399. [CrossRef]
165. Yoshida, K.; McCormack, S.; Espana, R.A.; Crocker, A.; Scammell, T.E. Afferents to the orexin neurons of the rat brain. *J. Comp. Neurol.* **2006**, *494*, 845–861. [CrossRef]
166. Avolio, E.; Alo, R.; Carelli, A.; Canonaco, M. Amygdalar orexinergic-GABAergic interactions regulate anxiety behaviors of the Syrian golden hamster. *Behav. Brain Res.* **2011**, *218*, 288–295. [CrossRef]
167. Steiner, M.A.; Lecourt, H.; Rakotoariniaina, A.; Jenck, F. Favoured genetic background for testing anxiolytics in the fear-potentiated and light-enhanced startle paradigms in the rat. *Behav. Brain Res.* **2011**, *221*, 34–42. [CrossRef]
168. Camina, E.; Guell, F. The Neuroanatomical, Neurophysiological and Psychological Basis of Memory: Current Models and Their Origins. *Front. Pharmacol.* **2017**, *8*, 438. [CrossRef] [PubMed]
169. Machaalani, R.; Hunt, N.J.; Waters, K.A. Effects of changes in energy homeostasis and exposure of noxious insults on the expression of orexin (hypocretin) and its receptors in the brain. *Brain Res.* **2013**, *1526*, 102–122. [CrossRef] [PubMed]

170. Elahdadi Salmani, M.; Sarfi, M.; Goudarzi, I. Hippocampal orexin receptors: Localization and function. *Vitam. Horm.* **2022**, *118*, 393–421. [CrossRef]
171. Bahramzadeh Zoeram, S.; Elahdadi Salmani, M.; Lashkarbolouki, T.; Goudarzi, I. Hippocampal orexin receptor blocking prevented the stress induced social learning and memory deficits. *Neurobiol. Learn. Mem.* **2019**, *157*, 12–23. [CrossRef] [PubMed]
172. Katzman, M.A.; Katzman, M.P. Neurobiology of the Orexin System and Its Potential Role in the Regulation of Hedonic Tone. *Brain Sci.* **2022**, *12*, 150. [CrossRef]
173. Piccoli, L.; Micioni Di Bonaventura, M.V.; Cifani, C.; Costantini, V.J.; Massagrande, M.; Montanari, D.; Martinelli, P.; Antolini, M.; Ciccocioppo, R.; Massi, M.; et al. Role of orexin-1 receptor mechanisms on compulsive food consumption in a model of binge eating in female rats. *Neuropsychopharmacology* **2012**, *37*, 1999–2011. [CrossRef]
174. Garcia-Garcia, F.; Juarez-Aguilar, E.; Santiago-Garcia, J.; Cardinali, D.P. Ghrelin and its interactions with growth hormone, leptin and orexins: Implications for the sleep-wake cycle and metabolism. *Sleep Med. Rev.* **2014**, *18*, 89–97. [CrossRef]
175. Toshinai, K.; Date, Y.; Murakami, N.; Shimada, M.; Mondal, M.S.; Shimbara, T.; Guan, J.L.; Wang, Q.P.; Funahashi, H.; Sakurai, T.; et al. Ghrelin-induced food intake is mediated via the orexin pathway. *Endocrinology* **2003**, *144*, 1506–1512. [CrossRef]
176. Quarta, D.; Smolders, I. Rewarding, reinforcing and incentive salient events involve orexigenic hypothalamic neuropeptides regulating mesolimbic dopaminergic neurotransmission. *Eur. J. Pharm. Sci.* **2014**, *57*, 2–10. [CrossRef]
177. Matzeu, A.; Martin-Fardon, R. Understanding the Role of Orexin Neuropeptides in Drug Addiction: Preclinical Studies and Translational Value. *Front. Behav. Neurosci.* **2021**, *15*, 787595. [CrossRef] [PubMed]
178. James, M.H.; Stopper, C.M.; Zimmer, B.A.; Koll, N.E.; Bowrey, H.E.; Aston-Jones, G. Increased Number and Activity of a Lateral Subpopulation of Hypothalamic Orexin/Hypocretin Neurons Underlies the Expression of an Addicted State in Rats. *Biol. Psychiatry* **2019**, *85*, 925–935. [CrossRef] [PubMed]
179. Shaw, J.K.; Ferris, M.J.; Locke, J.L.; Brodnik, Z.D.; Jones, S.R.; Espana, R.A. Hypocretin/orexin knock-out mice display disrupted behavioral and dopamine responses to cocaine. *Addict. Biol.* **2017**, *22*, 1695–1705. [CrossRef] [PubMed]
180. Steiner, N.; Rossetti, C.; Sakurai, T.; Yanagisawa, M.; de Lecea, L.; Magistretti, P.J.; Halfon, O.; Boutrel, B. Hypocretin/orexin deficiency decreases cocaine abuse liability. *Neuropharmacology* **2018**, *133*, 395–403. [CrossRef]
181. McGregor, R.; Thannickal, T.C.; Siegel, J.M. Pleasure, addiction, and hypocretin (orexin). *Handb. Clin. Neurol.* **2021**, *180*, 359–374. [CrossRef] [PubMed]
182. Mohammadkhani, A.; Fragale, J.E.; Pantazis, C.B.; Bowrey, H.E.; James, M.H.; Aston-Jones, G. Orexin-1 Receptor Signaling in Ventral Pallidum Regulates Motivation for the Opioid Remifentanil. *J. Neurosci.* **2019**, *39*, 9831–9840. [CrossRef] [PubMed]
183. Mohammadkhani, A.; James, M.H.; Pantazis, C.B.; Aston-Jones, G. Persistent effects of the orexin-1 receptor antagonist SB-334867 on motivation for the fast acting opioid remifentanil. *Brain Res.* **2020**, *1731*, 146461. [CrossRef] [PubMed]
184. Morganstern, I.; Chang, G.Q.; Barson, J.R.; Ye, Z.; Karatayev, O.; Leibowitz, S.F. Differential effects of acute and chronic ethanol exposure on orexin expression in the perifornical lateral hypothalamus. *Alcohol. Clin. Exp. Res.* **2010**, *34*, 886–896. [CrossRef]
185. Rotter, A.; Bayerlein, K.; Hansbauer, M.; Weiland, J.; Sperling, W.; Kornhuber, J.; Biermann, T. Orexin A expression and promoter methylation in patients with cannabis dependence in comparison to nicotine-dependent cigarette smokers and nonsmokers. *Neuropsychobiology* **2012**, *66*, 126–133. [CrossRef]
186. Bayerlein, K.; Kraus, T.; Leinonen, I.; Pilniok, D.; Rotter, A.; Hofner, B.; Schwitulla, J.; Sperling, W.; Kornhuber, J.; Biermann, T. Orexin A expression and promoter methylation in patients with alcohol dependence comparing acute and protracted withdrawal. *Alcohol.* **2011**, *45*, 541–547. [CrossRef]
187. Skofitsch, G.; Jacobowitz, D.M.; Zamir, N. Immunohistochemical localization of a melanin concentrating hormone-like peptide in the rat brain. *Brain Res. Bull.* **1985**, *15*, 635–649. [CrossRef]
188. Cowley, M.A.; Smith, R.G.; Diano, S.; Tschop, M.; Pronchuk, N.; Grove, K.L.; Strasburger, C.J.; Bidlingmaier, M.; Esterman, M.; Heiman, M.L.; et al. The distribution and mechanism of action of ghrelin in the CNS demonstrates a novel hypothalamic circuit regulating energy homeostasis. *Neuron* **2003**, *37*, 649–661. [CrossRef]
189. Ferrini, F.; Salio, C.; Lossi, L.; Merighi, A. Ghrelin in central neurons. *Curr. Neuropharmacol.* **2009**, *7*, 37–49. [CrossRef]
190. Mori, K.; Miyazato, M.; Ida, T.; Murakami, N.; Serino, R.; Ueta, Y.; Kojima, M.; Kangawa, K. Identification of neuromedin S and its possible role in the mammalian circadian oscillator system. *EMBO J.* **2005**, *24*, 325–335. [CrossRef] [PubMed]
191. Saito, Y.; Nagasaki, H. The melanin-concentrating hormone system and its physiological functions. *Results Probl. Cell Differ.* **2008**, *46*, 159–179. [CrossRef] [PubMed]
192. DiBona, G.F. Neuropeptide Y. *Am. J. Physiol. Regul. Integr. Comp. Physiol.* **2002**, *282*, R635–R636. [CrossRef] [PubMed]
193. Antushevich, H.; Wojcik, M. Review: Apelin in disease. *Clin. Chim. Acta* **2018**, *483*, 241–248. [CrossRef] [PubMed]
194. Telegdy, G.; Adamik, A.; Jaszberenyi, M. Involvement of neurotransmitters in the action of apelin-13 on passive avoidance learning in mice. *Peptides* **2013**, *39*, 171–174. [CrossRef]
195. Telegdy, G.; Jaszberenyi, M. Transmitter mediation of the anxiolytic action of apelin-13 in male mice. *Behav. Brain Res.* **2014**, *263*, 198–202. [CrossRef]
196. Kojima, M.; Kangawa, K. Ghrelin: Structure and function. *Physiol. Rev.* **2005**, *85*, 495–522. [CrossRef] [PubMed]
197. Malendowicz, L.K.; Rucinski, M. Neuromedins NMU and NMS: An Updated Overview of Their Functions. *Front. Endocrinol.* **2021**, *12*, 713961. [CrossRef] [PubMed]
198. Holland, P.R. Biology of Neuropeptides: Orexinergic Involvement in Primary Headache Disorders. *Headache* **2017**, *57* (Suppl. 2), 76–88. [CrossRef]

199. Horvath, T.L.; Diano, S.; van den Pol, A.N. Synaptic interaction between hypocretin (orexin) and neuropeptide Y cells in the rodent and primate hypothalamus: A novel circuit implicated in metabolic and endocrine regulations. *J. Neurosci.* **1999**, *19*, 1072–1087. [CrossRef]
200. Kageyama, H.; Takenoya, F.; Hirako, S.; Wada, N.; Kintaka, Y.; Inoue, S.; Ota, E.; Ogawa, T.; Shioda, S. Neuronal circuits involving neuropeptide Y in hypothalamic arcuate nucleus-mediated feeding regulation. *Neuropeptides* **2012**, *46*, 285–289. [CrossRef]
201. Russell, S.H.; Small, C.J.; Kennedy, A.R.; Stanley, S.A.; Seth, A.; Murphy, K.G.; Taheri, S.; Ghatei, M.A.; Bloom, S.R. Orexin A interactions in the hypothalamo-pituitary gonadal axis. *Endocrinology* **2001**, *142*, 5294–5302. [CrossRef]
202. Funahashi, H.; Yamada, S.; Kageyama, H.; Takenoya, F.; Guan, J.L.; Shioda, S. Co existence of leptin- and orexin-receptors in feeding-regulating neurons in the hypothalamic arcuate nucleus-a triple labeling study. *Peptides* **2003**, *24*, 687–694. [CrossRef] [PubMed]
203. Horvath, T.L.; Peyron, C.; Diano, S.; Ivanov, A.; Aston-Jones, G.; Kilduff, T.S.; van Den Pol, A.N. Hypocretin (orexin) activation and synaptic innervation of the locus coeruleus noradrenergic system. *J. Comp. Neurol.* **1999**, *415*, 145–159. [CrossRef]
204. Chen, B.; Xu, J.; Chen, S.; Mou, T.; Wang, Y.; Wang, H.; Zhang, Z.; Ren, F.; Wang, Z.; Jin, K.; et al. Dysregulation of striatal dopamine D2/D3 receptor-mediated by hypocretin induces depressive behaviors in rats. *J. Affect. Disord.* **2023**, *325*, 256–263. [CrossRef]
205. Kim, S.; Nam, Y.; Shin, S.J.; Park, Y.H.; Jeon, S.G.; Kim, J.I.; Kim, M.J.; Moon, M. The Potential Roles of Ghrelin in Metabolic Syndrome and Secondary Symptoms of Alzheimer's Disease. *Front. Neurosci.* **2020**, *14*, 583097. [CrossRef]
206. Scammell, T.E.; Winrow, C.J. Orexin receptors: Pharmacology and therapeutic opportunities. *Annu. Rev. Pharmacol. Toxicol.* **2011**, *51*, 243–266. [CrossRef] [PubMed]
207. Fronczek, R.; Schinkelshoek, M.; Shan, L.; Lammers, G.J. The orexin/hypocretin system in neuropsychiatric disorders: Relation to signs and symptoms. *Handb. Clin. Neurol.* **2021**, *180*, 343–358. [CrossRef] [PubMed]
208. Dauvilliers, Y.; Arnulf, I.; Mignot, E. Narcolepsy with cataplexy. *Lancet* **2007**, *369*, 499–511. [CrossRef]
209. Wang, W.; Pan, Y.; Li, Q.; Wang, L. Orexin: A potential role in the process of obstructive sleep apnea. *Peptides* **2013**, *42*, 48–54. [CrossRef] [PubMed]
210. Sakurai, S.; Nishijima, T.; Arihara, Z.; Takahashi, K. Plasma orexin-A levels in obstructive sleep apnea-hypopnea syndrome. *Chest* **2004**, *125*, 1963, author reply 1963–1964. [CrossRef]
211. Nishijima, T.; Sakurai, S.; Arihara, Z.; Takahashi, K. Plasma orexin-A-like immunoreactivity in patients with sleep apnea hypopnea syndrome. *Peptides* **2003**, *24*, 407–411. [CrossRef]
212. Seifinejad, A.; Ramosaj, M.; Shan, L.; Li, S.; Possovre, M.L.; Pfister, C.; Fronczek, R.; Garrett-Sinha, L.A.; Frieser, D.; Honda, M.; et al. Epigenetic silencing of selected hypothalamic neuropeptides in narcolepsy with cataplexy. *Proc. Natl. Acad. Sci. USA* **2023**, *120*, e2220911120. [CrossRef]
213. Partinen, M.; Kornum, B.R.; Plazzi, G.; Jennum, P.; Julkunen, I.; Vaarala, O. Narcolepsy as an autoimmune disease: The role of H1N1 infection and vaccination. *Lancet Neurol.* **2014**, *13*, 600–613. [CrossRef] [PubMed]
214. Rahman, Q.F.A.; Jufri, N.F.; Hamid, A. Hyperphagia in Prader-Willi syndrome with obesity: From development to pharmacological treatment. *Intractable Rare Dis. Res.* **2023**, *12*, 5–12. [CrossRef] [PubMed]
215. Mehr, J.B.; Mitchison, D.; Bowrey, H.E.; James, M.H. Sleep dysregulation in binge eating disorder and "food addiction": The orexin (hypocretin) system as a potential neurobiological link. *Neuropsychopharmacology* **2021**, *46*, 2051–2061. [CrossRef]
216. Berner, L.A.; Brown, T.A.; Lavender, J.M.; Lopez, E.; Wierenga, C.E.; Kaye, W.H. Neuroendocrinology of reward in anorexia nervosa and bulimia nervosa: Beyond leptin and ghrelin. *Mol. Cell Endocrinol.* **2019**, *497*, 110320. [CrossRef] [PubMed]
217. Pizza, F.; Barateau, L.; Dauvilliers, Y.; Plazzi, G. The orexin story, sleep and sleep disturbances. *J. Sleep Res.* **2022**, *31*, e13665. [CrossRef]
218. Wang, J.Y.; Han, F.; Dong, S.X.; Li, J.; An, P.; Zhang, X.Z.; Chang, Y.; Zhao, L.; Zhang, X.L.; Liu, Y.N.; et al. Cerebrospinal Fluid Orexin A Levels and Autonomic Function in Kleine-Levin Syndrome. *Sleep* **2016**, *39*, 855–860. [CrossRef]
219. Razzoli, M.; Bartolomucci, A. The Dichotomous Effect of Chronic Stress on Obesity. *Trends Endocrinol. Metab.* **2016**, *27*, 504–515. [CrossRef]
220. Yilmaz, E.; Celik, O.; Celik, N.; Celik, E.; Turkcuoglu, I.; Simsek, Y.; Minareci, Y.; Boz, M.; Aydin, S. Maternal and fetal serum orexin-A levels in gestational diabetes mellitus. *J. Obstet. Gynaecol. Res.* **2013**, *39*, 139–145. [CrossRef]
221. Yilmaz, E.; Celik, O.; Celik, N.; Simsek, Y.; Celik, E.; Yildirim, E. Serum orexin-A (OXA) level decreases in polycystic ovarian syndrome. *Gynecol. Endocrinol.* **2013**, *29*, 388–390. [CrossRef]
222. Celik, O.; Aydin, S.; Celik, N.; Yilmaz, M. Peptides: Basic determinants of reproductive functions. *Peptides* **2015**, *72*, 34–43. [CrossRef] [PubMed]
223. Jequier, E. Leptin signaling, adiposity, and energy balance. *Ann. N. Y. Acad. Sci.* **2002**, *967*, 379–388. [CrossRef] [PubMed]
224. Hopf, F.W. Recent perspectives on orexin/hypocretin promotion of addiction-related behaviors. *Neuropharmacology* **2020**, *168*, 108013. [CrossRef] [PubMed]
225. Zhou, Y.; Proudnikov, D.; Yuferov, V.; Kreek, M.J. Drug-induced and genetic alterations in stress-responsive systems: Implications for specific addictive diseases. *Brain Res.* **2010**, *1314*, 235–252. [CrossRef]
226. Berteotti, C.; Calvello, C.; Liguori, C. Role of the orexin system in the bidirectional relation between sleep and epilepsy: New chances for patients with epilepsy by the antagonism to orexin receptors? *Epilepsia* **2023**, *64*, 1991–2005. [CrossRef] [PubMed]

227. Gorka, S.M.; Khorrami, K.J.; Manzler, C.A.; Phan, K.L. Acute orexin antagonism selectively modulates anticipatory anxiety in humans: Implications for addiction and anxiety. *Transl. Psychiatry* **2022**, *12*, 308. [CrossRef] [PubMed]
228. Abreu, A.R.; Molosh, A.I.; Johnson, P.L.; Shekhar, A. Role of medial hypothalamic orexin system in panic, phobia and hypertension. *Brain Res.* **2020**, *1731*, 145942. [CrossRef] [PubMed]
229. Kaplan, G.B.; Lakis, G.A.; Zhoba, H. Sleep-wake and arousal dysfunctions in post-traumatic stress disorder: Role of orexin systems. *Brain Res. Bull.* **2022**, *186*, 106–122. [CrossRef]
230. Brundin, L.; Bjorkqvist, M.; Petersen, A.; Traskman-Bendz, L. Reduced orexin levels in the cerebrospinal fluid of suicidal patients with major depressive disorder. *Eur. Neuropsychopharmacol.* **2007**, *17*, 573–579. [CrossRef]
231. Salomon, R.M.; Ripley, B.; Kennedy, J.S.; Johnson, B.; Schmidt, D.; Zeitzer, J.M.; Nishino, S.; Mignot, E. Diurnal variation of cerebrospinal fluid hypocretin-1 (Orexin-A) levels in control and depressed subjects. *Biol. Psychiatry* **2003**, *54*, 96–104. [CrossRef]
232. Al-Kuraishy, H.M.; Abdulhadi, M.H.; Hussien, N.R.; Al-Niemi, M.S.; Rasheed, H.A.; Al-Gareeb, A.I. Involvement of orexinergic system in psychiatric and neurodegenerative disorders: A scoping review. *Brain Circ.* **2020**, *6*, 70–80. [CrossRef] [PubMed]
233. Toor, B.; Ray, L.B.; Pozzobon, A.; Fogel, S.M. Sleep, Orexin and Cognition. *Front. Neurol. Neurosci.* **2021**, *45*, 38–51. [CrossRef] [PubMed]
234. Mobarakeh, J.I.; Takahashi, K.; Sakurada, S.; Nishino, S.; Watanabe, H.; Kato, M.; Naghdi, N.; Yanai, K. Enhanced antinociception by intracerebroventricularly administered orexin A in histamine H1 or H2 receptor gene knockout mice. *Pain* **2005**, *118*, 254–262. [CrossRef]
235. Watanabe, S.; Kuwaki, T.; Yanagisawa, M.; Fukuda, Y.; Shimoyama, M. Persistent pain and stress activate pain-inhibitory orexin pathways. *Neuroreport* **2005**, *16*, 5–8. [CrossRef]
236. Li, S.B.; Jones, J.R.; de Lecea, L. Hypocretins, Neural Systems, Physiology, and Psychiatric Disorders. *Curr. Psychiatry Rep.* **2016**, *18*, 7. [CrossRef]
237. Kalliomaki, M.L.; Panula, P. Neuropeptide FF, but not prolactin-releasing peptide, mRNA is differentially regulated in the hypothalamic and medullary neurons after salt loading. *Neuroscience* **2004**, *124*, 81–87. [CrossRef]
238. Roehrs, T.; Withrow, D.; Koshorek, G.; Verkler, J.; Bazan, L.; Roth, T. Sleep and pain in humans with fibromyalgia and comorbid insomnia: Double-blind, crossover study of suvorexant 20 mg versus placebo. *J. Clin. Sleep Med.* **2020**, *16*, 415–421. [CrossRef]
239. Razavi, B.M.; Hosseinzadeh, H. A review of the role of orexin system in pain modulation. *Biomed. Pharmacother.* **2017**, *90*, 187–193. [CrossRef] [PubMed]
240. Navarro, V.M. Metabolic regulation of kisspeptin—The link between energy balance and reproduction. *Nat. Rev. Endocrinol.* **2020**, *16*, 407–420. [CrossRef]
241. Voisin, T.; Nicole, P.; Gratio, V.; Chassac, A.; Mansour, D.; Rebours, V.; Couvelard, A.; Couvineau, A. The Orexin-A/OX1R System Induces Cell Death in Pancreatic Cancer Cells Resistant to Gemcitabine and Nab-Paclitaxel Treatment. *Front. Oncol.* **2022**, *12*, 904327. [CrossRef] [PubMed]
242. Kotani, M.; Detheux, M.; Vandenbogaerde, A.; Communi, D.; Vanderwinden, J.M.; Le Poul, E.; Brezillon, S.; Tyldesley, R.; Suarez-Huerta, N.; Vandeput, F.; et al. The metastasis suppressor gene KiSS-1 encodes kisspeptins, the natural ligands of the orphan G protein-coupled receptor GPR54. *J. Biol. Chem.* **2001**, *276*, 34631–34636. [CrossRef] [PubMed]
243. Wahab, F.; Atika, B.; Shahab, M.; Behr, R. Kisspeptin signalling in the physiology and pathophysiology of the urogenital system. *Nat. Rev. Urol.* **2016**, *13*, 21–32. [CrossRef]
244. Ten-Blanco, M.; Flores, A.; Cristino, L.; Pereda-Perez, I.; Berrendero, F. Targeting the orexin/hypocretin system for the treatment of neuropsychiatric and neurodegenerative diseases: From animal to clinical studies. *Front. Neuroendocrinol.* **2023**, *69*, 101066. [CrossRef] [PubMed]
245. Liguori, C.; Spanetta, M.; Izzi, F.; Franchini, F.; Nuccetelli, M.; Sancesario, G.M.; Di Santo, S.; Bernardini, S.; Mercuri, N.B.; Placidi, F. Sleep-Wake Cycle in Alzheimer's Disease Is Associated with Tau Pathology and Orexin Dysregulation. *J. Alzheimers Dis.* **2020**, *74*, 501–508. [CrossRef] [PubMed]
246. Liguori, C.; Mercuri, N.B.; Nuccetelli, M.; Izzi, F.; Bernardini, S.; Placidi, F. Cerebrospinal Fluid Orexin Levels and Nocturnal Sleep Disruption in Alzheimer's Disease Patients Showing Neuropsychiatric Symptoms. *J. Alzheimers Dis.* **2018**, *66*, 993–999. [CrossRef] [PubMed]
247. Liguori, C. Orexin and Alzheimer's Disease. *Curr. Top. Behav. Neurosci.* **2017**, *33*, 305–322. [CrossRef] [PubMed]
248. Ropper, A.H.; Samuels, M.A.; Klein, J.; Prasad, S. *Adams and Victor's Principles of Neurology*; McGraw Hill: New York, NY, USA, 2023.
249. McKnight, R.; Price, J.; Geddes, J. *Psychiatry*, 5th ed.; Oxford University Press: New York, NY, USA, 2019.
250. Tiwari, S.B.; Amiji, M.M. A review of nanocarrier-based CNS delivery systems. *Curr. Drug Deliv.* **2006**, *3*, 219–232. [CrossRef]
251. Cummings, D.E. Ghrelin and the short- and long-term regulation of appetite and body weight. *Physiol. Behav.* **2006**, *89*, 71–84. [CrossRef]
252. Kastin, A.J.; Pan, W.; Maness, L.M.; Banks, W.A. Peptides crossing the blood-brain barrier: Some unusual observations. *Brain Res.* **1999**, *848*, 96–100. [CrossRef]
253. Bonifazi, A.; Del Bello, F.; Giorgioni, G.; Piergentili, A.; Saab, E.; Botticelli, L.; Cifani, C.; Micioni Di Bonaventura, E.; Micioni Di Bonaventura, M.V.; Quaglia, W. Targeting orexin receptors: Recent advances in the development of subtype selective or dual ligands for the treatment of neuropsychiatric disorders. *Med. Res. Rev.* **2023**, *43*, 1607–1667. [CrossRef]

254. Yukitake, H.; Fujimoto, T.; Ishikawa, T.; Suzuki, A.; Shimizu, Y.; Rikimaru, K.; Ito, M.; Suzuki, M.; Kimura, H. TAK-925, an orexin 2 receptor-selective agonist, shows robust wake-promoting effects in mice. *Pharmacol. Biochem. Behav.* **2019**, *187*, 172794. [CrossRef]
255. Dauvilliers, Y.; Mignot, E.; Del Rio Villegas, R.; Du, Y.; Hanson, E.; Inoue, Y.; Kadali, H.; Koundourakis, E.; Meyer, S.; Rogers, R.; et al. Oral Orexin Receptor 2 Agonist in Narcolepsy Type 1. *N. Engl. J. Med.* **2023**, *389*, 309–321. [CrossRef]
256. Brooks, S.; Jacobs, G.E.; de Boer, P.; Kent, J.M.; Van Nueten, L.; van Amerongen, G.; Zuiker, R.; Kezic, I.; Luthringer, R.; van der Ark, P.; et al. The selective orexin-2 receptor antagonist seltorexant improves sleep: An exploratory double-blind, placebo controlled, crossover study in antidepressant-treated major depressive disorder patients with persistent insomnia. *J. Psychopharmacol.* **2019**, *33*, 202–209. [CrossRef] [PubMed]
257. Coleman, P.J.; Gotter, A.L.; Herring, W.J.; Winrow, C.J.; Renger, J.J. The Discovery of Suvorexant, the First Orexin Receptor Drug for Insomnia. *Annu. Rev. Pharmacol. Toxicol.* **2017**, *57*, 509–533. [CrossRef] [PubMed]
258. Cox, C.D.; Breslin, M.J.; Whitman, D.B.; Schreier, J.D.; McGaughey, G.B.; Bogusky, M.J.; Roecker, A.J.; Mercer, S.P.; Bednar, R.A.; Lemaire, W.; et al. Discovery of the dual orexin receptor antagonist [(7R)-4-(5-chloro-1,3-benzoxazol-2-yl)-7-methyl-1,4-diazepan-1-yl][5-methyl-2-(2H-1,2,3-triazol-2-yl)phenyl]methanone (MK-4305) for the treatment of insomnia. *J. Med. Chem.* **2010**, *53*, 5320–5332. [CrossRef] [PubMed]
259. Yoshida, Y.; Naoe, Y.; Terauchi, T.; Ozaki, F.; Doko, T.; Takemura, A.; Tanaka, T.; Sorimachi, K.; Beuckmann, C.T.; Suzuki, M.; et al. Discovery of (1R,2S)-2-[(2,4-Dimethylpyrimidin-5-yl)oxy]methyl-2-(3-fluorophenyl)-N-(5-fluoropyridin-2-yl)cyclopropanecarboxamide (E2006): A Potent and Efficacious Oral Orexin Receptor Antagonist. *J. Med. Chem.* **2015**, *58*, 4648–4664. [CrossRef]
260. Kaufmann, P.; Ort, M.; Golor, G.; Kornberger, R.; Dingemanse, J. First-in-human study with ACT-539313, a novel selective orexin-1 receptor antagonist. *Br. J. Clin. Pharmacol.* **2020**, *86*, 1377–1386. [CrossRef]
261. Salvadore, G.; Bonaventure, P.; Shekhar, A.; Johnson, P.L.; Lord, B.; Shireman, B.T.; Lebold, T.P.; Nepomuceno, D.; Dugovic, C.; Brooks, S.; et al. Translational evaluation of novel selective orexin-1 receptor antagonist JNJ-61393215 in an experimental model for panic in rodents and humans. *Transl. Psychiatry* **2020**, *10*, 308. [CrossRef]
262. Battaglia, S.; Schmidt, A.; Hassel, S.; Tanaka, M. Editorial: Case reports in neuroimaging and stimulation. *Front. Psychiatry* **2023**, *14*, 1264669. [CrossRef]
263. Tanaka, M.; Diano, M.; Battaglia, S. Editorial: Insights into structural and functional organization of the brain: Evidence from neuroimaging and non-invasive brain stimulation techniques. *Front. Psychiatry* **2023**, *14*, 1225755. [CrossRef]
264. Borgomaneri, S.; Battaglia, S.; Sciamanna, G.; Tortora, F.; Laricchiuta, D. Memories are not written in stone: Re-writing fear memories by means of non-invasive brain stimulation and optogenetic manipulations. *Neurosci. Biobehav. Rev.* **2021**, *127*, 334–352. [CrossRef]
265. Milbank, E.; Lopez, M. Orexins/Hypocretins: Key Regulators of Energy Homeostasis. *Front. Endocrinol.* **2019**, *10*, 830. [CrossRef]
266. Singh, R.; Biswas, D.A. Physiological Role of Orexin/Hypocretin in the Human Body in Motivated Behavior: A Comprehensive Review. *Cureus* **2023**, *15*, e34009. [CrossRef]
267. Baimel, C.; Borgland, S.L. Orexin Signaling in the VTA Gates Morphine-Induced Synaptic Plasticity. *J. Neurosci.* **2015**, *35*, 7295–7303. [CrossRef] [PubMed]
268. Kang, X.; Tang, H.; Liu, Y.; Yuan, Y.; Wang, M. Research progress on the mechanism of orexin in pain regulation in different brain regions. *Open Life Sci.* **2021**, *16*, 46–52. [CrossRef]
269. Brundin, L.; Petersen, A.; Bjorkqvist, M.; Traskman-Bendz, L. Orexin and psychiatric symptoms in suicide attempters. *J. Affect. Disord.* **2007**, *100*, 259–263. [CrossRef]
270. Tanaka, M.; Vecsei, L. Editorial of Special Issue "Crosstalk between Depression, Anxiety, and Dementia: Comorbidity in Behavioral Neurology and Neuropsychiatry". *Biomedicines* **2021**, *9*, 517. [CrossRef]
271. Muehlan, C.; Roch, C.; Vaillant, C.; Dingemanse, J. The orexin story and orexin receptor antagonists for the treatment of insomnia. *J. Sleep Res.* **2023**, *32*, e13902. [CrossRef] [PubMed]
272. Mattar, P.; Uribe-Cerda, S.; Pezoa, C.; Guarnieri, T.; Kotz, C.M.; Teske, J.A.; Morselli, E.; Perez-Leighton, C. Brain site-specific regulation of hedonic intake by orexin and DYN peptides: Role of the PVN and obesity. *Nutr. Neurosci.* **2022**, *25*, 1105–1114. [CrossRef] [PubMed]
273. Butterick, T.A.; Billington, C.J.; Kotz, C.M.; Nixon, J.P. Orexin: Pathways to obesity resistance? *Rev. Endocr. Metab. Disord.* **2013**, *14*, 357–364. [CrossRef]
274. Perez-Leighton, C.E.; Butterick-Peterson, T.A.; Billington, C.J.; Kotz, C.M. Role of orexin receptors in obesity: From cellular to behavioral evidence. *Int. J. Obes.* **2013**, *37*, 167–174. [CrossRef]
275. Seale, P. Orexin turns up the heat on obesity. *Cell Metab.* **2011**, *14*, 441–442. [CrossRef]
276. Krause, A.; Lott, D.; Brussee, J.M.; Muehlan, C.; Dingemanse, J. Population pharmacokinetic modeling of daridorexant, a novel dual orexin receptor antagonist. *CPT Pharmacomet. Syst. Pharmacol.* **2023**, *12*, 74–86. [CrossRef] [PubMed]

biomedicines

MDPI

Review

Evaluating p-tau217 and p-tau231 as Biomarkers for Early Diagnosis and Differentiation of Alzheimer's Disease: A Narrative Review

Dorian Julian Jarek [1,*], Hubert Mizerka [1], Jarosław Nuszkiewicz [2] and Karolina Szewczyk-Golec [2,*]

1 Student Research Club of Medical Biology and Biochemistry, Department of Medical Biology and Biochemistry, Faculty of Medicine, Ludwik Rydygier Collegium Medicum in Bydgoszcz, Nicolaus Copernicus University in Toruń, 85-092 Bydgoszcz, Poland; 310894@stud.umk.pl

2 Department of Medical Biology and Biochemistry, Faculty of Medicine, Ludwik Rydygier Collegium Medicum in Bydgoszcz, Nicolaus Copernicus University in Toruń, 85-092 Bydgoszcz, Poland; jnuszkiewicz@cm.umk.pl

* Correspondence: 309897@stud.umk.pl (D.J.J.); karosz@cm.umk.pl (K.S.-G.)

Abstract: The escalating prevalence of Alzheimer's disease (AD) highlights the urgent need to develop reliable biomarkers for early diagnosis and intervention. AD is characterized by the pathological accumulation of amyloid-beta plaques and tau neurofibrillary tangles. Phosphorylated tau (p-tau) proteins, particularly p-tau217 and p-tau231, have been identified as promising biomarker candidates to differentiate the disease progression from preclinical stages. This narrative review is devoted to a critical evaluation of the diagnostic accuracy, sensitivity, and specificity of p-tau217 and p-tau231 levels in the detection of AD, measured in plasma, serum, and cerebrospinal fluid, compared to established biomarkers. Additionally, the efficacy of these markers in distinguishing AD from other neurodegenerative disorders is examined. The significant advances offered by p-tau217 and p-tau231 in AD diagnostics are highlighted, demonstrating their unique utility in early detection and differential diagnosis. This comprehensive analysis not only confirms the excellent diagnostic capabilities of these markers, but also deepens the understanding of the molecular dynamics of AD, contributing to the broader scientific discourse on neurodegenerative diseases. This review is aimed to provide key information for researchers and clinicians across disciplines, filling interdisciplinary gaps and highlighting the role of p-tau proteins in revolutionizing AD research and clinical practice.

Keywords: Alzheimer's disease; amyloid plaques; biomarker; diagnosis; neurodegenerative diseases; neurofibrillary tangles; p-tau; p-tau217; p-tau231; tau proteins

1. Introduction

Since the first diagnosis of Alzheimer's disease (AD), published by Alois Alzheimer [1,2] on 3 November 1906, more than a century has passed. AD is the most common cause of cognitive impairment among older adults. It affects approximately 3–4% of the population aged 60 years and older [3]. A global status report on the public health response to dementia issued by the World Health Organization (WHO) states that, in 2019, 55.2 million people worldwide were living with dementia [4]. However, a recent study estimated that 22% of individuals worldwide aged 50 years or older have AD [5]. When including patients in the earlier stages of the disease, this estimate rises to a total of 416 million people worldwide, with figures ranging between 327 and 525 million. According to the latest systematic literature review, numerous cases of AD might not be captured in studies including only individuals with a formal diagnosis of AD dementia [6]. The incidence of AD has been increasing in recent years, and it is estimated that this trend will continue [3]. The prevalence of dementia in Europe is expected to double by 2050 [7].

Currently, three main stages of AD are recognized as preclinical AD, AD with mild cognitive impairment (MCI), and dementia [3,8,9]. The earliest phase, preclinical AD, is clinically asymptomatic, but in this phase of the disease, it is possible to identify diagnostic biomarkers of the disease [10,11]. MCI is defined by the initial stage symptoms, which typically include the impairment of short-term memory, followed by a decline in additional cognitive domains [12,13]. The dementia stage is characterized by cognitive impairment severe enough to impact the daily life of a person with AD [7,14].

AD is related to age, and a greater risk of developing AD is observed in women [15], which is probably caused by menopause and the associated disruption of the functioning of estrogen-regulated systems [16,17]. Several genes are significantly associated with AD. Mutations in the amyloid protein precursor (*APP*) and the presenilin-1/2 (*PSEN1/2*) genes account for less than 5% of all AD cases [15,18]. Allelic variation of the apolipoprotein E (*APOE*) gene, specifically the type ε4 allele, is a major risk factor in sporadic AD [15,19]. This allele is 2–3 times more frequent in individuals with AD compared to normal control cases [15]. Modifiable risk factors for AD have also been identified [20–22]. Significant risk factors for developing AD include hyperhomocysteinemia and depression [23,24]. Other risk-enhancing factors include pre-existing diseases such as frailty, carotid atherosclerosis, hypertension, low diastolic blood pressure, and type 2 diabetes mellitus in the Asian population, as well as lifestyle factors like low education, increased body mass index (BMI) in mid-life, and low BMI in later life [22,25,26].

The molecular mechanism of AD is determined by the accumulation of both β-amyloid (Aβ) in the form of extracellular neuritic plaques and hyperphosphorylated tau protein in the form of intracellular neurofibrillary tangles (NFTs) [27,28]. Aβ plaques are produced by sequential cleavage of APP by β-secretase (BACE-1) and γ-secretase within cells [29,30]. This process results in the formation of Aβ monomers, which are secreted outside the cell into the intercellular space [31]. Then, they aggregate to form Aβ oligomers, protofibrils, and fibrils [32,33]. These aggregates lead to the hyperphosphorylation of tau, a decrease in cerebral capillary blood flow, and the impairment of the function of synapses [27,28]. In vitro studies have underscored the ability of tau proteins to promote the assembly and stabilization of axonal microtubules (MTs), a process vital for proper neuronal function and axonal transport [28]. Under normal conditions, the interaction between tau and MTs is precisely regulated by phosphorylation, which adjusts tau's binding affinity to MTs and its neuronal distribution. However, in AD and related tauopathies, tau undergoes aberrant hyperphosphorylation, significantly diminishing its affinity for MTs [28,34]. Consequently, hyperphosphorylated tau accumulates in the cytosol, leading to aggregation and fibrillization. This process results in the formation of NFTs, insoluble aggregates that are characteristic of AD pathology [28,34]. Such pathological aggregation disrupts MT stability and induces neuronal dysfunction by redistributing tau from axonal to somatodendritic compartments. This redistribution hinders essential neuronal processes, including glutamate receptor trafficking and synaptic anchoring, exacerbating synaptic dysfunction and contributing to the cognitive decline seen in AD [28]. Additionally, recent research indicates that the spread of tau aggregates might occur through a prion-like mechanism in which misfolded tau proteins catalyze the misfolding of normal tau, promoting the progression of pathology across neuronal networks [35,36]. The described mechanisms are associated with the clinical and neuropathological stages of AD, underscoring the critical role of tau pathology in the disease evolution and its potential as a therapeutic target. Moreover, NFTs can spread trans-synaptically to anatomically connected brain regions, causing further formation of NFTs in remote parts of the brain, spreading from the entorhinal cortex to the neocortex [28]. The process of NFT production appears to correlate with Aβ deposition [37]. The progression of hyperphosphorylated tau to other parts of the brain occurs only in the presence of Aβ, suggesting a mechanistic link [28]. However, the presence of Aβ, unlike the stage of tau pathology, does not correlate with the progression of cognitive impairment, indicating the significant role of tau hyperphosphorylation in inducing AD symptoms [28].

Given the critical need for advancements in the early detection and differentiation of AD amid its growing global prevalence, this narrative review sets forth to critically evaluate the diagnostic utility of phosphorylated-tau (p-tau) proteins, specifically p-tau

Thr217 (p-tau217) and p-tau Thr231 (p-tau231), as potential biomarkers for AD. This evaluation synthesizes findings from a broad spectrum of studies to elucidate the sensitivity, specificity, and overall diagnostic accuracy of these biomarkers across the various stages of AD, including the preclinical and prodromal phases. Furthermore, this review aims to contrast the effectiveness of p-tau217 and p-tau231 against other established biomarkers for AD, examine their potential in distinguishing AD from other neurodegenerative disorders, and explore the practical implications of their application in clinical settings. By delving into these areas, the review endeavors to fill existing gaps in interdisciplinary research and underscore the transformative role of p-tau proteins in revolutionizing AD research and clinical practice.

2. Current Diagnosis of AD

The diagnosis of AD is based on the 2011 recommendations of the National Institute on Aging–Alzheimer's Association (NIA-AA) workgroups on diagnostic guidelines for Alzheimer's disease [38]. Unlike the recommendations for diagnosing MCI due to AD and AD dementia stage, recommendations for preclinical AD are not intended for clinical diagnosis and are based only on the presence of biomarkers, due to the asymptomatic course of this phase of AD. The diagnosis of MCI due to AD requires the establishment of clinical and cognitive criteria. These criteria include a change in cognition reported by a patient, an informant, or a clinician; objective evidence of impairment in one or more cognitive domains—such as memory, executive function, attention, language, and visuospatial skills—obtained through testing; maintenance of the patient's independence in functional abilities; and no dementia in a patient [39]. Additionally, it is necessary to assess the etiology of MCI to ensure it is consistent with the AD pathophysiological process [39]. The diagnosis of AD dementia is based on symptoms of cognitive decline that develops over time and interferes with the patient's usual activities. The cognitive or behavioral impairment must involve at least two of the previously mentioned domains [40,41]. It is crucial to exclude other causes of dementia, such as delirium or major psychiatric disorders [40,42]. The cognitive impairment should be detected by history-taking from the patient and other informants, as well as objective forms of cognitive assessments by neurophysiological testing [40]. Additionally to the mentioned-above core criteria for the diagnosis of MCI due to AD and AD dementia, in the 2011 recommendations from the NIA-AA, biomarkers have been established to support the diagnosis of both stages [38–40]. Aβ deposition is the first biomarker, examined by the presence of the Aβ42 variant of Aβ in the cerebrospinal fluid (CSF) or by detection during positron emission tomography (PET) amyloid imaging [40,43]. The second set of biomarkers is related to neuronal injury and includes the presence of phosphorylated-tau in the CSF, volumetric measurements or visual assessments of hippocampal volume or medial temporal lobe atrophy, the rate of brain atrophy, fluorodeoxyglucose-18 (FDG)-PET imaging, and single-photon emission computed tomography (SPECT) perfusion imaging. Additionally, there are less validated methods such as functional magnetic resonance imaging (fMRI) activation studies, resting blood oxygen level-dependent (BOLD) functional connectivity, MRI perfusion, magnetic resonance spectroscopy, diffusion tensor imaging, and voxel-based and multivariate measures [39,40,43]. The biomarkers of the third type include inflammatory biomarkers (cytokines), oxidative stress biomarkers (isoprostanes), and other markers of synaptic damage and neurodegeneration such as cell death [39,40].

3. New 'Candidates' for AD Biomarkers

For diagnostic purposes, the currently used p-tau biomarker includes p-tau phosphorylated at Thr181 (p-tau181) [44–46]. Recently, new 'candidate' p-tau biomarkers have been proposed, namely p-tau217 and p-tau231 [44,47–49]. Studies have demonstrated that pre-screening with blood testing could significantly reduce the need for more invasive testing in AD, and that plasma p-tau may offer greater diagnostic power than plasma amyloid measures [47]. It has been shown that p-tau181 and p-tau217 can differentiate between amyloid-PET or tau-PET positive cases and amyloid-PET or tau-PET negative cases. Furthermore, the p-tau level allows us to distinguish patients with AD dementia from those with frontotemporal lobar degeneration [47]. Recent studies have revealed increased levels of p-tau217 in the plasma of individuals in the preclinical and early clinical stages of AD compared to a control group of healthy individuals [49]. This increase is also associated with a higher risk of progressing to AD dementia, a faster rate of cognitive decline, and thinning of the temporal cortex and hippocampus. The authors suggest the possibility of monitoring treatment responses over time by comparing p-tau217 levels in non-demented, amyloid-positive individuals and those without such pathology, as well as in non-demented individuals who later develop AD dementia compared to those who remain non-demented during follow-up, highlighting a greater increase in AD-related individuals [49]. They advocate for the use of p-tau217 in monitoring the disease progression. Studies have also demonstrated that plasma p-tau231, similarly to plasma p-tau181, could identify clinical stages and neuropathology, with the advantage of increasing earlier than p-tau181 in response to early brain tau deposition, even before the threshold for Aβ PET positivity is reached [48]. Research on plasma p-tau231 and p-tau217 concludes that these biomarkers more effectively capture the earliest cerebral Aβ changes, even before the observable presence of Aβ deposits, thus indicating plasma p-tau231 and p-tau217 as promising biomarkers for preclinical AD [48].

4. Characteristics of tau Protein

Tau protein is encoded by the MT-associated protein tau (*MAPT*) gene located on human chromosome 17 at band position 17q21 [50–53]. It was discovered in 1975 [51,54,55]. The *MAPT* gene contains 16 exons [51,56,57], although exon 1, being a part of the promoter, and exon 14 under transcription but not translation [56,57]. Exons 9–12 play a crucial role, encoding four highly conserved imperfect repeats that make up the MT-binding domain of tau [56]. Uniquely, tau mRNA is transported to the proximal axon for translation, which facilitates the establishment of neuronal polarity [51].

Tau protein is divided into four functional domains: the N-terminal projection domain (NTPD), proline-rich regions (PRRs), MT-binding domain (MTBD), and C-terminal domain (CTD) [50,51,56]. The protein exists in six isoforms [52,53,55,56], which result from the alternative splicing of exons 2, 3, and 10 [51–53,56]. These isoforms include 3R0N, 3R1N, 3R2N, 4R0N, 4R1N, and 4R2N. The first three are collectively referred to as 3R isoforms, and the latter three as 4R isoforms. The number of 'R's indicates the number of MTBDs included in an isoform, and 'N' indicates the number of NTPDs [50,52,53,55,56]. The isoforms range from 352 to 441 amino acid residues in a chain [50,52,57]. In the fetal human brain, only 3R isoforms are expressed [50,51,53,56]. In the adult human brain, the expression of tau isoforms varies between regions; for example, the cerebellum has an elevated amount of 3R0N, whereas in the globus pallidus, 4R isoforms dominate [56]. However, physiologically, the ratio of 3R to 4R tau isoforms in the adult human brain should be approximately one to one [51,52,56]. An abnormal ratio of these isoforms is a characteristic feature of tauopathies such as AD [51]. This is why the alternative splicing of exon 10, which determines the type of protein (3R or 4R), is the subject of intensive scientific research [50].

Compared to other proteins, 2N4R, the longest human tau isoform present in the central nervous system (441 amino acid residues), has a relatively low proportion of hydrophobic amino acid residues, making tau generally a hydrophilic protein [56]. Tau is a natively unfolded protein that maintains a highly flexible conformation with a low content of secondary structure [56]. However, this does not preclude the possibility of folding through intramolecular interactions between differently charged domains [56]. MTBD consists of four repeating motifs, separated by flanking regions. Notably, the second and third repeats of the MTBD have a tendency to form a β-sheet structure [56].

Tau protein is described as a scaffolding protein [50]. Its main function is the stabilization of MTs in the distal portions of axons, which are essential for axonal transport systems. These systems ensure the transport of organelles and signaling molecules, making tau protein crucial for the proper functioning of neurons [51]. In that way, tau is also responsible for the dynamics of axonal growth cones [52]. Furthermore, some studies have reported tau's interaction with actin, which influences actin polymerization and the interaction between actin filaments and MTs. Additionally, tau has other functions, such as binding to molecules like PSEN-1 and RNA [51].

The conformation of tau has a "paperclip" form, in which the CTD folds over MTBD and the NTPD folds back over the CTD, bringing the two termini in close proximity [56]. The association between CTD and NTPD is reduced when tau binds to MTs. NTPD projects away from MTs without binding to them directly; however, it plays a role in regulating MT dynamics by influencing the attachment and spacing between MTs and other cellular components. Additionally, the extreme N-terminal region of tau (residues 2–18) is involved in a signaling cascade that inhibits axonal transport in neurons [56]. However, the specific functions of NTPD are not yet well established, although it is hypothesized to influence tau distribution because the 0 N, 1 N, and 2 N isoforms exhibit distinct subcellular localizations in the mouse brain [56].

Tau protein can also be found in dendrites and at the post-synapse under both physiological and pathological conditions [50,51,53]. However, its physiological role in the mentioned compartments is less understood [50]. The binding of tau to MTs occurs through interactions between MTBD and α- and β-tubulin heterodimers [50] within specific pockets in the tubulin on the inner surface of MTs [51]. Because the MT surface is negatively charged, this binding is enhanced by the presence of positively charged PRRs [50,51]. The C-terminal domain likely plays a role in inhibiting tau polymerization [50].

Post-translational modifications, including phosphorylation, N- and O-glycosylation, ubiquitination, truncation, and oxidation, regulate the interaction between tau and MTs [50,55]. Among them, the most important role in the pathogenesis of tau is played by phosphorylation, which is directly related to the pathophysiology of AD [52].

5. Characteristics of Hyperphosphorylation Process of tau Protein

Phosphorylation is the primary post-translational modification regulating the binding of tau to MTs under physiological conditions. Approximately 85 putative phosphorylation sites have been predicted, with over 50 of these sites confirmed to be modified in tau [55]. Most of these phosphorylation sites are found in the C-terminal half of the amino acid sequence [55], although notable exceptions, such as Thr217 and Thr231, are situated in the N-terminal region [34].

In the physiological state, tau phosphorylation plays a crucial role, with phosphorylation at Ser396 and Ser404 stabilizing beta-catenin, rendering cells anti-apoptotic and providing neuronal protection [58]. This process also significantly contributes to adult hippocampal neurogenesis. Both aggregated and soluble tau found in the brain of AD patients show reactivity to antibodies detecting phosphorylated tau, as well as to an antibody reactive for non-phosphorylated tau following alkaline phosphatase digestion [55]. This has led to the conclusion that tau in its hyperphosphorylated form is associated with tau aggregation and toxicity, with a damaging effect on the brain [58]. In autopsied AD brains, tau phosphorylation level has been found 3–4 times higher than in healthy individuals [30], marking it as an early pathology in the development of AD [58]. Hyperphosphorylation of tau at sites such as Thr205, Thr231, Ser262, and Ser396 is known to attenuate endoplasmic reticulum stress and death-associated protein kinase-induced apoptosis [58]. It also reduces the affinity of tau for MTs, leading to the formation of highly toxic tau oligomers [58]. Critically, in the pathogenesis of AD, hyperphosphorylation leads to the dissociation of tau from MTs, contributing to the formation of NFTs, MT collapse, axon degeneration, and axoplasmic transport disorders [34]. This disrupts the distribution of neurotransmitters (including their synthesis, transport, release, and uptake), culminating in neurodegeneration [58].

Hyperphosphorylation results from the deregulation of Ser/Thr kinases (see Figure 1) [34]. A-kinase, C-kinase, calmodulin kinase II (CaMK II), cyclin-dependent kinase 5 (CDK-5), mitogen-activated protein kinase (MAPK), and glycogen synthase kinase-3β (GSK-3β) are responsible for the phosphorylation of Thr 217 and Thr 231 sites, among many other sites on tau protein [34]. Tau protein undergoes prephosphorylation at sites such as Ser262/Ser356 by C-kinase, CaMK II, and CDK-5, making it more susceptible to subsequent phosphorylation by GSK-3β [34]. The prephosphorylation at Ser262/Ser356 may induce a conformational change in tau, enabling GSK-3β to recognize Thr231 and other sites more readily [34]. GSK-3β is also directly involved in the phosphorylation of Thr217 [59]. The process of tau hyperphosphorylation is further accelerated by Aβ, which mediates the activation of CDK-5 and GSK-3β [34]. Deregulation of kinase activities may also result from a disruption in the expression of non-coding RNA genes. For instance, decreased activity of miRNA-195 in knock-out rat models has been found to activate Cdk5/p25 signaling, promoting the phosphorylation of tau at Ser202, Thr205, Ser262, and Ser422 sites, and, crucially for this discussion, at the Thr231 site [58,60]. Furthermore, overexpression of death-associated protein kinase 1 (DAPK1) has been shown to increase tau protein stability and phosphorylation, including the Thr231 site [58,61].

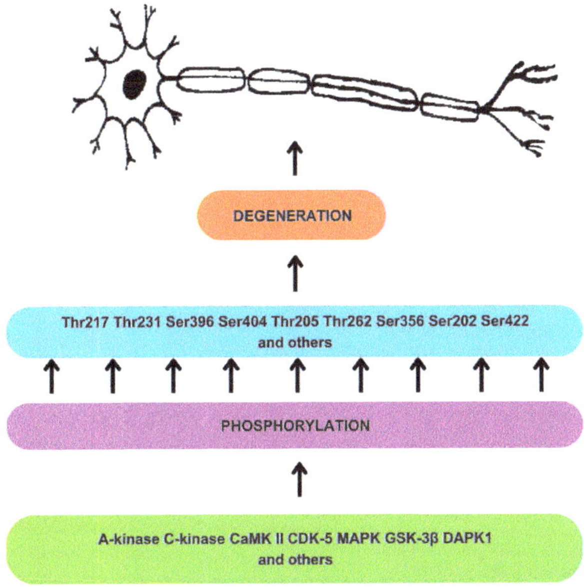

Figure 1. Mechanism of hyperphosphorylation of tau protein in the development of neuronal degeneration. Dysregulation of Ser/Thr kinases, including A-kinase, C-kinase, calmodulin kinase II (CaMK II), cyclin-dependent kinase 5 (CDK-5), mitogen-activated protein kinase (MAPK), glycogen synthase kinase-3β (GSK-3β), and death-associated protein kinase 1 (DAPK1) results in tau hyperphosphorylation, which contributes to tau dysfunction and neurodegeneration.

Protein phosphatase 2A (PP2A) plays a central role in tau dephosphorylation and is implicated in AD's pathogenesis [62]. PP2A accounts for the majority of tau phosphatase activity in the brain, and its activity is found to be reduced in AD, contributing to abnormal tau hyperphosphorylation and aggregation. In their review, Martin et al. [62] highlight the predominant role of PP2A in regulating tau phosphorylation sites, showing that disruptions in PP2A activity could significantly impact tau's pathological phosphorylation in AD. The involvement of other phosphatases, such as protein phosphatase 1 (PP1), protein phosphatase 5 (PP5), and phosphatase and tensin homolog deleted on chromosome 10 (PTEN), although less pronounced than PP2A, still contributes to the complex regulation of tau phosphorylation and has been observed to be altered in AD as well. The balance between kinase and phosphatase activities determines the phosphorylation status of tau, and the disruption of this balance leads to the tau pathology observed in AD.

In summary, tau hyperphosphorylation is a multifactorial and complex process that plays a key role in the pathomechanism of tauopathies, including AD. Undoubtedly, further research is necessary, which may bring a breakthrough in the treatment and prevention of neurodegenerative diseases related to the abnormal function of the tau protein.

6. From tau Phosphorylation to Neurofibrillary Tangle Formation

Tau, as a 'tubulin-associated unit' and a protein constituting over 80% of MT-associated proteins, primarily plays a physiological role in bundling and stabilizing axonal MTs through tubulin polymerization, a process that is disrupted by phosphorylation [63–65]. Additionally, phosphorylation, particularly by GSK-3β, results in reduced tau transport along the axon due to diminished interaction with kinesin [64,66]. The primary pathway for tau phosphorylation involves protein kinases such as GSK-3β, cAMP-dependent protein kinase, MT affinity-regulating kinase 4, and CDK-5. The phosphorylation by the mentioned kinases causes the destabilization of MTs. It has been demonstrated that the phosphorylation of tau is inversely correlated with its association with MTs [63–67]. Moreover, the specific consequences of tau phosphorylation depend on the site of modification [65,68]. For example, in contrast to the majority of the sites, phosphorylation at Ser208 leads to an increase in tau's affinity for binding MTs, but it does not reduce tau aggregation, as this modification is particularly found in late-stage NFTs [68]. Man et al. [65] found that phosphorylation at Ser289 and Ser293 leads to enhanced oligomerization and a change in the structure of the tau peptide chain from a helix to a coil [63]. Thus, this transformation to an unorganized structure may be a "driving force" for the aggregation of tau [65]. Unfortunately, the exact mechanism of NFT formation is not fully understood, and further studies on this subject are necessary [66,69]. Regardless of the exact mechanism, the diminished affinity for MTs through phosphorylation primarily leads to aggregation, which in turn plays a role in the formation of NFTs [64,65]. Furthermore, it has been stated in numerous studies that NFTs are present in AD pathology and are strictly correlated with neurodegeneration in the development of AD [63–68,70]. Higher concentrations of phosphorylated tau have been correlated with neuronal damage and death in the process of dementia. Emerging theories suggest that NFTs may have a role in AD that differs from the traditionally proposed one, with some suggesting a protective function [64]. Buée et al. [64] proposed that NFTs may have a protective role against toxic phosphorylated tau species during neurodegeneration. They argue that, while apoptosis takes 24 h to complete, the tau aggregation leading to cell death spans over 24 years. This suggests that NFTs might prolong the disease development by more than two decades before neurons ultimately succumb to the toxic effects of the protein's accumulation [64]. Regardless of the actual role of NFTs, their strong correlation with phosphorylated tau and neurodegeneration remains undisputed, advancing the field towards the better detection of AD pathology.

7. P-tau Isoforms as AD Biomarkers

7.1. P-tau Isoforms Are Effective AD Biomarkers

The first step in challenging the status of p-tau181 as the 'gold standard' biomarker is to demonstrate that p-tau181 and other p-tau species exhibit the necessary accuracy and correlations to qualify as biomarkers in AD [71]. P-tau181 has been proven to accurately discriminate between Aβ and tau stages and correlate with their PET statuses [71]. It has been confirmed in multiple studies that other tau species, such as p-tau217 and particularly p-tau231, are as effective or even more effective for early AD detection than p-tau181 [72–81]. What makes p-tau variants useful biomarkers is their specificity for the so-called "biological AD", which means a positive status for both Aβ PET (A+) and tau PET (T+). However, this correlation varies, as demonstrated by Therriault et al. [80], who, based on comparative analysis, found that p-tau biomarkers had a significantly higher correlation with Aβ PET than with tau PET. Accordingly, a study by Palmqvist et al. [82] states that the accumulation of Aβ promotes an increase in the production of soluble tau in neurons. This mechanism explains high levels of p-tau, especially p-tau217, in AD. Moreover, this mechanism is not present in other tauopathies. This finding has also been supported by Barthélemy et al. [79], who demonstrated an inverse correlation of the plasma p-tau217/tau217 ratio with the CSF Aβ42/Aβ40 ratio. This suggests that normal concentrations of Aβ are associated with reduced tau phosphorylation [79].

As it was previously mentioned, Aβ and p-tau show a strong correlation in AD pathogenesis. This also reflects the correlation in detecting the presence of Aβ with the higher levels of plasma p-tau217 [56]. Plasma p-tau217 mediates the association between accumulated Aβ and tau, and plasma p-tau217 may indicate the early accumulation of Aβ even before widespread tau aggregation occurs [56]. Other research studies report that p-tau217 and p-tau231 capture the earliest changes in cerebral Aβ imaged on PET [48] and that p-tau231 reaches abnormal levels with the lowest Aβ load [48]. To clarify, plasma levels of p-tau181 and p-tau217 are elevated in individuals with an A+T+ profile compared to A+T- and A−T-, and in A+T- compared to A−T- [81,83–85]. Importantly, the CSF exhibits a higher concentration of p-tau species, and as shown in the study by Barthélemy et al. [79], the p-tau/tau ratios are significantly higher in the CSF compared to the blood plasma. However, the use of blood-derived p-tau isoforms as AD biomarkers is still considered feasible because they reflect tau changes in the CSF. Moreover, peripheral phosphorylation of tau exhibits a distinct profile [79]. However, according to Palmqvist et al. [86], the accuracy of CSF and plasma biomarkers is similar in significance [86]. Plasma p-tau217 has been found to perform worse than its CSF counterpart [82]. However, due to the lower cost and the ease of testing, it may still serve as a viable biomarker in facilities with limited or no access to CSF or PET testing [82]. Blood serum is also considered a viable medium for measuring p-tau concentration, as its accuracy has been demonstrated to be similar to that of plasma [76].

Higher concentrations of p-tau181 and p-tau271 correlate with higher levels of AD neuropathological change (ADNC) and the *APOE* ε4 allele, which is directly involved in inherited AD [73,83,87]. However, the use of *APOE* ε4 as a prediction factor did not show a significant improvement in the effectiveness of the combination of plasma markers Aβ42/40 and plasma p-tau217 [88]. According to Woo et al. [84], p-tau181 and p-tau217 demonstrate the highest efficacy in differentiating T+ from T− patients. However, the accuracy of p-tau181 in determining tau PET status diminishes when considering only A+ patients, because only individuals with concurrent amyloid and tau pathologies can definitively be diagnosed with AD [84]. P-tau217 maintains a performance of over 85% in discriminating between T+ and T− even with the introduced change [84]. Additionally, p-tau217 correlates with common AD assessment scores, such as the Mini-Mental State Examination (MMSE) and clinical dementia rating (CDR), the scales typically used for evaluating a patient's mental capabilities and potential neuropathology [84]. According to Janelidze et al. [89], considering the tau PET prediction, CSF p-tau217 correlates better than CSF p-tau181 with CSF Aβ42 and the retention of [18F] flortaucipir and [18F] flutemetamol, two radiopharmaceuticals used to visualize brain pathologies in AD on PET scans [89]. P-tau217 also is more accurate when it comes to the identification of patients with a pathological increase in [18F] flortaucipir binding [89]. The results from the article by Mundada et al. [90] also indicate a strong correlation between p-tau217 and [18F] flortaucipir. These findings confirm the superiority of p-tau217 over p-tau181 in tau PET prediction [89].

The performance of p-tau species depends on their clinical status. P-tau217 is considered a versatile biomarker as it accurately differentiates A+ from A− in both cognitively unimpaired (CU) and MCI groups. It has also been shown to increase with age [49,84,87]. Woo et al. [84] established thresholds for p-tau217 levels indicative of tau PET positivity: levels above 0.09 pg/mL (sensitivity = 0.91, specificity = 0.9, accuracy = 0.91) for the general population and levels above 0.14 pg/mL (sensitivity = 0.90, specificity = 0.72, accuracy = 0.79) for Aβ+ individuals. This distinction highlights a higher threshold for A+ individuals, suggesting that Aβ accumulation can lead to an increase in p-tau not necessarily associated with tau PET positivity [84]. Moreover, the study by Mattsson-Carlgren et al. [49] confirmed a similar pattern of p-tau217 changes in different stages of AD development, including CU, MCI, and AD conversion, with a higher baseline for A+ with a significant increase, and a stable baseline for A− and other dementia converters [49]. Analogously, Jonaitis et al. [91] provided evidence that baseline levels of plasma p-tau217 correlate with the trajectory of cognition: higher levels are associated with a steeper, more negative trajectory, while lower levels correlate with a more stable, flatter trajectory [91]. Furthermore, studies by Brickman et al. [73] and Yu et al. [92] showed that higher concentrations of plasma p-tau, specifically p-tau217, were correlated with posthumously confirmed AD [73,92].

The ability of a biomarker to differentiate AD from other neurodegenerative diseases is a crucial aspect of its effectiveness. The study by Yu et al. [92] indicated that p-tau217 is not associated with neurodegenerative diseases other than AD, with the exception of cerebral amyloid angiopathy (CAA). It has been shown that patients with both AD and CAA, of which the latter is also closely related to Aβ, have significantly higher levels of p-tau217 [92,93]. Importantly, plasma p-tau has been found to distinguish AD from primary age-related tauopathy (PART) [92]. High levels of p-tau217 and p-tau181 have been correlated with a greater likelihood of AD rather than PART.

From a practical standpoint, comparing the levels of tau and p-tau proteins in serum and blood plasma is critically important. In the study by Kac et al. [76], the diagnostic potential of p-tau231 and p-tau181 levels in serum and plasma for AD has been explored. Conducted across three cohorts with a total of 115 participants, the study revealed that p-tau levels in both serum and plasma were significantly higher in AD patients than in controls, indicating good diagnostic performance in serum. Notably, p-tau231 was found at lower concentrations in serum compared to plasma. Despite this, the strong correlation between p-tau levels in serum and plasma underscored the viability of serum as a practical alternative for AD diagnostics and research. These results endorse the use of serum in environments that prefer it to plasma, emphasizing its effectiveness for p-tau analysis. However, the necessity for further validation in independent cohorts and across different p-tau assays should be emphasized.

There are some limitations to the studies described above on the use of p-tau variants as biomarkers. It should be emphasized that the findings cannot be generalized to all individuals due to insufficiently diverse ethnic representation in the research groups [81,82,94]. The need to extend the research to unselected primary care populations should be also underlined [82]. Moreover, using plasma p-tau as a biomarker has some outstanding challenges such as the need for analytical guidelines, inter-laboratory method comparison and standardization, cut-off value generation and validation, and appropriate use criteria for clinical implementation [82,95]. The higher cost of mass spectrometry tests, which have shown the best performance compared to currently used immunoassays, has also been indicated [94].

7.2. Diagnostic Performance of Various p-tau Assays

Several trials have examined assays for measuring different p-tau species in order to use them as diagnostic tools in AD. The performance of various p-tau assays in differentiating AD patients is summarized in Table 1. The trial conducted by Bayoumy et al. [96] utilized six different plasma immunoassays: the p-tau217 assay from Lilly Research Laboratories, Indianapolis, IN, USA (Lilly); p-tau181 assay from Lilly; p-tau181 assay from Adx Neurosciences, Ghent, Belgium (ADx); p-tau231 assay from ADx; p-tau181 assay from Quanterix, Billerica, MA, USA (Quan); and p-tau231 assay from University of Gothenburg, Gothenburg, Sweden (UGot). The study confirmed that p-tau levels were significantly higher in AD patients compared to controls. The increase ranged from 4.1-fold for p-tau217 Lilly to 1.3-fold for p-tau231 ADx. Notably, the p-tau217 Lilly assay, all p-tau181 assays, and the p-tau231 UGot assay demonstrated high diagnostic accuracy for AD [96]. A post hoc comparison of the receiver operating characteristic (ROC) analysis of the area under the curve (AUC) indicated that p-tau181 ADx and p-tau217 Lilly both performed well, outperforming p-tau181 Quan. Moreover, p-tau217 Lilly surpassed p-tau231 UGot in performance, with p-tau181 ADx showing a similar trend. Additionally, both p-tau217 Lilly and p-tau181 ADx had better performance than p-tau181 Lilly. The p-tau231 ADx assay was the least effective, being outperformed by all other assays.

Table 1. Diagnostic performance of various p-tau assays in distinguishing Alzheimer's disease (AD) patients from healthy controls [96], normal and abnormal Aβ42/40 ratio in the cerebrospinal fluid (CSF) [97], and non-AD (NAD) patients [98]. Data are shown as median and interquartile range (in brackets).

Assay	Fold Increase in CSF	AUC (95% CI) in CSF	Fold Increase in Plasma	AUC (95% CI) in Plasma	Ref.
p-tau 181 Lilly	-	-	1.8	0.938 (0.872–1.000)	[96]
	-	-	1.2–1.4	0.759 (0.676–0.841)	[97]
	3.29	0.95 (0.91–0.98)	2.59	0.91 (0.86–0.96)	[98]
p-tau217 Lilly	-	-	4.1	0.995 (0.987–1.000)	[96]
	-	-	2.0	0.886 (0.827–0.944)	[97]
	7.18	0.98 (0.96–1.00)	3.27	0.94 (0.90–0.98)	[98]
t-tau Lilly	1.97	0.85 (0.79–0.90)	1.36	0.73 (0.65–0.81)	[98]
p-tau181 ADx	-	-	2.9	0.988 (0.969–1.000)	[96]
	-	-	1.8	0.841 (0.768–0.913)	[97]
	4.77	0.96 (0.93–0.98)	3.48	0.94 (0.91–0.97)	[98]
p-tau231 ADx	-	-	1.3	0.719 (0.607–0.831)	[96]
	3.59	0.93 (0.88–0.97)	1.39	0.66 (0.58–0.74)	[98]
p-tau181 UGot	-	-	1.2–1.4	0.743 (0.652–0.833)	[97]
	2.1	0.94 (0.90–0.97)	1.38	0.80 (0.73–0.87)	[98]
p-tau231 UGot	-	-	1.5	0.943 (0.896–0.991)	[96]
	-	-	1.2–1.4	0.784 (0.703–0.864)	[97]
	-	0.91 (0.87–0.95)	1.95	0.88 (0.83–0.93)	[98]
p-tau181 WashU	-	-	1.2–1.4	0.835 (0.765–0.906)	[97]
p-tau217 WashU	-	-	3.6	0.947 (0.907–0.987)	[97]
p-tau181 Fuji	-	-	1.2–1.4	0.694 (0.604–0.784)	[97]
p-tau181 Splex	-	-	1.2–1.4	0.642 (0.533–0.751)	[97]
p-tau181 Quanterix	-	-	1.9	0.936 (0.885–0.987)	[96]
	5.02	0.96 (0.93–0.99)	1.66	0.80 (0.73–0.87)	[98]
p-tau217 Janss	-	-	2.7	0.858 (0.795–0.920)	[97]
	8.53	0.98 (0.96–1.00)	5.22	0.96 (0.93–0.99)	[98]

Abbreviations: AUC—area under the curve; CI—confidence interval; p-tau181—tau phosphorylated at threonine-181; p-tau217—tau phosphorylated at threonine-217; p-tau231—tau phosphorylated at threonine-231. The origin of the p-tau assays: ADx—ADx Neurosciences, Ghent, Belgium; Fuji—Fujirebio Inc, Tokyo, Japan; Janss—Janssen Research and Development, Raritan, NJ, USA; Lilly—Lilly Research Laboratories, Indianapolis, IN, USA; Quanterix—Quanterix Corp., Billerica, MA, USA; Splex—S-Plex immunoassay from Meso Scale Discovery, Rockville, MD, USA; UGot—University of Gothenburg, Gothenburg, Sweden; WashU—Washington University, Washington, DC, USA.

The study by Janelidze et al. [97] compared 10 assays: the p-tau181 assay from Washington University, Washington, DC, USA (WashU); p-tau181 ADx; p-tau181 Lilly; p-tau181 UGot; p-tau181 assay from Fujirebio Inc, Tokyo, Japan (Fuji); p-tau181 S-Plex immunoassay from Meso Scale Discovery, Rockville, MD, USA (Splex); p-tau217 WashU; p-tau217 Lilly; p-tau217 assay from Janssen Research and Development, Raritan, NJ, USA (Janss); and p-tau231 UGot. The results were in line with other findings, suggesting an increase in various p-tau species in A+ individuals compared to controls [97]. In this study, the best-performing assay was p-tau217 WashU, a mass spectrometry (MS)-based assay, followed by two immunoassays, namely p-tau217 Lilly and p-tau217 Janns [97]. On average, p-tau217 assays achieved higher AUCs than p-tau181 assays. In summary, the fold increase in p-tau species ranged from 1.2 to 3.6 [97]. When it comes to distinguishing MCI patients with progression to AD from those without AD, p-tau217 WashU was the best, followed by p-tau217 Lilly [97]. However, p-tau217 Janss, p-tau181 ADx, and p-tau181 WashU were not significantly worse than p-tau217 Lilly in that case, whereas other assays performed with significantly lower AUCs [97]. P-tau217 WashU performed with a higher AUC than other assays, which corroborated the superiority of MS-based assays for p-tau quantification [97]. It is worth noting that the concentration of p-tau217 in the CSF is approximately 5 times lower than that of p-tau181, which makes this quantification more difficult [99]. However, it should be concluded that p-tau217 has superior accuracy as a biomarker for AD compared to p-tau181 [97]. Expectedly, CSF p-tau measurements appeared to have AUC values unmatched by the corresponding plasma assays [97]. The strongest correlation was observed in the case of p-tau217 WashU. P-tau217 Lilly revealed a significant difference between the CSF and plasma correlation coefficients [97]. Other assays had moderate or weak correlations [97]. P-tau217 Lilly was found to be the immunoassay with the highest AUC; however, this was not the only assay with potentially useful accuracy [97]. P-tau217 Janss and p-tau181 ADx performed comparably in indicating Aβ deposition and possible progression to AD [97]. Additionally, a post hoc analysis revealed a significant increase in plasma p-tau217 levels in MCI to AD progressors in comparison to A+ non-progressors. This characteristic was not demonstrated by p-tau181 or p-tau231 [97].

The study by Ashton et al. [81] examined the plasma p-Tau217 immunoassay from ALZpath Inc., Carlsbad, CA, USA (ALZpath), and concluded that it predicts abnormal Aβ-PET and CSF Aβ42/40 with high accuracy. These results suggest that the performance of plasma p-tau217 ALZpath is comparable to that of CSF measurements and superior to that of brain atrophy assessments. Furthermore, its properties and accuracy significantly surpass those of other plasma biomarkers. In a long-term perspective, p-tau217 ALZpath levels tend to increase only when the Aβ accumulation is present and enhance further if tau pathology coexists [81].

Another study by Mielke et al. [100] found that, for the Meso Scale Discovery (MSD) p-tau181, MSD p-tau217, and single-molecule array (Simoa) p-tau231 platforms, p-tau levels were significantly higher in T+ compared to A− and T− groups. The study also highlighted that MSD p-tau217 exhibited the highest fold change and diagnostic performance among all evaluated platforms. Conversely, Simoa p-tau231 showed the lowest performance.

In the study by Ashton et al. [98], 18 immunoassays, including 9 plasma-based and 9 CSF-based, were examined. The plasma biomarker group included p-tau181 ADx, p-tau217 Janss, p-tau217 Lilly, p-tau181 Lilly, p-tau231 UGot, p-tau181 UGot, p-tau181 Quanterix, t-tau Lilly, and p-tau231 ADx. The CSF group comprised the CSF counterparts of these plasma assays. All biomarkers showed a significant increase in the AD CSF profile group compared to the non-AD (NAD) group, although the extent of change varied. The largest differences in plasma, categorized as 'large', were observed for p-tau181 Lilly, p-tau217 Lilly, p-tau181 ADx, p-tau217 Janss, and p-tau231 UGot. All CSF biomarkers were categorized as having a 'large' effect size. Further analysis revealed that the five mentioned plasma p-tau assays significantly outperformed the other plasma p-tau biomarkers in terms of differentiation accuracy. The study also found strong correlations between CSF and plasma immunoassays of the same type for p-tau181 ADx, p-tau217 Janss, p-tau181 Lilly, and p-tau217 Lilly. However, the discrimination accuracy of p-tau231 ADx, t-tau Lilly, p-tau181 Quanterix, and p-tau181 UGot was significantly weaker in plasma than in CSF.

In light of the aforementioned assays as a whole, a pattern emerges—tests from the same manufacturer for p-tau217 show higher AUC and fold increase than for p-tau181. These results lay a foundation for the conclusion that p-tau217 seems to be more accurate than p-tau181 and might be widely used as an AD biomarker.

7.3. P-tau217 Proves to Be Superior to p-tau181 and Other Isoforms

After proving the usefulness of p-tau-based biomarkers, several studies have focused on finding the most effective one. Generally, P-tau217 has been found to be a better option.

Ashton et al. [78] and Barthélemy et al. [101] reported that both CSF and plasma p-tau217 levels increased 6-fold in CU A+ individuals compared to CU A−, and in AD compared to NAD. This increase was significantly higher than in the case of other p-tau biomarkers. For instance, plasma p-tau181 exhibited only a 1.3-fold increase. Moreover, with CSF p-tau181, a decrease in performance was observed when distinguishing MCI from NAD or CU, an issue not observed with CSF p-tau217 [78]. Additionally, several studies have proclaimed that plasma p-tau217 and p-tau181 are elevated in AD groups compared to controls [73,78,102]. Thijssen et al. [102] presented that p-tau217 increased by 4.4-fold and p-tau181 by 2.8-fold in clinical AD compared to healthy people. In an AD group compared to a frontotemporal lobar degeneration (FTLD) group, plasma p-tau217 and p-tau181 levels were elevated. P-tau217 demonstrated a higher fold change than p-tau181 in distinguishing AD from clinical FTLD-spectrum disorders (3.5-fold vs. 2.4-fold), FTLD-tau (4.1-fold vs. 2.8-fold), and FTLD-TDP (5.6-fold vs. 3.7-fold) [102]. In addition to demonstrating the specificity of p-tau species for AD and the superiority of plasma p-tau217 in that matter, the study proved that p-tau can be used to differentiate AD from FTLD, again with p-tau217 clearly leading in terms of maximum accuracy [102]. Moreover, Barthélemy et al. [79] used the p-tau/t-tau ratio to normalize tau variability and evidenced that p-tau217/tau217 exhibited an almost 9-fold increase compared to p-tau181/tau181 (+220% vs. +25%). Moreover, p-tau217 reached a greater increase in Aβ+ than p-tau181 (from +230% to +340% vs. from +60% to +80%) [79]. These findings support the thesis that the p-tau217/tau217 ratio reasonably distinguishes Aβ+ and Aβ− CU, whereas the p-tau181/tau181 ratio is not so accurate [79]. Interestingly, Salvadó et al. [103] indicated that p-tau217, used in the study along with four other biomarkers for successfully staging AD, continued to increase even after reaching its threshold of positivity. However, according to Barthélemy et al. [99], there is a negative correlation between both mentioned-above ratios and neurodegeneration measured by MRI and longitudinal cognitive decline. This suggests a reversal in the rate of phosphorylation during the disease progression. Thijssen et al. [102] also found that plasma p-tau217 has slightly higher AUC than p-tau181 for differentiating T+ and T−. However, there was no significant difference in distinguishing positive tau-PET between p-tau217 and p-tau181 in subgroups of MCI and corticobasal syndrome [102]. These findings were not observed in A− participants but were present in A+ patients [78,102]. In summary, plasma p-tau217 has been found to perform better than p-tau181 in multiple ways such as a higher fold increase and therefore a higher AUC for differentiating AD from FTLD, A+ from A−, and T+ from T−, although the magnitudes of differences varied between studies. However, in several studies, the results have indicated no significant differences between p-tau217 and p-tau181 in terms of distinguishing Aβ-PET or tau-PET [78,87,89,102].

Nevertheless, Barthélemy et al. [101] suggested that p-tau217 may be significantly better at the differentiation of AD from NAD because of an overlap in the distribution of p-tau181 values between NAD and AD. The aforementioned overlap did not exist for p-tau217. P-tau181 levels in several conditions classified as NAD, such as FTLD, Lewy body dementia, and progressive supranuclear palsy, have been found to reach the range seen in AD, whereas p-tau217 levels in these cases have been found to be different to those in AD. These findings support the superior differential abilities of p-tau217. On the contrary, according to Palmqvist et al. [86], there were no significant differences between plasma p-tau217 and p-tau181 in the predictive accuracy for progression to AD within 4 years. They concluded that p-tau and its variants are highly accurate in predicting AD, and their predictive power can be enhanced by combining them with brief cognitive tests of memory and executive function, as well as the *APOE* genotype [23]. They also noted that p-tau217 outperforms clinical diagnostic predictions of AD, which include medical history, memory assessment, and MRI and CT imaging [23]. This underscores the significant value of p-tau biomarkers in supporting clinical assessments in the diagnosis of AD.

According to the study by Mattsson-Carlgren et al. [104], p-tau217 is the most potent individual biomarker in both plasma and CSF for predicting modified Preclinical Alzheimer Cognitive Composite (mPACC) and MMSE slopes, with the levels in CSF showing marginally better performance than those in plasma. Yu et al. [92] also stated that p-tau217 offers higher accuracy for differentiation than p-tau181. Moreover, according to Janelidze et al. [88], p-tau217 can be outperformed by a combination of plasma Aβ42/40 with plasma p-tau217; however, this combination does not always produce a significantly better result than p-tau217 alone. Another study by Palmqvist et al. [105] established a combination of three plasma biomarkers, namely Aβ42/40, p-tau181, and *APOE*. In this combination, p-tau181 was interchangeable with p-tau217 with no difference in AUC. However, the study ultimately identified plasma p-tau181 as the biomarker with the highest predictive value for AD.

The results from a study by Yu et al. [92] suggested that plasma p-tau217 was more strongly correlated with Aβ plaques and tau tangles than plasma p-tau181. Additionally, the risk of progressing to AD nearly quadruples with every fold increase in plasma p-tau217 levels, whereas it only triples with each fold increase in plasma p-tau181 [92]. Salvadó et al. [93] showed that plasma p-tau217 exhibited the highest correlations with plaques and tangles of all biomarkers tested, including plasma p-tau181, which significantly outclassed other biomarkers, except Aβ42/40 and glial fibrillary acid protein (GFAP) for plaques and tangles, respectively. However, it is worth noting that none of these biomarkers came close in terms of correlation with both plaques and tangles [93]. The strong association between p-tau217 and both Aβ plaques and tau tangles has been further confirmed by Mattsson-Carlgren et al. [106]. These findings make p-tau217 a versatile and accurate biomarker, with the ability to assess the status of both amyloid and tau at once [93]. In the same study, the authors developed parsimonious models for detecting amyloid plaques and neurofibrillary tangles. The models for plaques consisted of plasma p-tau217 and Aβ42/40, and the models for tangles included only plasma p-tau217 [93]. The efficacy of plasma p-tau217 as a sole biomarker, surpassing combinations of biomarkers, further corroborates its superiority [93].

The study by Therriault et al. [107] suggested that p-tau217 exhibits a significantly smaller degree of change between CSF and plasma levels compared to p-tau181 and p-tau231, with an effect size of 84% instead of a mere 50%. Additionally, the overlap of CSF and plasma p-tau217 levels was similar, making it much more accurate than those of p-tau181 and p-tau231. Moreover, the fold change of plasma p-tau217 was higher than in the case of the CSF p-tau181 and p-tau231, further corroborating its high utility [107]. The study also found that the agreement on positivity between CSF and plasma variants was highest for p-tau217, at 88.5% (58.7% both negative, 29.8% both positive, and 11.5% discordant), while p-tau181 had a lower agreement rate of 74.7% (55.1% both negative, 19.6% both positive, and 25.3% discordant). Notably, none of the discordant results for p-tau217 occurred in patients with CDR of 1 or higher, or with positive tau-PET [107]. Plasma p-tau217 had higher accuracy for identifying Aβ PET and biological AD (Aβ and tau PET positivity) than plasma p-tau181 and plasma p-tau231, with not significantly different results from CSF variations of these markers [107]. Moreover, according to Montoliu-Gaya et al. [108], plasma p-tau217 had the highest accuracy for differentiating Aβ status. Accordingly, a study by Horie et al. [109] states that CSF p-tau217/tau217 ratio had the strongest correlation with Aβ PET. Post hoc comparisons revealed that p-tau217 values were significantly elevated in subjects at advanced stages of brain pathology assessed during an autopsy, namely Thal phases 4–5, Braak stages 5–6, and The Consortium to Establish a Registry for Alzheimer's Disease (CERAD) frequent scores [102,110–112]. The specific locations of pathological changes in Thal phases and Braak stages are shown in Figure 2.

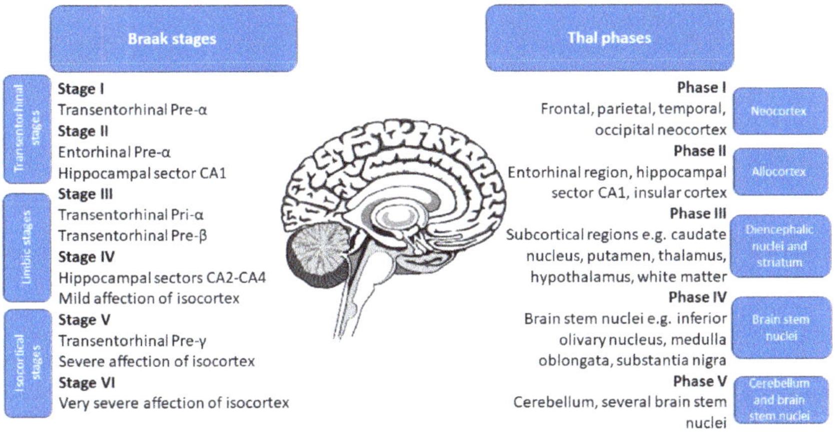

Figure 2. Location of pathological changes in Braak stages and Thal phases, used to classify the brain pathology in Alzheimer's disease assessed during an autopsy.

The superiority of p-tau217 as an AD biomarker is strengthened by the findings of Salvadó et al. [93] regarding the prediction of ADNC, CERAD classification, and Braak staging. According to their findings, p-tau217 achieves the highest accuracy for CERAD classification as an individual biomarker, comparable only to the Aβ42/40 ratio, and is not significantly inferior for CERAD classification and ADNC prediction, for which its combination with Aβ42/40 performed best. It also attained the highest accuracy for Braak staging, with only GFAP being similarly significant. According to Montoliu-Gaya et al. [108], plasma p-tau217 allows for distinguishing Braak I–IV from V–VI with decent accuracy [108]. Leuzy et al. [113] created a parsimonious model, using plasma p-tau217 and tau PET, which was associated with an annual change in the radioligand [^{18}F]RO948 standardized uptake value ratio (SUVR) and could facilitate the recruitment for clinical trials on AD.

Interestingly, Salvadó et al. [93] suggested the use of the p-tau217/Aβ42 ratio as a novel biomarker. This ratio outperforms other parameters in predicting the presence of plaques and tangles and shows significant differences between the absence and low levels of ADNC.

Overall, the results of the described studies indicate p-tau217 as the best-performing tau biomarker, and even the best of all available biomarkers. CSF p-tau217 has the highest accuracy, followed by CSF p-tau181 and plasma p-tau217, but their comparison gives ambiguous results. Few studies indicate that plasma p-tau217 may be more effective than CSF p-tau181, but there is not much evidence to definitely prove this.

7.4. Longitudinal Effectiveness and Change in p-tau217 Levels

A study by Mattsson-Carlgren et al. [49] focused on long-term changes in levels of plasma p-tau217 and their diagnostic value. According to the article, a longitudinal increase in p-tau217 was associated with cognitive decline in both CU and MCI, also within the subgroups of A+ participants [49]. Additionally, p-tau217 levels were linked to faster atrophy of the temporal cortex and hippocampus in A− CU, A+ CU, and the overall MCI group, although this correlation was not significant in the Aβ+ MCI subgroup. As proven by Ashton et al. [114], plasma p-tau217 levels increased over time in the preclinical and early clinical stages of AD but remained stable in control groups, including A− CU, A− MCI, and MCI that did not convert to AD. Over time, longitudinal increases in plasma p-tau217 levels were significantly associated with worsening MMSE and mPACC scores, impaired delayed recall memory, and accelerated cortical thickness atrophy over 6 and 8 years. Notably, p-tau217 was the only biomarker significantly linked to cognitive decline, including Aβ+ CU individuals, while p-tau181 demonstrated only modest performance [114]. Moreover, according to Suárez-Calvet et al. [74], the commonly used mid-region p-tau181 and t-tau in CSF were less useful than CSF N-terminal p-tau181, N-terminal p-tau217, and mid-region p-tau231, which showed more evident increases at the onset of AD. These markers reached higher levels before Aβ, the current gold standard, reached its threshold. Furthermore, in early AD, the annual rate of increase in p-tau217 in entorhinal PET SUVR was higher among individuals with higher baseline levels compared to those with lower levels [85]. Additionally, longitudinal increases in p-tau217 were correlated with the burden of plaques and tangle load, a correlation not found for p-tau181 [93]. Overall, these results demonstrated that the longitudinal increase in p-tau217 is significantly correlated with AD development.

7.5. P-tau231 Is Probably the Earliest AD Biomarker

An important part of the treatment of neurodegenerative disorders is their early detection. In several studies, p-tau231 has shown exceptionally high accuracy in early-stage AD. Yakoub et al. [83] proved that p-tau231 levels increased in A+T+ individuals compared to A− T−, confirming its specificity for AD pathology. P-tau231 levels increased in AD, measured in CSF, plasma, and serum [76]. The increase in its levels ranged from 2-fold in plasma and serum to up to 5-fold in CSF [76]. Lilek et al. [115] showed evidence that p-tau231 primarily accumulates at the postsynaptic density, and this occurs in an early, often presymptomatic stage of the disease. The study of Montoliu-Gaya et al. [108] indicated that p-tau231 increased significantly along the AD continuum and that its levels did not increase in MCI and demented patients without AD pathology. Furthermore, its levels did not significantly elevate after Braak III-IV, supporting the hypothesis that p-tau231 increases early on and that the rate of this increase then slows down.

Plasma p-tau231 shows a strong correlation with Aβ PET measured using the radioligand [18F]AZD4694, with a particularly strong association in the precuneus, frontal cortex, and striatum [44,77]. Interestingly, in CU individuals, the relationship between plasma p-tau231 and Aβ PET is observed in both A+ and A− groups. However, in cognitively impaired patients, the correlation between plasma p-tau231 and Aβ is limited to A+ individuals only [50]. Additionally, plasma p-tau231 accurately predicts a 1-year decline in MMSE scores and hippocampal atrophy [44].

Plasma p-tau231 demonstrates superior accuracy in distinguishing between CU A+ and A− individuals compared to plasma p-tau181, plasma p-tau217, and the Aβ42/40 ratio, showing significantly better performance than other plasma biomarkers, with the exception of Aβ42/40 [44,74,114]. However, it has lower accuracy in differentiating between elderly CU and MCI Aβ+ individuals, highlighting its increase in the preclinical stages of AD [44]. Moreover, p-tau231 is more effective at distinguishing elderly CU Aβ+ from MCI Aβ–, but less effective in separating CU Aβ+ from AD, supporting the idea that p-tau231 levels rise in the early stages of the disease [44,78]. Levels of p-tau231 progressively increase from CU in young individuals to elderly, MCI, and AD stages, and p-tau231 can differentiate AD from both young and elderly CU individuals but not from MCI [44].

Studies by Ashton et al. [44] and Milà-Alomà et al. [48] indicated that plasma p-tau231 levels increased earlier than plasma p-tau181 in relation to Aβ deposition load and before Aβ reached its positivity threshold. Similar observations were made for the CSF levels of these biomarkers [78]. However, plasma results suggest that p-tau231 may better characterize the earliest changes in AD. This is also supported by the fact that p-tau231 levels plateau at later stages of the disease, while p-tau217 and p-tau181 levels continue to increase with higher Aβ burden [114].

The research conducted by Smirnov et al. [116] and Ashton et al. [44], regarding plasma p-tau231, revealed that it increased and correlated with Aβ PET, often before Aβ PET showed positivity. This explains its earlier significant increase compared to plasma p-tau181 and its ability to detect tau accumulation, which plasma p-tau181 did not exhibit. Furthermore, according to the study of Therriault et al. [80], CSF p-tau231, CSF p-tau217, and plasma p-tau231 showed a strong correlation with Aβ PET.

The performance of CSF p-tau231 as a predictor of A+ is superior to that of p-tau181 and is as significant as that of CSF p-tau217 and CSF Aβ42/40 [78]. Studies by Ashton et al. [78] and Smirnov et al. [116] supported the finding that p-tau231 is the first p-tau marker to reach abnormal levels within the pre-Aβ phase, making it a valuable tool for the early detection of AD pathology.

Furthermore, p-tau231 is quite accurate in predicting tau PET, with a 76% concordance rate. However, a study by Tissot et al. [77] noted that 20% of patients had a p-tau231+/tau PET- result, leading to the conclusion that an increase in p-tau231 levels begins well before tau PET reaches the threshold of positivity. Similarly to CSF concentrations, plasma p-tau231 showed differences at earlier Braak stages, while plasma p-tau181 showed larger differences at later Braak stages [116,117]. Compared to CSF concentrations, plasma p-tau231 does not reach a plateau in the later stages of AD; thus, it has a significantly lower performance in identifying A+T+ individuals [107,117].

In summary, p-tau231 is highly correlated with Aβ pathology and demonstrates an early increase, often in the pre-clinical stage of the disease, even before Aβ PET positivity is detected. However, its accuracy and utility decrease in later stages, as it does not differentiate between advanced stages, though it can clearly distinguish between early and later stages. Together, these features make p-tau231 a valuable complementary biomarker to p-tau217 as an early indicator of emerging AD pathology.

8. Discussion

The best-known physiological role of the tau protein, as the main MT-associated protein and the so-called scaffolding protein, is MT stabilization [50,63–65]. However, tau has been found to have a multitude of functions, including maintaining structural integrity, axonal transport, and signaling within and between neurons [51,56]. It can be assumed that this multifunctionality of the tau protein makes it one of two main proteins involved in AD pathology [34,58–61,63–70]. Tau hyperphosphorylation seems to significantly participate in the process of aberrant assembly and functioning of tau and, consequently, in the development of neurodegeneration. This phosphorylation can take place in different loci. Thus, the levels of several p-tau variants may indicate the state of the disease or even predict it, as well as differentiating AD from other neurodegenerative disorders [49,71,73–84,86,87,89]. In this narrative review, we have tried to gather and organize studies that, through experimentation, achieved results regarding the efficacy and utility of p-tau species as biomarkers for AD. The review provides a broad overview of the subject of p-tau species as AD biomarkers, especially p-tau217 and p-tau231, both in CSF and plasma. This summary of the current state of knowledge may inspire future research by identifying known facts and previously unexplored areas, indicating an urgent need for further research on AD. The fundamental purpose of AD research is to develop methods to detect and treat the disease [71,73–80,82–89,91–93,96–105,107–109]. This goal could be achieved by deepening our understanding of tau's role in AD pathology, including identifying the feasibility of using p-tau species as biomarkers and potential therapeutic targets. Achieving these goals is difficult due to the late and expensive detection of AD, which impedes further research and requires the development of more accurate, less expensive, and easier-to-use markers in AD.

An important issue, which also requires further research, is the impact of disease comorbidities on tau changes in AD patients. Comorbidities seem to play a significant role in influencing the detection of tau and p-tau biomarkers, which is crucial for AD diagnostics. Studies indicate that systemic health conditions such as diabetes mellitus, kidney disease, and hypertension, along with demographic factors, may notably affect these biomarkers. Martínez-Dubarbie et al. [118] revealed renal function's impact on plasma Aβ levels and the association of hypertension with increased p-tau181 levels. Similarly, Pan et al. [119] demonstrated that demographic factors, especially age, and comorbidities like cardiovascular and metabolic disorders affect p-tau181 plasma levels in cognitively normal individuals. Zenuni et al. [120] further validated the significant linkage between comorbidities related to heart, vascular disorders, and diabetes mellitus and CSF biomarkers for neurodegeneration, including tau and p-tau. Furthermore, Ossenkoppele et al. [121] investigated tau PET status across a broad cohort, identifying a high tau PET positivity in AD dementia and MCI with Aβ+ status, notably lower in non-AD and CU groups. Key predictors of tau PET positivity across these studies included younger age, lower MMSE scores, and reduced cortical thickness in AD-related conditions, highlighting the complex interplay between systemic health, tau pathology, and AD diagnostics. These findings underscore the importance of considering both comorbidities and demographic factors for the accurate interpretation of AD biomarkers, spotlighting the complex relationship between systemic health conditions and neurodegenerative disease markers.

Interestingly, blood levels of tau and p-tau differ significantly among individuals with cognitive impairments, traumatic brain injury (TBI), or COVID-19. The study by Dang et al. [122] emphasizes the significant correlation between tau accumulation and cognitive decline, as well as neuropsychiatric symptoms, showcasing its diagnostic superiority over Aβ for distinguishing AD patients from cognitively normal controls. Notably, tau PET imaging demonstrates greater accuracy than Aβ in this differentiation, with pronounced tau deposition in the inferior temporal lobes strongly associated with the severity of cognitive impairments. These results indicate that tau could act as a more sensitive and specific biomarker for both the diagnosis of AD and the tracking of cognitive decline's progression, underscoring its value in clinical practice. The study by Rubenstein et al. [123] provides crucial insights into how blood levels of tau and p-tau differ among individuals with TBI. Its key findings indicate a significant increase in both t-tau and p-tau levels in serum and CSF within the first five days post-TBI, with a notably sharper rise in p-tau, suggesting a shift towards tau hyperphosphorylation. This hyperphosphorylation, marked by a substantial increase in the p-tau/t-tau ratio, points to an early and sustained alteration in tau dynamics post-injury. The study also reveals that higher chronic mean levels of p-tau, rather than t-tau, are associated with greater disability and worse outcomes up to 12 months post-TBI. This emphasizes the distinct and critical role of p-tau in the aftermath of TBI and its potential as a prognostic marker for long-term recovery and the development of tauopathies. The review by Sfera [124] explores the role of tau and p-tau blood levels in cognitive impairments among individuals with long COVID-19, also referred to as the post-acute sequelae of SARS-CoV-2. The authors suggest that chronic inflammation, triggered by viral remnants in specific body sites, results in the formation of pathological syncytia involving microglia and astrocytes. This, in turn, facilitates the seeding of hyperphosphorylated tau within the brain. This process is further exacerbated by the virus-induced increase in the permeability of the blood–brain barrier, enabling substances that can induce tau hyperphosphorylation, such as microbial components, to infiltrate the brain. Consequently, the review underscores the potential significance of blood levels of phosphorylated tau as biomarkers for cognitive dysfunctions in long COVID-19 patients, thereby establishing a link between SARS-CoV-2 infection and neurodegenerative processes.

9. Conclusions

Alzheimer's disease remains an unresolved challenge in medicine. Undoubtedly, successful biomarkers could significantly accelerate the process of recruiting trial participants for researchers looking for effective therapies. Through a comprehensive analysis, this review endeavored to provide insights into the pathophysiological significance of p-tau217 and p-tau231 as biomarkers in AD progression and their prospective role in enhancing diagnostic protocols, guiding therapeutic interventions, and potentially serving as targets for future treatments. While studies generally agree on the superiority of p-tau217 as the most effective tau isoform and overall AD biomarker, following studies are essential for its implementation and the identification of other potential early-detection biomarkers. Nevertheless, further research on plasma biomarkers is warranted, as they appear to be the future of AD detection and potential early screening. The development of specific assays for p-tau measurement, which would enable easy clinical application of the discussed biomarkers, seems to be of first importance. We believe that this review will be useful for researchers, clinicians, and students eager to explore the subject of state-of-the-art AD biomarkers.

Author Contributions: Conceptualization, D.J.J. and H.M.; writing—original draft preparation, D.J.J. and H.M.; writing—review and editing, J.N. and K.S.-G.; visualization, D.J.J., H.M., J.N., and K.S.-G.; supervision, J.N. and K.S.-G. All authors have read and agreed to the published version of the manuscript.

Funding: This research received no external funding.

Conflicts of Interest: The authors declare no conflicts of interest.

Abbreviations

Aβ	amyloid β
AD	Alzheimer's disease
ADNC	AD neuropathological change
APOE	apolipoprotein E
APP	amyloid protein precursor
AUC	area under the curve
BACE-1	β-secretase
BMI	body mass index
BOLD	resting blood oxygen level-dependent imaging
CAA	cerebral amyloid angiopathy
CAMK II	calmodulin kinase II
CDK-5	cyclin-dependent kinase 5
CDR	clinical dementia rating
CERAD	The Consortium to Establish a Registry for Alzheimer's Disease
CSF	cerebrospinal fluid
CTD	C-terminal domain
CU	cognitively unimpaired
FDG-PET	fluorodeoxyglucose-18 positron resonance imaging
fMRI	functional magnetic resonance imaging
FTLD	frontotemporal lobar degeneration
GFAP	glial fibrillary acid protein
GSK-3β	glycogen synthase kinase-3β
MAPT	microtubule-associated protein tau
MCI	mild cognitive impairment
MMSE	Mini-Mental State Examination
mPACC	modified Preclinical Alzheimer Cognitive Composite
MRI	magnetic resonance imaging
MS	mass spectrometry
MTBD	microtubule-binding domain
MT	Microtubule
NAD	non-Alzheimer's disease condition
NFTs	neurofibrillary tangles
NTA	N-terminal tau
NTPD	N-terminal projection domain
PART	primary age-related tauopathy
PET	positron emission tomography
PP1	protein phosphatase 1
PP2A	protein phosphatase 2A
PP5	protein phosphatase 5
PRR	proline-rich region
PSEN1/2	presenilin-1/2
p-tau	phosphorylated tau

p-tau217	tau phosphorylated at threonine-217
p-tau181	tau phosphorylated at threonine-181
p-tau231	tau phosphorylated at threonine-231
PTEN	phosphatase and tensin homolog deleted on chromosome 10
SPECT	single-photon emission computed tomography
SUVR	standardized uptake value ratio
t-tau	total tau
TBI	traumatic brain injury

References

1. Alzheimer, A. Über Einen Eigenartigen Schweren Erkrankungsprozeβ Der Hirnrincle. Neurol Central. *Neurol Cent.* **1906**, *25*, 1134.
2. Stelzmann, R.A.; Norman Schnitzlein, H.; Reed Murtagh, F. An English Translation of Alzheimer's 1907 Paper, "Über Eine Eigenartige Erkankung Der Hirnrinde". *Clin. Anat.* **1995**, *8*, 429–431. [CrossRef]
3. Tahami Monfared, A.A.; Byrnes, M.J.; White, L.A.; Zhang, Q. Alzheimer's Disease: Epidemiology and Clinical Progression. *Neurol. Ther.* **2022**, *11*, 553–569. [CrossRef] [PubMed]
4. World Health Organization Global Status Report on the Public Health Response to Dementia. Available online: https://www.who.int/publications/i/item/9789240033245 (accessed on 2 February 2024).
5. Gustavsson, A.; Norton, N.; Fast, T.; Frölich, L.; Georges, J.; Holzapfel, D.; Kirabali, T.; Krolak-Salmon, P.; Rossini, P.M.; Ferretti, M.T.; et al. Global Estimates on the Number of Persons across the Alzheimer's Disease Continuum. *Alzheimer's Dement.* **2023**, *19*, 658–670. [CrossRef] [PubMed]
6. Lanctôt, K.L.; Hviid Hahn-Pedersen, J.; Eichinger, C.S.; Freeman, C.; Clark, A.; Tarazona, L.R.S.; Cummings, J. Burden of Illness in People with Alzheimer's Disease: A Systematic Review of Epidemiology, Comorbidities and Mortality. *J. Prev. Alzheimer's Dis.* **2023**, *11*, 97–107. [CrossRef] [PubMed]
7. Scheltens, P.; De Strooper, B.; Kivipelto, M.; Holstege, H.; Chételat, G.; Teunissen, C.E.; Cummings, J.; van der Flier, W.M. Alzheimer's Disease. *Lancet* **2021**, *397*, 1577–1590. [CrossRef] [PubMed]
8. Khan, S.; Barve, K.H.; Kumar, M.S. Recent Advancements in Pathogenesis, Diagnostics and Treatment of Alzheimer's Disease. *Curr. Neuropharmacol.* **2020**, *18*, 1106–1125. [CrossRef] [PubMed]
9. Ossenkoppele, R.; van der Kant, R.; Hansson, O. Tau Biomarkers in Alzheimer's Disease: Towards Implementation in Clinical Practice and Trials. *Lancet Neurol.* **2022**, *21*, 726–734. [CrossRef] [PubMed]
10. Chatterjee, P.; Pedrini, S.; Ashton, N.J.; Tegg, M.; Goozee, K.; Singh, A.K.; Karikari, T.K.; Simrén, J.; Vanmechelen, E.; Armstrong, N.J.; et al. Diagnostic and Prognostic Plasma Biomarkers for Preclinical Alzheimer's Disease. *Alzheimer's Dement.* **2022**, *18*, 1141–1154. [CrossRef]
11. Prins, S.; de Kam, M.L.; Teunissen, C.E.; Groeneveld, G.J. Inflammatory Plasma Biomarkers in Subjects with Preclinical Alzheimer's Disease. *Alzheimers. Res. Ther.* **2022**, *14*, 106. [CrossRef]
12. Porsteinsson, A.P.; Isaacson, R.S.; Knox, S.; Sabbagh, M.N.; Rubino, I. Diagnosis of Early Alzheimer's Disease: Clinical Practice in 2021. *J. Prev. Alzheimer's Dis.* **2021**, *8*, 371–386. [CrossRef] [PubMed]
13. Kirova, A.-M.; Bays, R.B.; Lagalwar, S. Working Memory and Executive Function Decline across Normal Aging, Mild Cognitive Impairment, and Alzheimer's Disease. *BioMed Res. Int.* **2015**, *2015*, 748212. [CrossRef] [PubMed]
14. Kim, B.; Noh, G.O.; Kim, K. Behavioural and Psychological Symptoms of Dementia in Patients with Alzheimer's Disease and Family Caregiver Burden: A Path Analysis. *BMC Geriatr.* **2021**, *21*, 160. [CrossRef] [PubMed]
15. Trepson, W.L. Risk Factors for Alzheimer's Disease. *Sci. Insights* **2020**, *32*, 125–132. [CrossRef]
16. Scheyer, O.; Rahman, A.; Hristov, H.; Berkowitz, C.; Isaacson, R.S.; Diaz Brinton, R.; Mosconi, L. Female Sex and Alzheimer's Risk: The Menopause Connection. *J. Prev. Alzheimer's Dis.* **2018**, *5*, 225–230. [CrossRef]
17. Villaseca, P.; Cisternas, P.; Inestrosa, N.C. Menopause and Development of Alzheimer's Disease: Roles of Neural Glucose Metabolism and Wnt Signaling. *Front. Endocrinol.* **2022**, *13*, 1021796. [CrossRef] [PubMed]
18. Mishra, S.; Knupp, A.; Szabo, M.P.; Williams, C.A.; Kinoshita, C.; Hailey, D.W.; Wang, Y.; Andersen, O.M.; Young, J.E. The Alzheimer's Gene SORL1 Is a Regulator of Endosomal Traffic and Recycling in Human Neurons. *Cell. Mol. Life Sci.* **2022**, *79*, 162. [CrossRef] [PubMed]
19. Serrano-Pozo, A.; Das, S.; Hyman, B.T. APOE and Alzheimer's Disease: Advances in Genetics, Pathophysiology, and Therapeutic Approaches. *Lancet Neurol.* **2021**, *20*, 68–80. [CrossRef]
20. Zhang, X.-X.; Tian, Y.; Wang, Z.-T.; Ma, Y.-H.; Tan, L.; Yu, J.-T. The Epidemiology of Alzheimer's Disease Modifiable Risk Factors and Prevention. *J. Prev. Alzheimer's Dis.* **2021**, *8*, 313–321. [CrossRef]
21. Litke, R.; Garcharna, L.C.; Jiwani, S.; Neugroschl, J. Modifiable Risk Factors in Alzheimer Disease and Related Dementias: A Review. *Clin. Ther.* **2021**, *43*, 953–965. [CrossRef]
22. Xu, W.; Tan, L.; Wang, H.-F.; Jiang, T.; Tan, M.-S.; Tan, L.; Zhao, Q.-F.; Li, J.-Q.; Wang, J.; Yu, J.-T. Meta-Analysis of Modifiable Risk Factors for Alzheimer's Disease. *J. Neurol. Neurosurg. Psychiatry* **2015**, *86*, jnnp-2015-310548. [CrossRef] [PubMed]
23. Carey, A.; Fossati, S. Hypertension and Hyperhomocysteinemia as Modifiable Risk Factors for Alzheimer's Disease and Dementia: New Evidence, Potential Therapeutic Strategies, and Biomarkers. *Alzheimer's Dement.* **2023**, *19*, 671–695. [CrossRef] [PubMed]

24. Elsworthy, R.J.; Aldred, S. Depression in Alzheimer's Disease: An Alternative Role for Selective Serotonin Reuptake Inhibitors? *J. Alzheimer's Dis.* **2019**, *69*, 651–661. [CrossRef] [PubMed]
25. West, R.K.; Ravona-Springer, R.; Sharvit-Ginon, I.; Ganmore, I.; Manzali, S.; Tirosh, A.; Golan, S.; Boccara, E.; Heymann, A.; Beeri, M.S. Long-term Trajectories and Current BMI Are Associated with Poorer Cognitive Functioning in Middle-aged Adults at High Alzheimer's Disease Risk. *Alzheimer's Dement. Diagn. Assess. Dis. Monit.* **2021**, *13*, e12247. [CrossRef] [PubMed]
26. Zhao, T.; Zhong, T.; Zhang, M.; Xu, Y.; Zhang, M.; Chen, L. Alzheimer's Disease: Causal Effect between Obesity and APOE Gene Polymorphisms. *Int. J. Mol. Sci.* **2023**, *24*, 13531. [CrossRef] [PubMed]
27. Breijyeh, Z.; Karaman, R. Comprehensive Review on Alzheimer's Disease: Causes and Treatment. *Molecules* **2020**, *25*, 5789. [CrossRef] [PubMed]
28. Long, J.M.; Holtzman, D.M. Alzheimer Disease: An Update on Pathobiology and Treatment Strategies. *Cell* **2019**, *179*, 312–339. [CrossRef] [PubMed]
29. Chow, V.W.; Mattson, M.P.; Wong, P.C.; Gleichmann, M. An Overview of APP Processing Enzymes and Products. *NeuroMolecular Med.* **2010**, *12*, 1–12. [CrossRef] [PubMed]
30. Maia, M.; Sousa, E. BACE-1 and γ-Secretase as Therapeutic Targets for Alzheimer's Disease. *Pharmaceuticals* **2019**, *12*, 41. [CrossRef]
31. Chen, G.; Xu, T.; Yan, Y.; Zhou, Y.; Jiang, Y.; Melcher, K.; Xu, H.E. Amyloid Beta: Structure, Biology and Structure-Based Therapeutic Development. *Acta Pharmacol. Sin.* **2017**, *38*, 1205–1235. [CrossRef]
32. Taneja, V.; Verma, M.; Vats, A. Toxic Species in Amyloid Disorders: Oligomers or Mature Fibrils. *Ann. Indian Acad. Neurol.* **2015**, *18*, 138. [CrossRef] [PubMed]
33. Amin, L.; Harris, D.A. Aβ Receptors Specifically Recognize Molecular Features Displayed by Fibril Ends and Neurotoxic Oligomers. *Nat. Commun.* **2021**, *12*, 3451. [CrossRef] [PubMed]
34. Zhang, H.; Wei, W.; Zhao, M.; Ma, L.; Jiang, X.; Pei, H.; Cao, Y.; Li, H. Interaction between Aβ and Tau in the Pathogenesis of Alzheimer's Disease. *Int. J. Biol. Sci.* **2021**, *17*, 2181–2192. [CrossRef] [PubMed]
35. Jackson, N.A.; Guerrero-Muñoz, M.J.; Castillo-Carranza, D.L. The Prion-like Transmission of Tau Oligomers via Exosomes. *Front. Aging Neurosci.* **2022**, *14*, 974414. [CrossRef] [PubMed]
36. Mudher, A.; Colin, M.; Dujardin, S.; Medina, M.; Dewachter, I.; Alavi Naini, S.M.; Mandelkow, E.-M.; Mandelkow, E.; Buée, L.; Goedert, M.; et al. What Is the Evidence That Tau Pathology Spreads through Prion-like Propagation? *Acta Neuropathol. Commun.* **2017**, *5*, 99. [CrossRef] [PubMed]
37. Sadigh-Eteghad, S.; Sabermarouf, B.; Majdi, A.; Talebi, M.; Farhoudi, M.; Mahmoudi, J. Amyloid-Beta: A Crucial Factor in Alzheimer's Disease. *Med. Princ. Pract.* **2015**, *24*, 1–10. [CrossRef] [PubMed]
38. Jack, C.R.; Albert, M.S.; Knopman, D.S.; McKhann, G.M.; Sperling, R.A.; Carrillo, M.C.; Thies, B.; Phelps, C.H. Introduction to the Recommendations from the National Institute on Aging-Alzheimer's Association Workgroups on Diagnostic Guidelines for Alzheimer's Disease. *Alzheimer's Dement.* **2011**, *7*, 257–262. [CrossRef] [PubMed]
39. Albert, M.S.; DeKosky, S.T.; Dickson, D.; Dubois, B.; Feldman, H.H.; Fox, N.C.; Gamst, A.; Holtzman, D.M.; Jagust, W.J.; Petersen, R.C.; et al. The Diagnosis of Mild Cognitive Impairment Due to Alzheimer's Disease: Recommendations from the National Institute on Aging-Alzheimer's Association Workgroups on Diagnostic Guidelines for Alzheimer's Disease. *Alzheimer's Dement.* **2011**, *7*, 270–279. [CrossRef] [PubMed]
40. McKhann, G.M.; Knopman, D.S.; Chertkow, H.; Hyman, B.T.; Jack, C.R.; Kawas, C.H.; Klunk, W.E.; Koroshetz, W.J.; Manly, J.J.; Mayeux, R.; et al. The Diagnosis of Dementia Due to Alzheimer's Disease: Recommendations from the National Institute on Aging-Alzheimer's Association Workgroups on Diagnostic Guidelines for Alzheimer's Disease. *Alzheimer's Dement.* **2011**, *7*, 263–269. [CrossRef]
41. Jiang, F.; Cheng, C.; Huang, J.; Chen, Q.; Le, W. Mild Behavioral Impairment: An Early Sign and Predictor of Alzheimer's Disease Dementia. *Curr. Alzheimer Res.* **2022**, *19*, 407–419. [CrossRef]
42. Mo, M.; Zacarias-Pons, L.; Hoang, M.T.; Mostafaei, S.; Jurado, P.G.; Stark, I.; Johnell, K.; Eriksdotter, M.; Xu, H.; Garcia-Ptacek, S. Psychiatric Disorders Before and After Dementia Diagnosis. *JAMA Netw. Open* **2023**, *6*, e2338080. [CrossRef] [PubMed]
43. Jack, C.R.; Bennett, D.A.; Blennow, K.; Carrillo, M.C.; Dunn, B.; Haeberlein, S.B.; Holtzman, D.M.; Jagust, W.; Jessen, F.; Karlawish, J.; et al. NIA-AA Research Framework: Toward a Biological Definition of Alzheimer's Disease. *Alzheimer's Dement.* **2018**, *14*, 535–562. [CrossRef] [PubMed]
44. Ashton, N.J.; Pascoal, T.A.; Karikari, T.K.; Benedet, A.L.; Lantero-Rodriguez, J.; Brinkmalm, G.; Snellman, A.; Schöll, M.; Troakes, C.; Hye, A.; et al. Plasma P-Tau231: A New Biomarker for Incipient Alzheimer's Disease Pathology. *Acta Neuropathol.* **2021**, *141*, 709–724. [CrossRef] [PubMed]
45. Kurihara, M.; Komatsu, H.; Sengoku, R.; Shibukawa, M.; Morimoto, S.; Matsubara, T.; Arakawa, A.; Orita, M.; Ishibashi, K.; Mitsutake, A.; et al. CSF P-Tau181 and Other Biomarkers in Patients With Neuronal Intranuclear Inclusion Disease. *Neurology* **2023**, *100*, e1009–e1019. [CrossRef] [PubMed]
46. Batzu, L.; Rota, S.; Hye, A.; Heslegrave, A.; Trivedi, D.; Gibson, L.L.; Farrell, C.; Zinzalias, P.; Rizos, A.; Zetterberg, H.; et al. Plasma P-Tau181, Neurofilament Light Chain and Association with Cognition in Parkinson's Disease. *npj Park. Dis.* **2022**, *8*, 154. [CrossRef]
47. Teunissen, C.E.; Thijssen, E.H.; Verberk, I.M.W. Plasma P-Tau217: From 'New Kid' to Most Promising Candidate for Alzheimer's Disease Blood Test. *Brain* **2020**, *143*, 3170–3172. [CrossRef] [PubMed]

48. Milà-Alomà, M.; Ashton, N.J.; Shekari, M.; Salvadó, G.; Ortiz-Romero, P.; Montoliu-Gaya, L.; Benedet, A.L.; Karikari, T.K.; Lantero-Rodriguez, J.; Vanmechelen, E.; et al. Plasma P-Tau231 and p-Tau217 as State Markers of Amyloid-β Pathology in Preclinical Alzheimer's Disease. *Nat. Med.* **2022**, *28*, 1797–1801. [CrossRef]
49. Mattsson-Carlgren, N.; Janelidze, S.; Palmqvist, S.; Cullen, N.; Svenningsson, A.L.; Strandberg, O.; Mengel, D.; Walsh, D.M.; Stomrud, E.; Dage, J.L.; et al. Longitudinal Plasma P-Tau217 Is Increased in Early Stages of Alzheimer's Disease. *Brain* **2020**, *143*, 3234–3241. [CrossRef]
50. Schutgens, F.; Clevers, H. Human Organoids: Tools for Understanding Biology and Treating Diseases. *Annu. Rev. Pathol. Mech. Dis.* **2020**, *15*, 211–234. [CrossRef]
51. Muralidar, S.; Ambi, S.V.; Sekaran, S.; Thirumalai, D.; Palaniappan, B. Role of Tau Protein in Alzheimer's Disease: The Prime Pathological Player. *Int. J. Biol. Macromol.* **2020**, *163*, 1599–1617. [CrossRef]
52. Pîrşcoveanu, D.F.V.; Pirici, I.; Tudorică, V.; Bălşeanu, T.A.; Albu, V.C.; Bondari, S.; Bumbea, A.M.; Pîrşcoveanu, M. Tau Protein in Neurodegenerative Diseases—A Review. *Rom. J. Morphol. Embryol.* **2017**, *58*, 1141–1150. [PubMed]
53. Ittner, A.; Ittner, L.M. Dendritic Tau in Alzheimer's Disease. *Neuron* **2018**, *99*, 13–27. [CrossRef] [PubMed]
54. Weingarten, M.D.; Lockwood, A.H.; Hwo, S.Y.; Kirschner, M.W. A Protein Factor Essential for Microtubule Assembly. *Proc. Natl. Acad. Sci. USA* **1975**, *72*, 1858–1862. [CrossRef] [PubMed]
55. Wegmann, S.; Biernat, J.; Mandelkow, E. A Current View on Tau Protein Phosphorylation in Alzheimer's Disease. *Curr. Opin. Neurobiol.* **2021**, *69*, 131–138. [CrossRef] [PubMed]
56. Guo, T.; Noble, W.; Hanger, D.P. Roles of Tau Protein in Health and Disease. *Acta Neuropathol.* **2017**, *133*, 665–704. [CrossRef] [PubMed]
57. Buée, L.; Bussière, T.; Buée-Scherrer, V.; Delacourte, A.; Hof, P.R. Tau Protein Isoforms, Phosphorylation and Role in Neurodegenerative Disorders11These Authors Contributed Equally to This Work. *Brain Res. Rev.* **2000**, *33*, 95–130. [CrossRef] [PubMed]
58. Yu, C.-C.; Jiang, T.; Yang, A.-F.; Du, Y.-J.; Wu, M.; Kong, L.-H. Epigenetic Modulation on Tau Phosphorylation in Alzheimer's Disease. *Neural Plast.* **2019**, *2019*, 6856327. [CrossRef] [PubMed]
59. Hirota, Y.; Sakakibara, Y.; Ibaraki, K.; Takei, K.; Iijima, K.M.; Sekiya, M. Distinct Brain Pathologies Associated with Alzheimer's Disease Biomarker-Related Phospho-Tau 181 and Phospho-Tau 217 in App Knock-in Mouse Models of Amyloid-β Amyloidosis. *Brain Commun.* **2022**, *4*, fcac286. [CrossRef] [PubMed]
60. Sun, L.; Ban, T.; Liu, C.; Chen, Q.; Wang, X.; Yan, M.; Hu, X.; Su, X.; Bao, Y.; Sun, L.; et al. Activation of Cdk5/P25 and Tau Phosphorylation Following Chronic Brain Hypoperfusion in Rats Involves Micro RNA -195 Down-regulation. *J. Neurochem.* **2015**, *134*, 1139–1151. [CrossRef]
61. Kim, B.M.; You, M.-H.; Chen, C.-H.; Lee, S.; Hong, Y.; Hong, Y.; Kimchi, A.; Zhou, X.Z.; Lee, T.H. Death-Associated Protein Kinase 1 Has a Critical Role in Aberrant Tau Protein Regulation and Function. *Cell Death Dis.* **2014**, *5*, e1237. [CrossRef]
62. Martin, L.; Latypova, X.; Wilson, C.M.; Magnaudeix, A.; Perrin, M.-L.; Terro, F. Tau Protein Phosphatases in Alzheimer's Disease: The Leading Role of PP2A. *Ageing Res. Rev.* **2013**, *12*, 39–49. [CrossRef] [PubMed]
63. Man, V.H.; He, X.; Han, F.; Cai, L.; Wang, L.; Niu, T.; Zhai, J.; Ji, B.; Gao, J.; Wang, J. Phosphorylation at Ser289 Enhances the Oligomerization of Tau Repeat R2. *J. Chem. Inf. Model.* **2023**, *63*, 1351–1361. [CrossRef] [PubMed]
64. Buée, L.; Troquier, L.; Burnouf, S.; Belarbi, K.; Van der Jeugd, A.; Ahmed, T.; Fernandez-Gomez, F.; Caillierez, R.; Grosjean, M.-E.; Begard, S.; et al. From Tau Phosphorylation to Tau Aggregation: What about Neuronal Death? *Biochem. Soc. Trans.* **2010**, *38*, 967–972. [CrossRef] [PubMed]
65. Man, V.H.; He, X.; Gao, J.; Wang, J. Phosphorylation of Tau R2 Repeat Destabilizes Its Binding to Microtubules: A Molecular Dynamics Simulation Study. *ACS Chem. Neurosci.* **2023**, *14*, 458–467. [CrossRef] [PubMed]
66. Song, L.; Oseid, D.E.; Wells, E.A.; Robinson, A.S. The Interplay between GSK3β and Tau Ser262 Phosphorylation during the Progression of Tau Pathology. *Int. J. Mol. Sci.* **2022**, *23*, 11610. [CrossRef] [PubMed]
67. Oba, T.; Saito, T.; Asada, A.; Shimizu, S.; Iijima, K.M.; Ando, K. Microtubule Affinity–Regulating Kinase 4 with an Alzheimer's Disease-Related Mutation Promotes Tau Accumulation and Exacerbates Neurodegeneration. *J. Biol. Chem.* **2020**, *295*, 17138–17147. [CrossRef] [PubMed]
68. Xia, Y.; Prokop, S.; Gorion, K.-M.M.; Kim, J.D.; Sorrentino, Z.A.; Bell, B.M.; Manaois, A.N.; Chakrabarty, P.; Davies, P.; Giasson, B.I. Tau Ser208 Phosphorylation Promotes Aggregation and Reveals Neuropathologic Diversity in Alzheimer's Disease and Other Tauopathies. *Acta Neuropathol. Commun.* **2020**, *8*, 88. [CrossRef] [PubMed]
69. Brion, J.-P.; Anderton, B.H.; Authelet, M.; Dayanandan, R.; Leroy, K.; Lovestone, S.; Octave, J.-N.; Pradier, L.; Touchet, N.; Tremp, G. Neurofibrillary Tangles and Tau Phosphorylation. *Biochem. Soc. Symp.* **2001**, *67*, 81–88. [CrossRef]
70. Drummond, E.; Pires, G.; MacMurray, C.; Askenazi, M.; Nayak, S.; Bourdon, M.; Safar, J.; Ueberheide, B.; Wisniewski, T. Phosphorylated Tau Interactome in the Human Alzheimer's Disease Brain. *Brain* **2020**, *143*, 2803–2817. [CrossRef]
71. Jack, C.R.; Wiste, H.J.; Algeciras-Schimnich, A.; Figdore, D.J.; Schwarz, C.G.; Lowe, V.J.; Ramanan, V.K.; Vemuri, P.; Mielke, M.M.; Knopman, D.S.; et al. Predicting Amyloid PET and Tau PET Stages with Plasma Biomarkers. *Brain* **2023**, *146*, 2029–2044. [CrossRef]
72. Xiao, Z.; Wu, W.; Ma, X.; Wu, J.; Liang, X.; Zhou, X.; Cao, Y.; Zhao, Q.; Ding, D. Plasma P-tau217, P-tau181, and NfL as Early Indicators of Dementia Risk in a Community Cohort: The Shanghai Aging Study. *Alzheimer's Dement. Diagn. Assess. Dis. Monit.* **2023**, *15*, e12514. [CrossRef] [PubMed]

73. Brickman, A.M.; Manly, J.J.; Honig, L.S.; Sanchez, D.; Reyes-Dumeyer, D.; Lantigua, R.A.; Lao, P.J.; Stern, Y.; Vonsattel, J.P.; Teich, A.F.; et al. Plasma P-tau181, P-tau217, and Other Blood-based Alzheimer's Disease Biomarkers in a Multi-ethnic, Community Study. *Alzheimer's Dement.* **2021**, *17*, 1353–1364. [CrossRef] [PubMed]
74. Suárez-Calvet, M.; Karikari, T.K.; Ashton, N.J.; Lantero Rodríguez, J.; Milà-Alomà, M.; Gispert, J.D.; Salvadó, G.; Minguillon, C.; Fauria, K.; Shekari, M.; et al. Novel Tau Biomarkers Phosphorylated at T181, T217 or T231 Rise in the Initial Stages of the Preclinical Alzheimer's Continuum When Only Subtle Changes in Aβ Pathology Are Detected. *EMBO Mol. Med.* **2020**, *12*, e12921. [CrossRef] [PubMed]
75. Gauthier, S.; Therriault, J.; Pascoal, T.; Rosa-Neto, P. Impact of P-Tau181 and p-Tau217 Levels on Enrollment for Randomized Clinical Trials and Future Use of Anti-Amyloid and Anti-Tau Drugs. *Expert Rev. Neurother.* **2020**, *20*, 1211–1213. [CrossRef] [PubMed]
76. Kac, P.R.; Gonzalez-Ortiz, F.; Simrén, J.; Dewit, N.; Vanmechelen, E.; Zetterberg, H.; Blennow, K.; Ashton, N.J.; Karikari, T.K. Diagnostic Value of Serum versus Plasma Phospho-Tau for Alzheimer's Disease. *Alzheimers. Res. Ther.* **2022**, *14*, 65. [CrossRef] [PubMed]
77. Tissot, C.; Therriault, J.; Kunach, P.; L Benedet, A.; Pascoal, T.A.; Ashton, N.J.; Karikari, T.K.; Servaes, S.; Lussier, F.Z.; Chamoun, M.; et al. Comparing Tau Status Determined via Plasma PTau181, PTau231 and [18F]MK6240 Tau-PET. *eBioMedicine* **2022**, *76*, 103837. [CrossRef] [PubMed]
78. Ashton, N.J.; Benedet, A.L.; Pascoal, T.A.; Karikari, T.K.; Lantero-Rodriguez, J.; Brum, W.S.; Mathotaarachchi, S.; Therriault, J.; Savard, M.; Chamoun, M.; et al. Cerebrospinal Fluid P-Tau231 as an Early Indicator of Emerging Pathology in Alzheimer's Disease. *eBioMedicine* **2022**, *76*, 103836. [CrossRef] [PubMed]
79. Barthélemy, N.R.; Horie, K.; Sato, C.; Bateman, R.J. Blood Plasma Phosphorylated-Tau Isoforms Track CNS Change in Alzheimer's Disease. *J. Exp. Med.* **2020**, *217*, e20200861. [CrossRef] [PubMed]
80. Therriault, J.; Vermeiren, M.; Servaes, S.; Tissot, C.; Ashton, N.J.; Benedet, A.L.; Karikari, T.K.; Lantero-Rodriguez, J.; Brum, W.S.; Lussier, F.Z.; et al. Association of Phosphorylated Tau Biomarkers With Amyloid Positron Emission Tomography vs Tau Positron Emission Tomography. *JAMA Neurol.* **2023**, *80*, 188. [CrossRef] [PubMed]
81. Ashton, N.J.; Brum, W.S.; Di Molfetta, G.; Benedet, A.L.; Arslan, B.; Jonaitis, E.; Langhough, R.E.; Cody, K.; Wilson, R.; Carlsson, C.M.; et al. Diagnostic Accuracy of a Plasma Phosphorylated Tau 217 Immunoassay for Alzheimer Disease Pathology. *JAMA Neurol.* **2024**, *81*, 255. [CrossRef]
82. Palmqvist, S.; Janelidze, S.; Quiroz, Y.T.; Zetterberg, H.; Lopera, F.; Stomrud, E.; Su, Y.; Chen, Y.; Serrano, G.E.; Leuzy, A.; et al. Discriminative Accuracy of Plasma Phospho-Tau217 for Alzheimer Disease vs Other Neurodegenerative Disorders. *JAMA* **2020**, *324*, 772. [CrossRef] [PubMed]
83. Yakoub, Y.; Ashton, N.J.; Strikwerda-Brown, C.; Montoliu-Gaya, L.; Karikari, T.K.; Kac, P.R.; Gonzalez-Ortiz, F.; Gallego-Rudolf, J.; Meyer, P.; St-Onge, F.; et al. Longitudinal Blood Biomarker Trajectories in Preclinical Alzheimer's Disease. *Alzheimer's Dement.* **2023**, *19*, 5620–5631. [CrossRef] [PubMed]
84. Woo, M.S.; Tissot, C.; Lantero-Rodriguez, J.; Snellman, A.; Therriault, J.; Rahmouni, N.; Macedo, A.C.; Servaes, S.; Wang, Y.; Arias, J.F.; et al. Plasma PTau-217 and N-terminal Tau (NTA) Enhance Sensitivity to Identify Tau PET Positivity in Amyloid-β Positive Individuals. *Alzheimer's Dement.* **2024**, *20*, 1166–1174. [CrossRef] [PubMed]
85. Janelidze, S.; Berron, D.; Smith, R.; Strandberg, O.; Proctor, N.K.; Dage, J.L.; Stomrud, E.; Palmqvist, S.; Mattsson-Carlgren, N.; Hansson, O. Associations of Plasma Phospho-Tau217 Levels With Tau Positron Emission Tomography in Early Alzheimer Disease. *JAMA Neurol.* **2021**, *78*, 149. [CrossRef] [PubMed]
86. Palmqvist, S.; Tideman, P.; Cullen, N.; Zetterberg, H.; Blennow, K.; Dage, J.L.; Stomrud, E.; Janelidze, S.; Mattsson-Carlgren, N.; Hansson, O. Prediction of Future Alzheimer's Disease Dementia Using Plasma Phospho-Tau Combined with Other Accessible Measures. *Nat. Med.* **2021**, *27*, 1034–1042. [CrossRef] [PubMed]
87. Mielke, M.M.; Dage, J.L.; Frank, R.D.; Algeciras-Schimnich, A.; Knopman, D.S.; Lowe, V.J.; Bu, G.; Vemuri, P.; Graff-Radford, J.; Jack, C.R.; et al. Performance of Plasma Phosphorylated Tau 181 and 217 in the Community. *Nat. Med.* **2022**, *28*, 1398–1405. [CrossRef] [PubMed]
88. Janelidze, S.; Palmqvist, S.; Leuzy, A.; Stomrud, E.; Verberk, I.M.W.; Zetterberg, H.; Ashton, N.J.; Pesini, P.; Sarasa, L.; Allué, J.A.; et al. Detecting Amyloid Positivity in Early Alzheimer's Disease Using Combinations of Plasma Aβ42/Aβ40 and P-tau. *Alzheimer's Dement.* **2022**, *18*, 283–293. [CrossRef] [PubMed]
89. Janelidze, S.; Stomrud, E.; Smith, R.; Palmqvist, S.; Mattsson, N.; Airey, D.C.; Proctor, N.K.; Chai, X.; Shcherbinin, S.; Sims, J.R.; et al. Cerebrospinal Fluid P-Tau217 Performs Better than p-Tau181 as a Biomarker of Alzheimer's Disease. *Nat. Commun.* **2020**, *11*, 1683. [CrossRef]
90. Mundada, N.S.; Rojas, J.C.; Vandevrede, L.; Thijssen, E.H.; Iaccarino, L.; Okoye, O.C.; Shankar, R.; Soleimani-Meigooni, D.N.; Lago, A.L.; Miller, B.L.; et al. Head-to-Head Comparison between Plasma p-Tau217 and Flortaucipir-PET in Amyloid-Positive Patients with Cognitive Impairment. *Alzheimers. Res. Ther.* **2023**, *15*, 157. [CrossRef]
91. Jonaitis, E.M.; Janelidze, S.; Cody, K.A.; Langhough, R.; Du, L.; Chin, N.A.; Mattsson-Carlgren, N.; Hogan, K.J.; Christian, B.T.; Betthauser, T.J.; et al. Plasma Phosphorylated Tau 217 in Preclinical Alzheimer's Disease. *Brain Commun.* **2023**, *5*, 1–11. [CrossRef]
92. Yu, L.; Boyle, P.A.; Janelidze, S.; Petyuk, V.A.; Wang, T.; Bennett, D.A.; Hansson, O.; Schneider, J.A. Plasma P-Tau181 and p-Tau217 in Discriminating PART, AD and Other Key Neuropathologies in Older Adults. *Acta Neuropathol.* **2023**, *146*, 1–11. [CrossRef]

93. Salvadó, G.; Ossenkoppele, R.; Ashton, N.J.; Beach, T.G.; Serrano, G.E.; Reiman, E.M.; Zetterberg, H.; Mattsson-Carlgren, N.; Janelidze, S.; Blennow, K.; et al. Specific Associations between Plasma Biomarkers and Postmortem Amyloid Plaque and Tau Tangle Loads. *EMBO Mol. Med.* **2023**, *15*, e17123. [CrossRef]
94. Barthélemy, N.R.; Salvadó, G.; Schindler, S.E.; He, Y.; Janelidze, S.; Collij, L.E.; Saef, B.; Henson, R.L.; Chen, C.D.; Gordon, B.A.; et al. Highly Accurate Blood Test for Alzheimer's Disease Is Similar or Superior to Clinical Cerebrospinal Fluid Tests. *Nat. Med.* 2024; *in press*. [CrossRef]
95. Karikari, T.K.; Ashton, N.J.; Brinkmalm, G.; Brum, W.S.; Benedet, A.L.; Montoliu-Gaya, L.; Lantero-Rodriguez, J.; Pascoal, T.A.; Suárez-Calvet, M.; Rosa-Neto, P.; et al. Blood Phospho-Tau in Alzheimer Disease: Analysis, Interpretation, and Clinical Utility. *Nat. Rev. Neurol.* **2022**, *18*, 400–418. [CrossRef]
96. Bayoumy, S.; Verberk, I.M.W.; den Dulk, B.; Hussainali, Z.; Zwan, M.; van der Flier, W.M.; Ashton, N.J.; Zetterberg, H.; Blennow, K.; Vanbrabant, J.; et al. Clinical and Analytical Comparison of Six Simoa Assays for Plasma P-Tau Isoforms P-Tau181, P-Tau217, and P-Tau231. *Alzheimers. Res. Ther.* **2021**, *13*, 198. [CrossRef]
97. Janelidze, S.; Bali, D.; Ashton, N.J.; Barthélemy, N.R.; Vanbrabant, J.; Stoops, E.; Vanmechelen, E.; He, Y.; Dolado, A.O.; Triana-Baltzer, G.; et al. Head-to-Head Comparison of 10 Plasma Phospho-Tau Assays in Prodromal Alzheimer's Disease. *Brain* **2023**, *146*, 1592–1601. [CrossRef]
98. Ashton, N.J.; Puig-Pijoan, A.; Milà-Alomà, M.; Fernández-Lebrero, A.; García-Escobar, G.; González-Ortiz, F.; Kac, P.R.; Brum, W.S.; Benedet, A.L.; Lantero-Rodriguez, J.; et al. Plasma and CSF Biomarkers in a Memory Clinic: Head-to-head Comparison of Phosphorylated Tau Immunoassays. *Alzheimer's Dement.* **2023**, *19*, 1913–1924. [CrossRef]
99. Barthélemy, N.R.; Li, Y.; Joseph-Mathurin, N.; Gordon, B.A.; Hassenstab, J.; Benzinger, T.L.S.; Buckles, V.; Fagan, A.M.; Perrin, R.J.; Goate, A.M.; et al. A Soluble Phosphorylated Tau Signature Links Tau, Amyloid and the Evolution of Stages of Dominantly Inherited Alzheimer's Disease. *Nat. Med.* **2020**, *26*, 398–407. [CrossRef]
100. Mielke, M.M.; Frank, R.D.; Dage, J.L.; Jeromin, A.; Ashton, N.J.; Blennow, K.; Karikari, T.K.; Vanmechelen, E.; Zetterberg, H.; Algeciras-Schimnich, A.; et al. Comparison of Plasma Phosphorylated Tau Species With Amyloid and Tau Positron Emission Tomography, Neurodegeneration, Vascular Pathology, and Cognitive Outcomes. *JAMA Neurol.* **2021**, *78*, 1108. [CrossRef] [PubMed]
101. Barthélemy, N.R.; Bateman, R.J.; Hirtz, C.; Marin, P.; Becher, F.; Sato, C.; Gabelle, A.; Lehmann, S. Cerebrospinal Fluid Phospho-Tau T217 Outperforms T181 as a Biomarker for the Differential Diagnosis of Alzheimer's Disease and PET Amyloid-Positive Patient Identification. *Alzheimers. Res. Ther.* **2020**, *12*, 26. [CrossRef] [PubMed]
102. Thijssen, E.H.; La Joie, R.; Strom, A.; Fonseca, C.; Iaccarino, L.; Wolf, A.; Spina, S.; Allen, I.E.; Cobigo, Y.; Heuer, H.; et al. Plasma Phosphorylated Tau 217 and Phosphorylated Tau 181 as Biomarkers in Alzheimer's Disease and Frontotemporal Lobar Degeneration: A Retrospective Diagnostic Performance Study. *Lancet Neurol.* **2021**, *20*, 739–752. [CrossRef]
103. Salvadó, G.; Horie, K.; Barthélemy, N.R.; Vogel, J.W.; Binette, A.P.; Chen, C.D.; Aschenbrenner, A.J.; Gordon, B.A.; Benzinger, T.L.S.; Holtzman, D.M.; et al. Novel CSF Tau Biomarkers Can Be Used for Disease Staging of Sporadic Alzheimer's. *Alzheimer's Dement.* **2023**, *19*, e075367. [CrossRef]
104. Mattsson-Carlgren, N.; Salvadó, G.; Ashton, N.J.; Tideman, P.; Stomrud, E.; Zetterberg, H.; Ossenkoppele, R.; Betthauser, T.J.; Cody, K.A.; Jonaitis, E.M.; et al. Prediction of Longitudinal Cognitive Decline in Preclinical Alzheimer Disease Using Plasma Biomarkers. *JAMA Neurol.* **2023**, *80*, 360. [CrossRef]
105. Palmqvist, S.; Stomrud, E.; Cullen, N.; Janelidze, S.; Manuilova, E.; Jethwa, A.; Bittner, T.; Eichenlaub, U.; Suridjan, I.; Kollmorgen, G.; et al. An Accurate Fully Automated Panel of Plasma Biomarkers for Alzheimer's Disease. *Alzheimer's Dement.* **2023**, *19*, 1204–1215. [CrossRef]
106. Mattsson-Carlgren, N.; Janelidze, S.; Bateman, R.J.; Smith, R.; Stomrud, E.; Serrano, G.E.; Reiman, E.M.; Palmqvist, S.; Dage, J.L.; Beach, T.G.; et al. Soluble P-tau217 Reflects Amyloid and Tau Pathology and Mediates the Association of Amyloid with Tau. *EMBO Mol. Med.* **2021**, *13*, e14022. [CrossRef]
107. Therriault, J.; Servaes, S.; Tissot, C.; Rahmouni, N.; Ashton, N.J.; Benedet, A.L.; Karikari, T.K.; Macedo, A.C.; Lussier, F.Z.; Stevenson, J.; et al. Equivalence of Plasma P-tau217 with Cerebrospinal Fluid in the Diagnosis of Alzheimer's Disease. *Alzheimer's Dement.* **2023**, *19*, 4967–4977. [CrossRef]
108. Montoliu-Gaya, L.; Benedet, A.L.; Tissot, C.; Vrillon, A.; Ashton, N.J.; Brum, W.S.; Lantero-Rodriguez, J.; Stevenson, J.; Nilsson, J.; Sauer, M.; et al. Mass Spectrometric Simultaneous Quantification of Tau Species in Plasma Shows Differential Associations with Amyloid and Tau Pathologies. *Nat. Aging* **2023**, *3*, 661–669. [CrossRef] [PubMed]
109. Horie, K.; Salvadó, G.; Barthélemy, N.R.; Janelidze, S.; Li, Y.; He, Y.; Saef, B.; Chen, C.D.; Jiang, H.; Strandberg, O.; et al. CSF MTBR-Tau243 Is a Specific Biomarker of Tau Tangle Pathology in Alzheimer's Disease. *Nat. Med.* **2023**, *29*, 1954–1963. [CrossRef] [PubMed]
110. Braak, H.; Braak, E. Neuropathological Stageing of Alzheimer-Related Changes. *Acta Neuropathol.* **1991**, *82*, 239–259. [CrossRef] [PubMed]
111. Thal, D.R.; Rüb, U.; Orantes, M.; Braak, H. Phases of Aβ-Deposition in the Human Brain and Its Relevance for the Development of AD. *Neurology* **2002**, *58*, 1791–1800. [CrossRef]
112. Moms, J.C.; Heyman, A.; Mohs, R.C.; Hughes, J.P.; van Belle, G.; Fillenbaum, G.; Mellits, E.D.; Clark, C. The Consortium to Establish a Registry for Alzheimer's Disease (CERAD). Part I. Clinical and Neuropsychological Assesment of Alzheimer's Disease. *Neurology* **1989**, *39*, 1159. [CrossRef] [PubMed]

113. Leuzy, A.; Smith, R.; Cullen, N.C.; Strandberg, O.; Vogel, J.W.; Binette, A.P.; Borroni, E.; Janelidze, S.; Ohlsson, T.; Jögi, J.; et al. Biomarker-Based Prediction of Longitudinal Tau Positron Emission Tomography in Alzheimer Disease. *JAMA Neurol.* **2022**, *79*, 149. [CrossRef]
114. Ashton, N.J.; Janelidze, S.; Mattsson-Carlgren, N.; Binette, A.P.; Strandberg, O.; Brum, W.S.; Karikari, T.K.; González-Ortiz, F.; Di Molfetta, G.; Meda, F.J.; et al. Differential Roles of Aβ42/40, p-Tau231 and p-Tau217 for Alzheimer's Trial Selection and Disease Monitoring. *Nat. Med.* **2022**, *28*, 2555–2562. [CrossRef]
115. Lilek, J.; Ajroud, K.; Feldman, A.Z.; Krishnamachari, S.; Ghourchian, S.; Gefen, T.; Spencer, C.L.; Kawles, A.; Mao, Q.; Tranovich, J.F.; et al. Accumulation of PTau231 at the Postsynaptic Density in Early Alzheimer's Disease. *J. Alzheimer's Dis.* **2023**, *92*, 241–260. [CrossRef]
116. Smirnov, D.S.; Ashton, N.J.; Blennow, K.; Zetterberg, H.; Simrén, J.; Lantero-Rodriguez, J.; Karikari, T.K.; Hiniker, A.; Rissman, R.A.; Salmon, D.P.; et al. Plasma Biomarkers for Alzheimer's Disease in Relation to Neuropathology and Cognitive Change. *Acta Neuropathol.* **2022**, *143*, 487–503. [CrossRef]
117. Therriault, J.; Pascoal, T.A.; Lussier, F.Z.; Tissot, C.; Chamoun, M.; Bezgin, G.; Servaes, S.; Benedet, A.L.; Ashton, N.J.; Karikari, T.K.; et al. Biomarker Modeling of Alzheimer's Disease Using PET-Based Braak Staging. *Nat. Aging* **2022**, *2*, 526–535. [CrossRef] [PubMed]
118. Martínez-Dubarbie, F.; Guerra-Ruiz, A.; López-García, S.; Irure-Ventura, J.; Lage, C.; Fernández-Matarrubia, M.; Pozueta-Cantudo, A.; García-Martínez, M.; Corrales-Pardo, A.; Bravo, M.; et al. Influence of Physiological Variables and Comorbidities on Plasma Aβ40, Aβ42, and p-Tau181 Levels in Cognitively Unimpaired Individuals. *Int. J. Mol. Sci.* **2024**, *25*, 1481. [CrossRef]
119. Pan, F.; Lu, Y.; Huang, Q.; Xie, F.; Yang, J.; Guo, Q. The Potential Impact of Clinical Factors on Blood-Based Biomarkers for Alzheimer's Disease. *Transl. Neurodegener.* **2023**, *12*, 39. [CrossRef] [PubMed]
120. Zenuni, H.; Grillo, P.; Sancesario, G.M.; Bernardini, S.; Mercuri, N.B.; Schirinzi, T. How Comorbidity Reflects on Cerebrospinal Fluid Biomarkers of Neurodegeneration in Aging. *J. Alzheimer's Dis. Reports* **2021**, *5*, 87–92. [CrossRef]
121. Ossenkoppele, R.; Leuzy, A.; Cho, H.; Sudre, C.H.; Strandberg, O.; Smith, R.; Palmqvist, S.; Mattsson-Carlgren, N.; Olsson, T.; Jögi, J.; et al. The Impact of Demographic, Clinical, Genetic, and Imaging Variables on Tau PET Status. *Eur. J. Nucl. Med. Mol. Imaging* **2021**, *48*, 2245–2258. [CrossRef]
122. Dang, M.; Chen, Q.; Zhao, X.; Chen, K.; Li, X.; Zhang, J.; Lu, J.; Ai, L.; Chen, Y.; Zhang, Z. Tau as a Biomarker of Cognitive Impairment and Neuropsychiatric Symptom in Alzheimer's Disease. *Hum. Brain Mapp.* **2023**, *44*, 327–340. [CrossRef] [PubMed]
123. Rubenstein, R.; McQuillan, L.; Wang, K.K.W.; Robertson, C.; Chang, B.; Yang, Z.; Xu, H.; Williamson, J.; Wagner, A.K. Temporal Profiles of P-Tau, T-Tau, and P-Tau:Tau Ratios in Cerebrospinal Fluid and Blood from Moderate-Severe Traumatic Brain Injury Patients and Relationship to 6–12 Month Global Outcomes. *J. Neurotrauma* **2024**, *41*, 369–392. [CrossRef] [PubMed]
124. Sfera, A.; Rahman, L.; Zapata-Martín del Campo, C.M.; Kozlakidis, Z. Long COVID as a Tauopathy: Of "Brain Fog" and "Fusogen Storms". *Int. J. Mol. Sci.* **2023**, *24*, 12648. [CrossRef]

biomedicines

MDPI

Review

TAARs as Novel Therapeutic Targets for the Treatment of Depression: A Narrative Review of the Interconnection with Monoamines and Adult Neurogenesis

Taisiia S. Shemiakova [1], Evgeniya V. Efimova [1] and Raul R. Gainetdinov [1,2,*]

[1] Institute of Translational Biomedicine, Saint-Petersburg State University, 199034 St. Petersburg, Russia; st035112@student.spbu.ru (T.S.S.); e.v.efimova@mail.ru (E.V.E.)

[2] Saint-Petersburg University Hospital, Saint-Petersburg State University, 199034 St. Petersburg, Russia

* Correspondence: r.gainetdinov@spbu.ru

Abstract: Depression is a common mental illness of great concern. Current therapy for depression is only suitable for 80% of patients and is often associated with unwanted side effects. In this regard, the search for and development of new antidepressant agents remains an urgent task. In this review, we discuss the current available evidence indicating that G protein-coupled trace amine-associated receptors (TAARs) might represent new targets for depression treatment. The most frequently studied receptor TAAR1 has already been investigated in the treatment of schizophrenia, demonstrating antidepressant and anxiolytic properties. In fact, the TAAR1 agonist Ulotaront is currently undergoing phase 2/3 clinical trials testing its safety and efficacy in the treatment of major depressive disorder and generalized anxiety disorder. Other members of the TAAR family (TAAR2, TAAR5, TAAR6, TAAR8, and TAAR9) are not only involved in the innate olfaction of volatile amines, but are also expressed in the limbic brain areas. Furthermore, animal studies have shown that TAAR2 and TAAR5 regulate emotional behaviors and thus may hold promise as potential antidepressant targets. Of particular interest is their connection with the dopamine and serotonin systems of the brain and their involvement in the regulation of adult neurogenesis, known to be affected by the antidepressant drugs currently in use. Further non-clinical and clinical studies are necessary to validate TAAR1 (and potentially other TAARs) as novel therapeutic targets for the treatment of depression.

Keywords: depression; antidepressant; neurogenesis; TAAR; TAAR1; monoamines; glutamate; dopamine; serotonin; SEP-363856

1. Introduction: Pharmacotherapy of Depression

Major depressive disorder is the most common mental illness with more than 280 million cases worldwide [1,2]. The clinical picture of depression is characterized by mental disorders—anhedonia, low mood and motivation, and loss of interest and pleasure, which can lead to suicide in severe cases [3]. The disease has a huge effect on people's standard of living, and some patients even become incapacitated and need constant care [4,5]. Apart from changes in mental state, depression in patients can be associated with cognitive impairment [6], sleep disorders [7], metabolic changes (hypercortisolemia, insulin, and leptin resistance leading to obesity, diabetes, and hypertension) [8,9]. The high prevalence of the disease, together with a negative effect on the patient's life, makes depression a socially significant disorder, and treatment of the disease is very important in modern psychiatry.

Treatment of depression in the world of psychiatry began in the 1950s with the accidental discovery of the first substances with a positive effect on mood—iproniazid [10] and imipramine [11]. Iproniazid and imipramine are able to increase 5-hydroxytryptamine (5-HT, serotonin) and norepinephrine (NE) brain level, which is what their antidepressant effect was associated with. The increase in 5-HT and NE concentration caused by iproniazid is achieved by inhibiting monoamine oxidase (MAO), an enzyme that metabolizes these biogenic amines, and by imipramine through the non-selective reuptake inhibition of these neurotransmitters [12]. Further, other antidepressants (ADs) were discovered with similar mechanisms of action and were combined into the MAO inhibitor (MAOI) and tricyclic antidepressant (TCA) groups. MAOIs and TCAs are the first-generation ADs. Today, first-generation ADs are practically not used in psychiatry, primarily due to the severe side effects. However, their discovery served as a foundation for the monoamine theory of depression, according to which monoamine depletion leads to the development of depression [13].

Since then, other ADs have been discovered that likewise affect the activity of monoamines. They are monoamine reuptake inhibitors (MRIs) that selectively block the reverse transport of the mediator into the neuron [12]: selective 5-HT reuptake inhibitors (SSRIs), e.g., fluoxetine; selective NE reuptake inhibitors (sNRIs), e.g., maprotiline; and selective dopamine (DA) reuptake inhibitors (SDRIs), e.g., bupropion. The other agents affect the metabolism of monoamines through the inhibition of MAO-A, e.g., moclobemide. So-called atypical ADs act mainly as ligands of monoamine receptors, e.g., mirtazapine or agomelatine [14]. Also, the antagonists of presynaptic 5-HT and NE receptors (e.g., mianserin) blocking the negative feedback regulatory mechanism of synaptic levels of monoamines are used in clinics.

The monoamine theory of depression has been dominant in psychiatry for decades. Not only classical monoamines themselves, but even other metabolites of their precursor amino acids, such as kynurenines originating from tryptophan, were implicated in depression [15,16]. Monoamine ADs are widely used in clinics and for a long time remained the leaders in terms of prescription [17]. However, the experimental basis for this hypothesis remains controversial [18]. Several studies show reduced levels of monoamines and their metabolites in the blood and cerebrospinal fluid of depressed patients [19–21], but post-mortem brain studies of patients and healthy individuals do not always correlate with these data [22]. Currently, a reliably confirmed point of the monoamine hypothesis is that the lack of 5-HT, DA, and NE does indeed worsen the course of the disease in depressed patients or those in remission, but is not capable of leading to depression, especially without burdened heredity [23]. In 2022, a comprehensive umbrella review was published refuting the link between 5-HT and depression and demonstrating no support for the hypothesis that depression is caused by lowered 5-HT activity or concentrations [24].

In addition, unresolved issues remain in the work of monoamine ADs. First of all, there is a clinical effect in the several weeks following the onset of drug taking. Second, a lot of patients (20–30%) with depression are resistant to treatment with these medications [15]. Moreover, even in the case of successful therapy, there is no guarantee that the patient will not develop resistance following long-term treatment [25].

These problems were solved by introducing ADs with a non-monoamine mechanism of action into clinical practice. In the 1990s, it became known that antagonists of the N-methyl-D-aspartate (NMDA) receptor, an ionotropic glutamate receptor, exhibit antidepressant activity [26]. Later, ketamine and esketamine, as well as other NMDA receptor antagonists, demonstrated rapid and long-lasting antidepressant effects for treatment-resistant depression [27].

In 2019 the first-in-class rapid-acting AD esketamine was approved by the Food and Drug Administration (FDA). The esketamine mechanism of action as well as ketamine (used off-label as AD) and dextromethorphan in combination with bupropion, recently approved by the FDA under the brand name Auvelity, seems to be associated with the blockade of NMDA receptors. These ADs are effective in the case of many patients resistant to the "traditional" ADs. These ADs are characterized by a fast onset of action and can be used in patients with a high risk of suicide. Despite the success of NMDA antagonists, it is important to understand that these agents can induce serious adverse reactions including addiction [28] and toxicity [29].

There is no universal treatment for depression, nor a mechanism that explains all aspects today. Due to this, the search for new drug targets and the study of pathogenesis still remains a relevant task. Currently, several substances are being tested in clinical trials for depression treatment. These include both agents affecting monoamine neurotransmission and those involving other systems [30]. As can be seen, pharmacotherapy for depression is gradually moving beyond the monoamine hypothesis, and unresolved difficulties stimulate the creation of new drugs.

In this review, we propose to consider trace amine-associated receptors (TAARs) as new promising pharmacological targets for the treatment of depression. Today, the study of TAARs is at the peak of its popularity, so it is very important to systematize existing information and provide new hypotheses. While there are excellent reviews showing the great potential of TAAR1 agonists in the treatment of depression [31,32], we extend these observations by including the most recent data on TAAR1 agonists and showing the potential of other TAARs as novel targets for the treatment of depression.

Here, we focused on the relationship of TAARs not only to monoamines, but also to adult neurogenesis, showing that all three systems mutually influence each other and contribute to the development and/or treatment of depression. Thus, we propose to direct further research in this area, considering it very promising. In addition, we go beyond the usual study of TAAR1 and show the potential of other receptors.

2. Neurogenesis and Its Association with Depression

Some gaps in the existing depression hypothesis can be filled by a theory linking altered hippocampal neurogenesis with the development of depression (Figure 1). Increasingly, the hippocampus is considered an area involved in the pathogenesis of depression and associated with cognitive and emotion formation processes. Moreover, healthy neurogenesis is required for depression treatment [33]. A lack of response to both drug therapy for depression (fluoxetine and imipramine) and alternative therapy (electroconvulsive antidepressant therapy [34], intermittent hypobaric hypoxia [35]) during neurogenesis ablation in animal models has been shown [36,37]. AD treatment (5-HT and NE reverse inhibitors) promotes neurogenesis by increasing cell proliferation, maturation, cell survival, dendritic growth, and neuronal plasticity [38]. In addition, neurogenesis can directly exert an antidepressant effect. The protective potential of activating and maintaining neurogenesis agents has been shown in mouse models of depression. For example, baicalin, a flavonoid with anti-inflammatory, anti-apoptotic, and neuroprotective functions, has demonstrated an antidepressant effect in the chronic unpredictable mild stress model [39].

The link between hippocampal neurogenesis and depression can be inferred in humans as well. It is known that cognitive dysfunction, in particular memory impairment, is a clear sign of depression. Studies of patients suffering from depression have revealed a decrease in the volume of the hippocampus, correlated with the severity and duration of the disease [40–42]. With stress-induced atrophy of the hippocampus, a decrease in the number of cells can contribute to the development of depression.

Having discussed the main points of the connection between depression and neurogenesis, it is important to note the role of monoamine systems in both of these processes. Monoamines are able to up- or downregulate neurogenesis by activating the corresponding G protein-coupled receptor (GPCR). As a rule, a decrease in cyclic adenosine monophosphate (cAMP) level through the activation of the Gi protein or an increase of phospholipase C through the activation of Gq leads to proliferative processes, while the stimulation of receptors associated with the activation of the Gs protein directs cells to the path of differentiation [43]. More recent studies show that the regulation of neurogenesis is related to the balance, or the ratio of up- and downregulating receptors involved in neurogenesis [44,45]. Receptors that stimulate different stages of neurogenesis include NE receptors (α1 [46], β3 [47]), DA receptors (D2-like receptors) [48], and 5-HT receptors (5-HT1A) [49].

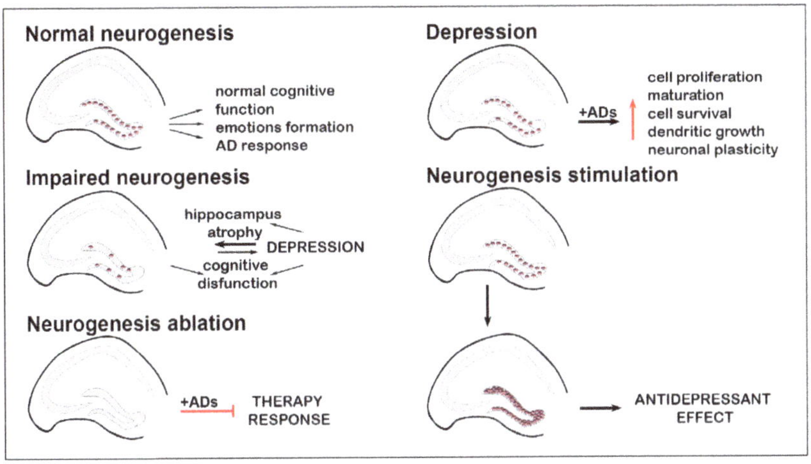

Figure 1. Interconnection between neurogenic processes and depression. Adult hippocampal neurogenesis is associated with emotion formation and cognitive function. Moreover, healthy adult neurogenesis is essential for response to antidepressant treatment. Impaired adult neurogenesis is associated with depression and cognitive decline. The priority of the processes is not yet clear. In the complete absence of adult neurogenesis, treatment with antidepressants is not effective. Antidepressant treatment enhances adult neurogenesis by increasing cell proliferation, maturation, and survival. The stimulation of adult neurogenesis leads to an antidepressant effect.

Neurogenic responses to ADs are also associated with the activation of certain monoamine GPCRs. Fluoxetine upregulates 5-HT1A receptors together with neurogenesis, suggesting that these processes could be related [33]. Rivastigmine activates neurogenesis and alleviates symptoms of depression in a mouse bulbectomy model by engaging the serotonin 5-HT1A receptor [50]. The β3-adrenergic receptor promotes the activation of neurogenic progenitors and stem cells [47]. During the activation of the D1 receptor by agonists, a neurogenic effect was observed, namely the increased proliferation and the survival of progenitor cells in the hippocampus of adult rats [51].

It is important to note that it is a chronic, but not acute, antidepressant treatment that has a neurogenic effect, which is consistent with the dynamics of human recovery. Moreover, the progress of the neurogenic process correlates with the success of therapy (rats). It has been shown that it is chronic rather than acute and subchronic, fluoxetine treatment which produces both antidepressant and neurogenic effects [52].

Together, the described data indicate the relationship between the development of depression and a decrease in neurogenesis. However, information is not yet sufficient to establish if neurogenesis is the cause of the development of depression or a consequence or just a coincidence. The neurogenic theory of depression may fill in the gaps in the monoamine theory. For example, to explain the delayed effect of ADs, it takes time to turn on neurogenic processes. It is possible that new hippocampal cells are able to overcome depression-induced atrophy [53] and serve as a new resource for the activation of brain plasticity and relearning, thus being the missing link in the response to ADs.

As depression is a complicated and heterogeneous disease with a complex etiology, more than one system is likely involved in its development. With further studies, more information is gathered suggesting that the monoamines and neurogenesis are not the only systems that are altered in depression and there could be other brain processes involved, possibly by influencing both those systems.

3. The Family of TAARs—A New Target for Depression Therapy?

3.1. Trace Amines

One of the intriguing players potentially involved in mood regulation is an endogenous compound's group of trace amines (TAs). TAs such as beta-phenylethylamine, tyramine, tryptamine, octopamine, synephrine, and many other biogenic amines are present in mammalian tissues at nanomolar (0.1–10 nM) trace concentrations [54,55]. Generally, many TAs are the products of decarboxylation of precursor amino acids by the enzyme aromatic L-amino acid decarboxylase and are metabolized by MAO-A and MAO-B [56]. In addition to being structurally similar to classical biogenic amines (DA, 5-HT, and NE), TAs are metabolically closely related to these neurotransmitter systems, where they are widely present. Along with these mediators, TAs seem to participate in the regulation of emotional behaviors, mood, thoughts, or perception [57–59].

TAs can function as neurotransmitters within their own unique signal transduction system, but in the aspect of depression, the work of TAs as co-transmitters and modulators of classical monoamines is intriguing [52]. At their physiological concentration, TAs are able to change a cell's responses to other neurotransmitters [56]. The modulation of postsynaptic transmission of NE and DA by beta-phenylethylamine and the potentiation of NE and DA responses in neurons by tryptamine are already well known [59,60]. Due to the ability of TAs to affect monoamine neurotransmission and their presence in monoamine regions of the mammalian brain, they are of great interest to psychiatry.

To clarify the role of TAs in the pathogenesis of depression, a number of studies were conducted to study the content of TAs and their metabolites. Thus, several studies have demonstrated that in depressed patients suffering from bipolar affective disorder, urinary excretion of beta-phenylethylamine is reduced [61–64], while in patients in the manic phase, on the contrary, it is increased [65]. Phenylethylamine deficiency in people with depression was confirmed by examining their cerebrospinal fluid. A reduced content of phenylacetic acid, a metabolite of beta-phenylethylamine, was found in the cerebrospinal fluid [66]. A similar decrease in the content of some other TAs in the blood plasma, cerebrospinal fluid, and urine of patients with depression is also known [67–69]. In turn, treatment with TCAs (clomipramine) in depressed patients who had reduced renal excretion of phenylethylamine led to both the disappearance of clinical symptoms and an increase in beta-phenylethylamine levels to normal values [62,65]. Furthermore, the use of beta-phenylethylamine precursor phenylalanine alone or in combination with other ADs led to progress in therapy in previously unresponsive patients [70]. It is worth noting that there are a sufficient number of studies in which researchers were unable to detect a connection between affective diseases and the TA content in biological fluids [71]. For example, renal excretion of tryptamine increased during treatment with imipramine in patients with depression, but it was not possible to identify a correlation between an increase in the level of this amine and an improvement in the clinical picture [72]. Based on these data, one can speculate about the role of TAs in the pathogenesis of depression. These data even gave rise to a hypothesis about the involvement of beta-phenylethylamine, and later other TAs, in the formation of depression [71]. However, these research projects were carried out in the second half of last century, and the results are multidirectional and contradictory, so a comprehensive, uniform, and detailed study of this issue is required.

3.2. TAAR1 Agonists Are New Generation Antipsychotics

The study of TAs reached a new level after the discovery of the so-called trace amine-associated receptors, TAARs. TAARs are a family of GPCR receptors that induce the classical cAMP cascade and activation of downstream targets. In vertebrates, there are nine TAAR subfamilies expressed both in the central nervous system and in the periphery [49]. TAARs have functional interspecies differences due to pseudogenization events and species-specific expansions. In humans, there are six functional types of TAARs—TAAR1, TAAR2, TAAR5, TAAR6, TAAR8, and TAAR9 receptors, with TAAR3, TAAR4, and TAAR7 receptors being pseudogenes [73]. The genes encoding TAARs form a cluster on chromosome 6 at band q23.2, which has been identified as a susceptibility locus for schizophrenia in humans [74].

The best known and most frequently studied of those, TAAR1, is already being actively investigated in the aspect of mental and neuropsychiatric disorders [75]. The ability of TAAR1 to regulate DA and 5-HT as well as glutamatergic neurotransmission formed the basis of this interest [55]. Moreover, TAAR1 is widely represented in the limbic and monoamine systems of the brain, which are responsible for psychotic states, mood, attention, memory, fear, and addiction [73]. In addition, *taar1* mutations disrupting the receptor's function were found in people diagnosed with schizophrenia [76]. It is possible that carriers of such genes are more at risk of schizophrenia and require activation of the subfunctional receptor [77].

The discovery of selective TAAR1 agonists made it possible to elucidate the functional significance and therapeutic potential of the receptor in more detail. Starting with RO5256390, new partial or full TAAR1 agonists with high affinity and selectivity for TAAR1 have been created and studied [78]. Initially, TAAR1 agonists were considered for the treatment of schizophrenia [79,80]. Researchers have already shown their effectiveness against the positive, negative (lack of motivation, anhedonia), and cognitive symptoms of schizophrenia, which are often overlooked by typical antipsychotics [64]. The most successful new psychotropic drug is SEP-363856 (SEP-856, trade name Ulotaront), a TAAR1 receptor agonist with low 5-HT1A activity [81]. Ulotaront has already passed the second phase of clinical trials in the treatment of schizophrenia, which led to FDA designation as a Breakthrough Therapy for this indication [82]. The unique mechanism of action avoids the side effects of typical D2 antagonist antipsychotics (extrapyramidal symptoms, weight gain), reduces substance abuse cravings, and relieves depressive symptoms [83]. Thus, therapy based on TAAR1 activation has proven to be an excellent alternative to antipsychotics for patients who do not respond to therapy or refuse it due to the severe side effects. Early evidence suggests that TAAR1 activation does not cause the side effects associated with typical antipsychotics [84]. However, more studies are needed to ascertain their safety and tolerability.

3.3. TAAR1 Agonists Are New Generation Antidepressants

Today, TAAR1 agonists have already been comprehensively studied and are of great value in the aspect of drug addiction, mental and metabolic diseases. Interestingly, it was found that TAAR1 agonists also exhibit useful properties for the treatment of depression [31]. For instance, TAAR1 agonists RO5256390, RO5203648, and RO5263397, in addition to antipsychotic actions, have demonstrated in vivo improvement in the sleep–wake cycle [85,86], reduction in drug cravings [87,88], and procognitive properties [89–91]. The direct antidepressant potential is indicated by work on the forced swimming test in rodents. It was shown that RO5263397 and RO5203648 treatment led to dose-dependent immobility time reduction in forced swimming tests [86–88]. The TAAR1 full agonist RO5256390 was not found to have any effects on depressive-like behavior in the same test [92].

It is significant that Ulotaront has also demonstrated an antidepressant effect in rodent and non-human primate tests [93]. In rats, behavioral tests of Ulotaront have shown that its efficacy in attenuated social withdrawal is comparable to that of clozapine. In forced swimming tests, mice have demonstrated immobility time reduction. On par with the above-mentioned agonists, Ulotaront exerts REM sleep suppression, improving the sleep–wake cycle [94]. Ulotaront is currently undergoing a phase 2/3 clinical trial testing its safety and efficacy in the treatment of major depressive disorder and generalized anxiety disorder and in adults [95]. In addition to the good isolated effect of Ulotaront, in combination with Duloxetine (5-HT and NE dual reuptake inhibitor), tests showed better results in experimental animals. Therefore, the synergy of TAAR1 and monoamines can be a powerful tool to improve AD action [96].

Another TAAR1 agonist, o-PIT (o-phenyl-iodotyramine), also confirms the antidepressant potential of TAAR1. In forced swimming tests, wild-type mice (but not TAAR1 knockout (KO) mice) have demonstrated immobility time reduction in a dose-dependent manner [97].

Based on data from the acute and chronic administration of RO5256390, the TAAR1 activation antidepressant effect is supposed to be associated with increased 5-HT and DA neurotransmission in the dorsal raphe nucleus and the ventral tegmental area, respectively. During acute exposure of RO5256390, an increased extracellular 5-HT and DA leads to activation of the 5-HT1A and D2 receptors, and during chronic exposure, desensitization of these receptors occurs [98]. Interestingly, the same mechanism of action is characteristic of monoamine ADs. For example, the acute administration of SSRIs also inhibits, and chronic administration stimulates, the firing rate of 5-HT neurons [99].

In addition, convincing evidence is emerging that TAAR1 is involved in the regulation of neurogenesis. According to transcriptomic data, TAAR1 is expressed in the murine and human hippocampus [100]. The ligands of TAAR1, beta-phenylethylamine and T1AM (3-Iodothyronamine), were shown to have a positive effect on neurogenesis [101,102]. Phenylethylamine is able to regulate BDNF levels and restore the number of hippocampal dendritic spines in the cortisol-induced depression mouse model [103].

Another piece of evidence comes from recent work showing a connection between TAAR1, neurogenesis, and depression [104]. The study demonstrated that TAAR1 in the hippocampal dentate gyrus mediates the effects of chronic stress on neurogenesis, hippocampal plasticity, and cognitive function in mice. Mice in the chronic social defeat stress model had reduced levels of TAAR1 mRNA and impairments in hippocampal neurogenesis and cognitive function. Interestingly, the effects of stress were neutralized by the administration of the TAAR1 agonist, RO5263397. Moreover, selective knockout of the taar1 gene in the dentate gyrus mimicked cognitive and neurogenic deficits caused by chronic stress [104].

In summary, although TAAR1 agonists are primarily considered antipsychotics, they have significant antidepressant potential. As the direct antidepressant effect has been shown in a few tests, they have demonstrated a line of useful properties for depression treatment. Among them are procognitive functions and improved sleep. Moreover, TAAR1 agonists attract the attention of clinicians due to the absence of severe side effects. Therefore, it is advisable to continue studying the antidepressant properties of TAAR1 and other TAARs.

3.4. *"Olfactory" TAARs in the Treatment of Depression: Perspectives*

The remaining TAARs (TAAR2-TAAR9) are primarily known as olfactory receptors sensing innate odors mediated by volatile amines originating from the decarboxylation of amino acids [105]. They are found in the olfactory epithelium and olfactory bulbs of mammals and activate innate behaviors. However, as studies progress, it becomes clear that the effect of "olfactory" TAARs is not limited to the detection of volatile and aversive amines from outside of the body and, along with TAAR1, can become a target for the treatment of mental illness, in particular depression (Figure 2).

Gradually accumulating transcriptomic data makes it possible to associate TAARs with the regulation of emotions, as they were shown to be expressed in the limbic areas [100]. Also, based on transcriptome data, it is hypothesized that TAARs may be involved in the pathogenesis of mental illness [100,106]. Several studies have identified the association of not only *taar1* but also *taar2*, *taar5*, and *taar6* SNPs (single nucleotide polymorphisms) with schizophrenia and bipolar disorder [77]. Mutations in the *taar6* gene may be associated with the severity of depression and the effectiveness of response to therapy [107]. Moreover, it turned out that TAAR5 expression in the prefrontal cortex may be impaired in patients with depression [108]. Thus, "olfactory" TAARs are of great interest for a more detailed and large-scale study in the context of mental illness.

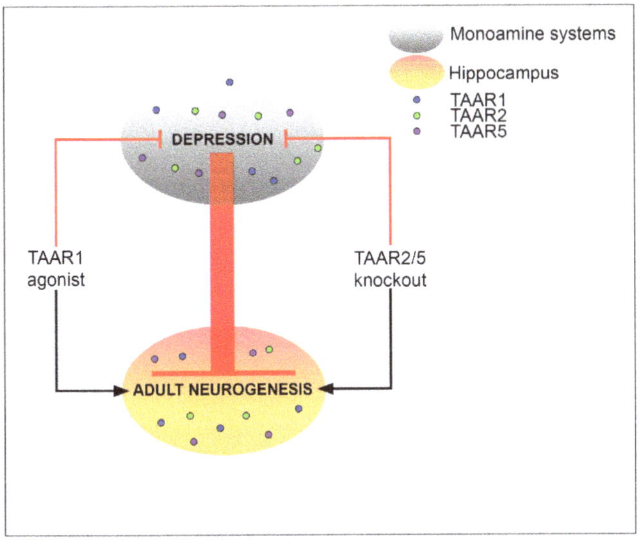

Figure 2. TAARs in depression and adult hippocampal neurogenesis. The pathogenesis of depression is closely related to the monoamine systems of the brain. TAAR1, TAAR2, and TAAR5 were found in the monoamine nuclei of the brain and in the hippocampus, the center of neurogenesis. Depression inhibits adult neurogenesis. TAAR1 agonists have an antidepressant effect and promote neurogenesis. TAAR2 and TAAR5 knockout animals exhibit decreased depressive-like behavior and increased adult neurogenesis.

TAAR2 and TAAR5 are currently the most studied of the "olfactory" TAARs and appear to have similar functional significance. To date, TAAR2 and TAAR5 have been found not only in the olfactory system but also in the limbic region of the mammalian brain and some monoamine nuclei. Histochemical methods have shown that both TAAR2 and TAAR5 are expressed in the hippocampus, the nuclei of the thalamus and hypothalamus, and the piriform cortex. In addition, TAAR5 was found in the amygdala, orbitofrontal cortex, nucleus accumbens, entorhinal cortex [109], and neurogenic niches—the subventricular zone [110]. TAAR2 was found in the lateral habenula and raphe nuclei [111]. The expression of other TAARs (most prominently TAAR5 and TAAR6) in the murine and human hippocampus and other limbic regions was also documented based on the analysis of public transcriptomic data [100,108,112]. In further studies in knockout (KO) mice, other properties of TAAR2 and TAAR5 were found that bring them closer to the pathogenesis of depression. There is accumulating evidence of a relationship between the TAARs and the monoamine system. Of particular interest is the increased DA level and its metabolites in the striatum in TAAR2-KO and TAAR5-KO mice, as well as the increased number of tyrosine hydroxylase-positive neurons in the substantia nigra pars compacta. These changes complement the increase in the content of growth factors: BDNF in the striatum in TAAR2-KO and GDNF in TAAR5-KO [110,111]. Behavioral changes in TAAR KO mice also support their emotional role and association with monoamines. In particular, TAAR5-KO and TAAR2-KO mice exhibited less anxious and depressive behavior in several behavioral tests [109,110]. Behavioral changes might also be connected to the 5-HT system. In TAAR5-KO mice, the level of 5-HT in the striatum and hippocampus is reduced, and 5-hydroxyindoleacetic acid is reduced in the hippocampus and hypothalamus. It is thus possible that the lack of TAAR5 affects the functional state of the brain 5-HT system [109]. This relationship is confirmed by the altered cognitive profile of TAAR5-KO. TAAR5-KO mice showed fewer errors, better execution speed, and higher learning progress [113].

Perhaps the most intriguing characteristic of TAAR2-KO and TAAR5-KO mice is the increased adult neurogenesis. In both models, an increased number of neurogenic markers, namely proliferating cell nuclear antigen (PCNA), and doublecortin (DCX) in the subventricular and the subgranular zone, were found compared to wild-type [107,108]. Intriguingly, the expression of several TAARs including TAAR2 and TAAR5 was found during the differentiation of human pluripotent stem cells to dopaminergic neurons [114].

The discovery of TAAR expression in the limbic and monoamine regions opens up new possibilities for their use for therapeutic purposes. However, one should not forget about their predominantly olfactory localization. It is the simultaneous representation of TAARs in both the olfactory and limbic systems that may be a key advantage for the treatment of mental illness, primarily depression. The olfactory system plays an important role in the functioning of the limbic system. By receiving olfactory inputs, the limbic region of the brain corrects emotional responses and species-specific behavior [115,116]. The relationship of these two systems is also indicated by the consequences of bulbectomy in mice. Removal of the olfactory bulbs leads to the manifestation of depression-like behavior and a decrease in neurogenesis [117]. At the same time, anosmia in humans is an early prognostic sign of various neurodegenerative and mental diseases and their symptoms [118]. Interestingly, TAAR2- and TAAR5-KO mice exhibit anti-anxiety and antidepressant behavior concomitantly with increased neurogenesis. The only non-selective TAAR5 agonist known to date, α-NETA, induces psychotic-like episodes in mice [119]. Such consequences of the absence of TAARs suggest the antidepressant potential of their antagonists. The search for such TAAR5 antagonists has already started [120].

Together, these data can be justification for considering "olfactory" TAARs and related neurotransmitter systems a new target for depression therapy and the further study of them in terms of this disease [121].

4. Conclusions

The accumulated data allow us to consider TAARs a promising new target for the treatment of mental and nervous diseases. Agonists of TAAR1, the most frequently studied of the receptors, are already in clinical trials as an antipsychotic, antidepressant, and anxiolytic drug. Exposure to TAAR1 agonists causes an antipsychotic effect but is not accompanied by serious side effects characteristic of typical antipsychotics. In addition, they have shown high efficacy against the negative and cognitive symptoms of schizophrenia, including the antidepressant effect. Other members of the TAAR family, the so-called "olfactory" TAARs, have also shown antidepressant potential. Animal studies have shown that TAAR2-KO and TAAR5-KO have an anti-anxiety and antidepressant phenotype and, like TAAR1, have a modulating effect on the brain's monoamine systems. In addition, the localization of TAARs in the limbic and monoamine systems of the mammalian brain, which are associated with the formation of emotions and mood, motivation, and cognitive functions, has recently become known. Against the background of these facts, changes in neurogenic processes during the blockade of TAAR1, TAAR2, and TAAR5 seem to be an extremely intriguing and promising detail. In summary, a detailed study of TAARs could help clarify aspects of depression pathogenesis and identify cause-and-effect relationships in its development. Probably, TAARs are in fact the missing link between depression, neurogenesis, and the monoamine system.

In addition, drugs based on TAAR agonists could become a panacea for vulnerable groups of the population, adolescents, the elderly, and pregnant women. For these groups, mental disease therapy is associated with risks and remains poorly studied. Given the good tolerability of TAAR1 agonists, it is necessary to expand the study of their use. The absence of serious side effects makes these drugs extremely attractive. Thus, it is necessary to continue the study of TAARs, and to look for TAAR agonists and antagonists to better understand their therapeutic properties.

Author Contributions: Conceptualization, T.S.S. and R.R.G.; formal analysis, T.S.S., E.V.E. and R.R.G.; investigation, T.S.S. and R.R.G.; writing—original draft preparation, T.S.S.; writing—review and editing, T.S.S., E.V.E. and R.R.G.; supervision, R.R.G.; project administration, R.R.G.; funding acquisition, R.R.G. All authors have read and agreed to the published version of the manuscript.

Funding: This research was funded by the Russian Science Foundation grant 19-75-30008-P (to R.R.G.).

Data Availability Statement: Not applicable.

Acknowledgments: We are grateful to Accellena LLC (Russia) for the continuous support of our research. The authors have no affiliation with this organization, nor hold any shares therein, and received no compensation for the present review article.

Conflicts of Interest: The authors declare no conflicts of interest.

References

1. Ferrari, A.J.; Charlson, F.J.; Norman, R.E.; Patten, S.B.; Freedman, G.; Murray, C.J.L.; Vos, T.; Whiteford, H.A. Burden of Depressive Disorders by Country, Sex, Age, and Year: Findings from the Global Burden of Disease Study 2010. *PLoS Med.* **2013**, *10*, e1001547. [CrossRef] [PubMed]
2. Abdallah, C.G.; Adams, T.G.; Kelmendi, B.; Esterlis, I.; Sanacora, G.; Krystal, J.H. Ketamine's mechanism of action: A path to rapid-acting antidepressants. *Depress. Anxiety* **2016**, *33*, 689–697. [CrossRef] [PubMed]
3. Ruderfer, D.M.; Walsh, C.G.; Aguirre, M.W.; Tanigawa, Y.; Ribeiro, J.D.; Franklin, J.C.; Rivas, M.A. Significant Shared Heritability Underlies Suicide Attempt and Clinically Predicted Probability of Attempting Suicide. *Mol. Psychiatry* **2020**, *25*, 2422–2430. [CrossRef] [PubMed]
4. Lindeman, L.M.; Abramson, L.Y. The Mental Simulation of Motor Incapacity in Depression. *J. Cogn. Psychother.* **2008**, *22*, 228–249. [CrossRef]
5. Millward, L.J.; Lutte, A.; Purvis, R.G. Depression and the Perpetuation of an Incapacitated Identity as an Inhibitor of Return to Work. *J. Psychiatr. Ment. Health Nurs.* **2005**, *12*, 565–573. [CrossRef] [PubMed]
6. Fehnel, S.E.; Forsyth, B.H.; DiBenedetti, D.B.; Danchenko, N.; François, C.; Brevig, T. Patient-Centered Assessment of Cognitive Symptoms of Depression. *CNS Spectr.* **2016**, *21*, 43–52. [CrossRef]
7. Nutt, D.; Wilson, S.; Paterson, L. Sleep Disorders as Core Symptoms of Depression. *Dialogues Clin. Neurosci.* **2008**, *10*, 329–336. [CrossRef] [PubMed]
8. Skilton, M.R.; Moulin, P.; Terra, J.-L.; Bonnet, F. Associations Between Anxiety, Depression, and the Metabolic Syndrome. *Biol. Psychiatry* **2007**, *62*, 1251–1257. [CrossRef] [PubMed]
9. Marazziti, D.; Rutigliano, G.; Baroni, S.; Landi, P.; Dell'Osso, L. Metabolic Syndrome and Major Depression. *CNS Spectr.* **2014**, *19*, 293–304. [CrossRef]
10. Loomer, H.P.; Saunders, J.C.; Kline, N.S. A Clinical and Pharmacodynamic Evaluation of Iproniazid as a Psychic Energizer. *Psychiatr. Res. Rep. Am. Psychiatr. Assoc.* **1957**, *8*, 129–141.
11. Kuhn, R. The Treatment of Depressive States with g 22355 (Imipramine Hydrochloride). *Am. J. Psychiatry* **1958**, *115*, 459–464. [CrossRef] [PubMed]
12. Ramachandraih, C.T.; Subramanyam, N.; Bar, K.J.; Baker, G.; Yeragani, V.K. Antidepressants: From MAOIs to SSRIs and More. *Indian J. Psychiatry* **2011**, *53*, 180–182. [CrossRef] [PubMed]
13. Delgado, P.L. Depression: The Case for a Monoamine Deficiency. *J. Clin. Psychiatry* **2000**, *61*, 7–11. [PubMed]
14. Mantas, I.; Saarinen, M.; Xu, Z.-Q.D.; Svenningsson, P. Update on GPCR-Based Targets for the Development of Novel Antidepressants. *Mol. Psychiatry* **2022**, *27*, 534–558. [CrossRef] [PubMed]
15. Tanaka, M.; Bohár, Z.; Martos, D.; Telegdy, G.; Vécsei, L. Antidepressant-like Effects of Kynurenic Acid in a Modified Forced Swim Test. *Pharmacol. Rep. PR* **2020**, *72*, 449–455. [CrossRef]
16. Tanaka, M.; Szabó, Á.; Spekker, E.; Polyák, H.; Tóth, F.; Vécsei, L. Mitochondrial Impairment: A Common Motif in Neuropsychiatric Presentation? The Link to the Tryptophan-Kynurenine Metabolic System. *Cells* **2022**, *11*, 2607. [CrossRef]
17. Al-Harbi, K.S. Treatment-Resistant Depression: Therapeutic Trends, Challenges, and Future Directions. Patient Prefer. *Adherence* **2012**, *6*, 369–388. [CrossRef] [PubMed]
18. Cowen, P.J.; Browning, M. What Has Serotonin to Do with Depression? *World Psychiatry* **2015**, *14*, 158–160. [CrossRef]
19. Paul-Savoie, É.; Potvin, S.; Daigle, K.; Normand, E.; Corbin, J.-F.; Gagnon, R.; Marchand, S. A Deficit in Peripheral Serotonin Levels in Major Depressive Disorder but Not in Chronic Widespread Pain. *Clin. J. Pain* **2011**, *27*, 529–534. [CrossRef]
20. Ogawa, S.; Tsuchimine, S.; Kunugi, H. Cerebrospinal Fluid Monoamine Metabolite Concentrations in Depressive Disorder: A Meta-Analysis of Historic Evidence. *J. Psychiatr. Res.* **2018**, *105*, 137–146. [CrossRef]
21. Pech, J.; Forman, J.; Kessing, L.V.; Knorr, U. Poor Evidence for Putative Abnormalities in Cerebrospinal Fluid Neurotransmitters in Patients with Depression versus Healthy Non-Psychiatric Individuals: A Systematic Review and Meta-Analyses of 23 Studies. *J. Affect. Disord.* **2018**, *240*, 6–16. [CrossRef] [PubMed]

22. Rajkowska, G. Postmortem Studies in Mood Disorders Indicate Altered Numbers of Neurons and Glial Cells. *Biol. Psychiatry* **2000**, *48*, 766–777. [CrossRef] [PubMed]
23. Ruhé, H.G.; Mason, N.S.; Schene, A.H. Mood Is Indirectly Related to Serotonin, Norepinephrine and Dopamine Levels in Humans: A Meta-Analysis of Monoamine Depletion Studies. *Mol. Psychiatry* **2007**, *12*, 331–359. [CrossRef] [PubMed]
24. Moncrieff, J.; Cooper, R.E.; Stockmann, T.; Amendola, S.; Hengartner, M.P.; Horowitz, M.A. The Serotonin Theory of Depression: A Systematic Umbrella Review of the Evidence. *Mol. Psychiatry* **2022**, *28*, 3243–3256. [CrossRef] [PubMed]
25. Souery, D.; Serretti, A.; Calati, R.; Oswald, P.; Massat, I.; Konstantinidis, A.; Linotte, S.; Bollen, J.; Demyttenaere, K.; Kasper, S.; et al. Switching Antidepressant Class Does Not Improve Response or Remission in Treatment-Resistant Depression. *J. Clin. Psychopharmacol.* **2011**, *31*, 512–516. [CrossRef] [PubMed]
26. Trullas, R.; Skolnick, P. Functional Antagonists at the NMDA Receptor Complex Exhibit Antidepressant Actions. *Eur. J. Pharmacol.* **1990**, *185*, 1–10. [CrossRef] [PubMed]
27. Berman, R.M.; Cappiello, A.; Anand, A.; Oren, D.A.; Heninger, G.R.; Charney, D.S.; Krystal, J.H. Antidepressant Effects of Ketamine in Depressed Patients. *Biol. Psychiatry* **2000**, *47*, 351–354. [CrossRef] [PubMed]
28. Liu, Y.; Lin, D.; Wu, B.; Zhou, W. Ketamine Abuse Potential and Use Disorder. *Brain Res. Bull.* **2016**, *126*, 68–73. [CrossRef] [PubMed]
29. Schep, L.J.; Slaughter, R.J.; Watts, M.; Mackenzie, E.; Gee, P. The Clinical Toxicology of Ketamine. *Clin. Toxicol.* **2023**, *61*, 415–428. [CrossRef]
30. Chen, T.; Cheng, L.; Ma, J.; Yuan, J.; Pi, C.; Xiong, L.; Chen, J.; Liu, H.; Tang, J.; Zhong, Y.; et al. Molecular Mechanisms of Rapid-Acting Antidepressants: New Perspectives for Developing Antidepressants. *Pharmacol. Res.* **2023**, *194*, 106837. [CrossRef]
31. Alnefeesi, Y.; Tamura, J.K.; Lui, L.M.W.; Jawad, M.Y.; Ceban, F.; Ling, S.; Nasri, F.; Rosenblat, J.D.; McIntyre, R.S. Trace Amine-Associated Receptor 1 (TAAR1): Potential Application in Mood Disorders: A Systematic Review. *Neurosci. Biobehav. Rev.* **2021**, *131*, 192–210. [CrossRef] [PubMed]
32. Le, G.H.; Gillissie, E.S.; Rhee, T.G.; Cao, B.; Alnefeesi, Y.; Guo, Z.; Di Vincenzo, J.D.; Jawad, M.Y.; March, A.M.; Ramachandra, R.; et al. Efficacy, Safety, and Tolerability of Ulotaront (SEP-363856, a Trace Amine-Associated Receptor 1 Agonist) for the Treatment of Schizophrenia and Other Mental Disorders: A Systematic Review of Preclinical and Clinical Trials. Expert Opin. *Investig. Drugs* **2023**, *32*, 401–415. [CrossRef]
33. Santarelli, L.; Saxe, M.; Gross, C.; Surget, A.; Battaglia, F.; Dulawa, S.; Weisstaub, N.; Lee, J.; Duman, R.; Arancio, O.; et al. Requirement of Hippocampal Neurogenesis for the Behavioral Effects of Antidepressants. *Science* **2003**, *301*, 805–809. [CrossRef] [PubMed]
34. Schloesser, R.J.; Orvoen, S.; Jimenez, D.V.; Hardy, N.F.; Maynard, K.R.; Sukumar, M.; Manji, H.K.; Gardier, A.M.; David, D.J.; Martinowich, K. Antidepressant-like Effects of Electroconvulsive Seizures Require Adult Neurogenesis in a Neuroendocrine Model of Depression. *Brain Stimul.* **2015**, *8*, 862–867. [CrossRef] [PubMed]
35. Zhu, X.-H.; Yan, H.-C.; Zhang, J.; Qu, H.-D.; Qiu, X.-S.; Chen, L.; Li, S.-J.; Cao, X.; Bean, J.C.; Chen, L.-H.; et al. Intermittent Hypoxia Promotes Hippocampal Neurogenesis and Produces Antidepressant-Like Effects in Adult Rats. *J. Neurosci.* **2010**, *30*, 12653–12663. [CrossRef] [PubMed]
36. Surget, A.; Saxe, M.; Leman, S.; Ibarguen-Vargas, Y.; Chalon, S.; Griebel, G.; Hen, R.; Belzung, C. Drug-Dependent Requirement of Hippocampal Neurogenesis in a Model of Depression and of Antidepressant Reversal. *Biol. Psychiatry* **2008**, *64*, 293–301. [CrossRef] [PubMed]
37. Perera, T.D.; Dwork, A.J.; Keegan, K.A.; Thirumangalakudi, L.; Lipira, C.M.; Joyce, N.; Lange, C.; Higley, J.D.; Rosoklija, G.; Hen, R.; et al. Necessity of Hippocampal Neurogenesis for the Therapeutic Action of Antidepressants in Adult Nonhuman Primates. *PLoS ONE* **2011**, *6*, e17600. [CrossRef] [PubMed]
38. Pechnick, R.N.; Zonis, S.; Wawrowsky, K.; Cosgayon, R.; Farrokhi, C.; Lacayo, L.; Chesnokova, V. Antidepressants Stimulate Hippocampal Neurogenesis by Inhibiting P21 Expression in the Subgranular Zone of the Hipppocampus. *PLoS ONE* **2011**, *6*, e27290. [CrossRef] [PubMed]
39. Xiao, Z.; Cao, Z.; Yang, J.; Jia, Z.; Du, Y.; Sun, G.; Lu, Y.; Pei, L. Baicalin Promotes Hippocampal Neurogenesis via the Wnt/β-Catenin Pathway in a Chronic Unpredictable Mild Stress-Induced Mouse Model of Depression. *Biochem. Pharmacol.* **2021**, *190*, 114594. [CrossRef]
40. Svanum, S.; Ehrmann, L.C. Screening for Maladjustment in College Students: An Application of Receiver Operating Characteristic Curve to MMPI Scales. *J. Pers. Assess.* **1993**, *60*, 397–410. [CrossRef]
41. Videbech, P. Hippocampal Volume and Depression: A Meta-Analysis of MRI Studies. *Am. J. Psychiatry* **2004**, *161*, 1957–1966. [CrossRef] [PubMed]
42. Campbell, S.; Marriott, M.; Nahmias, C.; MacQueen, G.M. Lower Hippocampal Volume in Patients Suffering from Depression: A Meta-Analysis. Am. *J. Psychiatry* **2004**, *161*, 598–607. [CrossRef] [PubMed]
43. Lauder, J.M. Neurotransmitters as Growth Regulatory Signals: Role of Receptors and Second Messengers. *Trends Neurosci.* **1993**, *16*, 233–240. [CrossRef] [PubMed]
44. Doze, V.A.; Perez, D.M. G-Protein-Coupled Receptors in Adult Neurogenesis. *Pharmacol. Rev.* **2012**, *64*, 645–675. [CrossRef] [PubMed]

45. Jhaveri, D.J.; Nanavaty, I.; Prosper, B.W.; Marathe, S.; Husain, B.F.A.; Kernie, S.G.; Bartlett, P.F.; Vaidya, V.A. Opposing Effects of A2- and β-Adrenergic Receptor Stimulation on Quiescent Neural Precursor Cell Activity and Adult Hippocampal Neurogenesis. *PLoS ONE* **2014**, *9*, e98736. [CrossRef] [PubMed]
46. Hiramoto, T.; Ihara, Y.; Watanabe, Y. α-1 Adrenergic Receptors Stimulation Induces the Proliferation of Neural Progenitor Cells in Vitro. *Neurosci. Lett.* **2006**, *408*, 25–28. [CrossRef] [PubMed]
47. Jhaveri, D.J.; Mackay, E.W.; Hamlin, A.S.; Marathe, S.V.; Nandam, L.S.; Vaidya, V.A.; Bartlett, P.F. Norepinephrine Directly Activates Adult Hippocampal Precursors via 3-Adrenergic Receptors. *J. Neurosci.* **2010**, *30*, 2795–2806. [CrossRef] [PubMed]
48. Kim, Y.; Wang, W.-Z.; Comte, I.; Pastrana, E.; Tran, P.B.; Brown, J.; Miller, R.J.; Doetsch, F.; Molnár, Z.; Szele, F.G. Dopamine Stimulation of Postnatal Murine Subventricular Zone Neurogenesis via the D3 Receptor: D3R Promotes SVZ Neurogenesis. *J. Neurochem.* **2010**, *114*, 750–760. [CrossRef] [PubMed]
49. Grabiec, M.; Turlejski, K.; Djavadian, R.L. The Partial 5-HT1A Receptor Agonist Buspirone Enhances Neurogenesis in the Opossum (Monodelphis Domestica). *Eur. Neuropsychopharmacol.* **2009**, *19*, 431–439. [CrossRef]
50. Islam, M.R.; Moriguchi, S.; Tagashira, H.; Fukunaga, K. Rivastigmine Improves Hippocampal Neurogenesis and Depression-like Behaviors via 5-HT1A Receptor Stimulation in Olfactory Bulbectomized Mice. *Neuroscience* **2014**, *272*, 116–130. [CrossRef]
51. Takamura, N.; Nakagawa, S.; Masuda, T.; Boku, S.; Kato, A.; Song, N.; An, Y.; Kitaichi, Y.; Inoue, T.; Koyama, T.; et al. The Effect of Dopamine on Adult Hippocampal Neurogenesis. *Prog. Neuropsychopharmacol. Biol. Psychiatry* **2014**, *50*, 116–124. [CrossRef] [PubMed]
52. Marcussen, A.B.; Flagstad, P.; Kristjansen, P.E.G.; Johansen, F.F.; Englund, U. Increase in Neurogenesis and Behavioural Benefit after Chronic Fluoxetine Treatment in Wistar Rats. *Acta Neurol. Scand.* **2007**, *117*, 94–100. [CrossRef] [PubMed]
53. Malberg, J.E.; Eisch, A.J.; Nestler, E.J.; Duman, R.S. Chronic Antidepressant Treatment Increases Neurogenesis in Adult Rat Hippocampus. *J. Neurosci.* **2000**, *20*, 9104–9110. [CrossRef] [PubMed]
54. Boulton, A.A.; Juorio, A.V. Brain Trace Amines. In *Chemical and Cellular Architecture*; Lajtha, A., Ed.; Springer: Boston, MA, USA, 1982; pp. 189–222, ISBN 978-1-4757-0616-1.
55. Berry, M.D.; Gainetdinov, R.R.; Hoener, M.C.; Shahid, M. Pharmacology of Human Trace Amine-Associated Receptors: Therapeutic Opportunities and Challenges. *Pharmacol. Ther.* **2017**, *180*, 161–180. [CrossRef] [PubMed]
56. Yang, H.-Y.T.; Neff, N.H. β-Phenylethylamine: A Specific Substrate for Type B Monoamine Oxidase Of Brain. *J. Pharmacol. Exp. Ther.* **1973**, *187*, 365–371. Available online: https://jpet.aspetjournals.org/content/187/2/365.short (accessed on 31 December 2022). [PubMed]
57. Philips, S.R.; Rozdilsky, B.; Boulton, A.A. Evidence for the Presence of M-Tyramine, p-Tyramine, Tryptamine, and Phenylethylamine in the Rat Brain and Several Areas of the Human Brain. *Biol. Psychiatry* **1978**, *13*, 51–57. [PubMed]
58. Philips, S.R. Analysis of Trace Amines: Endogenous Levels and the Effects of Various Drugs on Tissue Concentrations in the Rat. In *Neurobiology of the Trace Amines: Analytical, Physiological, Pharmacological, Behavioral, and Clinical Aspects*; Boulton, A.A., Baker, G.B., Dewhurst, W.G., Sandler, M., Eds.; Humana Press: Totowa, NJ, USA, 1984; pp. 127–143, ISBN 978-1-4612-5312-9.
59. Burchett, S.A.; Hicks, T.P. The Mysterious Trace Amines: Protean Neuromodulators of Synaptic Transmission in Mammalian Brain. *Prog. Neurobiol.* **2006**, *79*, 223–246. [CrossRef] [PubMed]
60. Jones, R.S.G. Specific Enhancement of Neuronal Responses to Catecholamine by P-Tyramine. *J. Neurosci. Res.* **1981**, *6*, 49–61. [CrossRef]
61. Boulton, A.A.; Milward, L. Separation, Detection and Quantitative, Analysis of Urinary β-Phenylethylamine. *J. Chromatogr. A* **1971**, *57*, 287–296. [CrossRef]
62. Mosnaim, A.D.; Inwang, E.E. A Spectrophotometric Method for the Quantification of 2-Phenylethylamine in Biological Specimens. *Anal. Biochem.* **1973**, *54*, 561–577. [CrossRef]
63. Sabelli, H.C.; Mosnaim, A.D. Phenylethylamine Hypothesis of Affective Behavior. *Am. J. Psychiatry* **1974**, *131*, 695–699. [CrossRef] [PubMed]
64. Sandler, M.; Ruthven, C.R.J.; Goodwin, B.L.; Coppen, A. Decreased Cerebrospinal Fluid Concentration of Free Phenylacetic Acid in Depressive Illness. *Clin. Chim. Acta* **1979**, *93*, 169–171. [CrossRef] [PubMed]
65. Fischer, E.; Spatz, H.; Heller, B.; Reggiani, H. Phenethylamine Content of Human Urine and Rat Brain, Its Alterations in Pathological Conditions and after Drug Administration. *Experientia* **1972**, *28*, 307–308. [CrossRef] [PubMed]
66. Ruthven, C.R.J.; Goodwin, B.L.; Reynolds, G.P.; Coppen, A.; Sandler, M. Trace amines in depression: Tyramine and octopamine deficit. In *Catecholamines: Basic and Clinical Frontiers*; Elsevier: Amsterdam, The Netherlands, 1979; pp. 1872–1874, ISBN 978-1-4832-8363-0.
67. Coppen, A.; Shaw, D.M.; Malleson, A.; Eccleston, E.; Gundy, G. Tryptamine Metabolism in Depression. *Br. J. Psychiatry* **1965**, *111*, 993–998. [CrossRef] [PubMed]
68. Kobayashi, K.; Koide, Y.; Yoshino, K.; Shohmori, T. P-hydroxyphenylacetic acid concentrations in cerebrospinal fluid. *No To Shinkei* **1982**, *34*, 769–774. [PubMed]
69. Sandler, M.; Ruthven, C.R.J.; Goodwin, B.L.; Reynolds, G.P.; Rao, V.A.R.; Coppen, A. Deficient Production of Tyramine and Octopamine in Cases of Depression. *Nature* **1979**, *278*, 357–358. [CrossRef] [PubMed]
70. Fischer, E.; Heller, B.; Nachon, M.; Spatz, H. Therapy of Depression by Phenylalanine. Preliminary Note. *Arzneimittelforschung* **1975**, *25*, 132. [PubMed]

71. Davis, B.A.; Boulton, A.A. The Trace Amines and Their Acidic Metabolites in Depression—An Overview. *Prog. Neuropsychopharmacol. Biol. Psychiatry* **1994**, *18*, 17–45. [CrossRef] [PubMed]
72. LaBrosse, E.H.; Kopin, I.; Felix, W.; Westlake, R. Urinary Tryptamine and Indole-3-Acetic Acid Excretion by Schizophrenic Patients: Use of the Tryptamine/Indole Acetic Acid Ratio as an Index of Monoamine Oxidase Inhibition. *J. Psychiatr. Res.* **1964**, *2*, 185–197. [CrossRef]
73. Lindemann, L.; Ebeling, M.; Kratochwil, N.A.; Bunzow, J.R.; Grandy, D.K.; Hoener, M.C. Trace Amine-Associated Receptors Form Structurally and Functionally Distinct Subfamilies of Novel G Protein-Coupled Receptors. *Genomics* **2005**, *85*, 372–385. [CrossRef]
74. Schizophrenia Working Group of the Psychiatric Genomics Consortium. Biological Insights from 108 Schizophrenia-Associated Genetic Loci. *Nature* **2014**, *511*, 421–427. [CrossRef]
75. Kuvarzin, S.R.; Sukhanov, I.; Onokhin, K.; Zakharov, K.; Gainetdinov, R.R. Unlocking the Therapeutic Potential of Ulotaront as a Trace Amine-Associated Receptor 1 Agonist for Neuropsychiatric Disorders. *Biomedicines* **2023**, *11*, 1977. [CrossRef] [PubMed]
76. John, J.; Kukshal, P.; Bhatia, T.; Chowdari, K.V.; Nimgaonkar, V.L.; Deshpande, S.N.; Thelma, B.K. Possible Role of Rare Variants in Trace Amine Associated Receptor 1 in Schizophrenia. *Schizophr. Res.* **2017**, *189*, 190–195. [CrossRef]
77. Rutigliano, G.; Zucchi, R. Molecular Variants in Human Trace Amine-Associated Receptors and Their Implications in Mental and Metabolic Disorders. *Cell. Mol. Neurobiol.* **2020**, *40*, 239–255. [CrossRef]
78. Cichero, E. Opportunities and Challenges in the Design of Selective TAAR1 Agonists: An Editorial. *Expert Opin. Ther. Pat.* **2018**, *28*, 437–440. [CrossRef]
79. Schwartz, M.D.; Canales, J.J.; Zucchi, R.; Espinoza, S.; Sukhanov, I.; Gainetdinov, R.R. Trace Amine-Associated Receptor 1: A Multimodal Therapeutic Target for Neuropsychiatric Diseases. Expert Opin. *Ther. Targets* **2018**, *22*, 513–526. [CrossRef]
80. Espinoza, S.; Gainetdinov, R.R. Neuronal Functions and Emerging Pharmacology of TAAR1. In *Taste and Smell*; Krautwurst, D., Ed.; Topics in Medicinal Chemistry; Springer International Publishing: Cham, Switzerland, 2014; Volume 23, pp. 175–194, ISBN 978-3-319-48925-4.
81. Synan, C.; Bowen, C.; Heal, D.J.; Froger-Colléaux, C.; Beardsley, P.M.; Dedic, N.; Hopkins, S.C.; Campbell, U.; Koblan, K.S. Ulotaront, a Novel TAAR1 Agonist with 5-HT1A Agonist Activity, Lacks Abuse Liability and Attenuates Cocaine Cue-Induced Relapse in Rats. *Drug Alcohol Depend.* **2022**, *231*, 109261. [CrossRef] [PubMed]
82. Højlund, M.; Correll, C.U. Ulotaront: A TAAR1/5-HT1A Agonist in Clinical Development for the Treatment of Schizophrenia. Expert Opin. *Investig. Drugs* **2022**, *31*, 1279–1290. [CrossRef]
83. Correll, C.U.; Koblan, K.S.; Hopkins, S.C.; Li, Y.; Dworak, H.; Goldman, R.; Loebel, A. Safety and Effectiveness of Ulotaront (SEP-363856) in Schizophrenia: Results of a 6-Month, Open-Label Extension Study. *Npj Schizophr.* **2021**, *7*, 63. [CrossRef] [PubMed]
84. Revel, F.G.; Moreau, J.-L.; Pouzet, B.; Mory, R.; Bradaia, A.; Buchy, D.; Metzler, V.; Chaboz, S.; Groebke Zbinden, K.; Galley, G.; et al. A New Perspective for Schizophrenia: TAAR1 Agonists Reveal Antipsychotic- and Antidepressant-like Activity, Improve Cognition and Control Body Weight. *Mol. Psychiatry* **2013**, *18*, 543–556. [CrossRef]
85. Black, S.W.; Schwartz, M.D.; Chen, T.-M.; Hoener, M.C.; Kilduff, T.S. Trace Amine-Associated Receptor 1 Agonists as Narcolepsy Therapeutics. *Biol. Psychiatry* **2017**, *82*, 623–633. [CrossRef] [PubMed]
86. Schwartz, M.D.; Black, S.W.; Fisher, S.P.; Palmerston, J.B.; Morairty, S.R.; Hoener, M.C.; Kilduff, T.S. Trace Amine-Associated Receptor 1 Regulates Wakefulness and EEG Spectral Composition. *Neuropsychopharmacology* **2017**, *42*, 1305–1314. [CrossRef] [PubMed]
87. Xue, Z.; Siemian, J.N.; Johnson, B.N.; Zhang, Y.; Li, J.-X. Methamphetamine-Induced Impulsivity during Chronic Methamphetamine Treatment in Rats: Effects of the TAAR 1 Agonist RO5263397. *Neuropharmacology* **2018**, *129*, 36–46. [CrossRef] [PubMed]
88. Hiranita, T. Trace Amine-Associated Receptor Type 1 as A Target for The Development of Treatments for Stimulant Abuse. *J. Alcohol. Drug Depend.* **2015**, *3*, e122. [CrossRef] [PubMed]
89. Dorotenko, A.; Tur, M.; Dolgorukova, A.; Bortnikov, N.; Belozertseva, I.V.; Zvartau, E.E.; Gainetdinov, R.R.; Sukhanov, I. The Action of TAAR1 Agonist RO5263397 on Executive Functions in Rats. *Cell. Mol. Neurobiol.* **2020**, *40*, 215–228. [CrossRef] [PubMed]
90. Wu, R.; Liu, J.; Seaman, R.; Johnson, B.; Zhang, Y.; Li, J.-X. The Selective TAAR1 Partial Agonist RO5263397 Promoted Novelty Recognition Memory in Mice. *Psychopharmacology* **2021**, *238*, 3221–3228. [CrossRef] [PubMed]
91. Revel, F.G.; Moreau, J.-L.; Gainetdinov, R.R.; Ferragud, A.; Velázquez-Sánchez, C.; Sotnikova, T.D.; Morairty, S.R.; Harmeier, A.; Groebke Zbinden, K.; Norcross, R.D.; et al. Trace Amine-Associated Receptor 1 Partial Agonism Reveals Novel Paradigm for Neuropsychiatric Therapeutics. *Biol. Psychiatry* **2012**, *72*, 934–942. [CrossRef]
92. Ferragud, A.; Howell, A.D.; Moore, C.F.; Ta, T.L.; Hoener, M.C.; Sabino, V.; Cottone, P. The Trace Amine-Associated Receptor 1 Agonist RO5256390 Blocks Compulsive, Binge-like Eating in Rats. *Neuropsychopharmacology* **2017**, *42*, 1458–1470. [CrossRef]
93. Dedic, N.; Dworak, H.; Zeni, C.; Rutigliano, G.; Howes, O.D. Therapeutic Potential of TAAR1 Agonists in Schizophrenia: Evidence from Preclinical Models and Clinical Studies. *Int. J. Mol. Sci.* **2021**, *22*, 13185. [CrossRef]
94. Dedic, N.; Jones, P.G.; Hopkins, S.C.; Lew, R.; Shao, L.; Campbell, J.E.; Spear, K.L.; Large, T.H.; Campbell, U.C.; Hanania, T.; et al. SEP-363856, a Novel Psychotropic Agent with a Unique, Non-D 2 Receptor Mechanism of Action. *J. Pharmacol. Exp. Ther.* **2019**, *371*, 1–14. [CrossRef]
95. Study Details | A Trial of the Safety and Efficacy of SEP-363856 in the Treatment of Adults with Major Depressive Disorder | ClinicalTrials.Gov. Available online: https://clinicaltrials.gov/study/NCT05593029?cond=Depression&intr=SEP363856&rank=1 (accessed on 28 February 2024).

96. Ren, X.; Xiong, J.; Liang, L.; Chen, Y.; Zhang, G. The Potential Antidepressant Action of Duloxetine Co-Administered with the TAAR1 Receptor Agonist SEP-363856 in Mice. *Molecules* **2022**, *27*, 2755. [CrossRef] [PubMed]
97. Mantas, I.; Millan, M.J.; Di Cara, B.; Groenink, L.; Veiga, S.; Cistarelli, L.; Brocco, M.; Bertrand, M.; Svenningsson, P.; Zhang, X. Trace Amine-Associated Receptor 1 Contributes to Diverse Functional Actions of O-Phenyl-Iodotyramine in Mice but Not to the Effects of Monoamine-Based Antidepressants. *Int. J. Mol. Sci.* **2021**, *22*, 8907. [CrossRef] [PubMed]
98. Grinchii, D.; Hoener, M.C.; Khoury, T.; Dekhtiarenko, R.; Nejati Bervanlou, R.; Jezova, D.; Dremencov, E. Effects of Acute and Chronic Administration of Trace Amine-Associated Receptor 1 (TAAR1) Ligands on in Vivo Excitability of Central Monoamine-Secreting Neurons in Rats. *Mol. Psychiatry* **2022**, *27*, 4861–4868. [CrossRef]
99. de Montigny, C.; Chaput, Y.; Blier, P. Modification of Serotonergic Neuron Properties by Long-Term Treatment with Serotonin Reuptake Blockers. *J. Clin. Psychiatry* **1990**, *51*, 4–8.
100. Katolikova, N.V.; Vaganova, A.N.; Efimova, E.V.; Gainetdinov, R.R. Expression of Trace Amine-Associated Receptors in the Murine and Human Hippocampus Based on Public Transcriptomic Data. *Cells* **2022**, *11*, 1813. [CrossRef]
101. Dinter, J.; Mühlhaus, J.; Wienchol, C.L.; Yi, C.-X.; Nürnberg, D.; Morin, S.; Grüters, A.; Köhrle, J.; Schöneberg, T.; Tschöp, M.; et al. Inverse Agonistic Action of 3-Iodothyronamine at the Human Trace Amine-Associated Receptor 5. *PLoS ONE* **2015**, *10*, e0117774. [CrossRef]
102. Lee, S.-S.; Kim, C.-J.; Shin, M.-S.; Lim, B.-V. Treadmill Exercise Ameliorates Memory Impairment through ERK-Akt-CREB-BDNF Signaling Pathway in Cerebral Ischemia Gerbils. *J. Exerc. Rehabil.* **2020**, *16*, 49–57. [CrossRef] [PubMed]
103. Borowsky, B.; Adham, N.; Jones, K.A.; Raddatz, R.; Artymyshyn, R.; Ogozalek, K.L.; Durkin, M.M.; Lakhlani, P.P.; Bonini, J.A.; Pathirana, S.; et al. Trace Amines: Identification of a Family of Mammalian G Protein-Coupled Receptors. *Proc. Natl. Acad. Sci. USA* **2001**, *98*, 8966–8971. [CrossRef]
104. Zhang, Y.; Zhang, X.-Q.; Niu, W.-P.; Sun, M.; Zhang, Y.; Li, J.-T.; Si, T.-M.; Su, Y.-A. TAAR1 in Dentate Gyrus Is Involved in Chronic Stress-Induced Impairments in Hippocampal Plasticity and Cognitive Function. *Prog. Neuropsychopharmacol. Biol. Psychiatry* **2024**, *132*, 110995. [CrossRef]
105. Liberles, S.D. Trace Amine-associated Receptors Are Olfactory Receptors in Vertebrates. *Ann. N. Y. Acad. Sci.* **2009**, *1170*, 168–172. [CrossRef]
106. Gaudel, F.; Guiraudie-Capraz, G.; Féron, F. Limbic Expression of mRNA Coding for Chemoreceptors in Human Brain—Lessons from Brain Atlases. *Int. J. Mol. Sci.* **2021**, *22*, 6858. [CrossRef] [PubMed]
107. Pae, C.-U.; Drago, A.; Kim, J.-J.; Patkar, A.A.; Jun, T.-Y.; De Ronchi, D.; Serretti, A. TAAR6 Variations Possibly Associated with Antidepressant Response and Suicidal Behavior. *Psychiatry Res.* **2010**, *180*, 20–24. [CrossRef] [PubMed]
108. Vaganova, A.N.; Katolikova, N.V.; Murtazina, R.Z.; Kuvarzin, S.R.; Gainetdinov, R.R. Public Transcriptomic Data Meta-Analysis Demonstrates TAAR6 Expression in the Mental Disorder-Related Brain Areas in Human and Mouse Brain. *Biomolecules* **2022**, *12*, 1259. [CrossRef]
109. Espinoza, S.; Sukhanov, I.; Efimova, E.V.; Kozlova, A.; Antonova, K.A.; Illiano, P.; Leo, D.; Merkulyeva, N.; Kalinina, D.; Musienko, P.; et al. Trace Amine-Associated Receptor 5 Provides Olfactory Input into Limbic Brain Areas and Modulates Emotional Behaviors and Serotonin Transmission. *Front. Mol. Neurosci.* **2020**, *13*, 18. [CrossRef]
110. Efimova, E.V.; Kozlova, A.A.; Razenkova, V.; Katolikova, N.V.; Antonova, K.A.; Sotnikova, T.D.; Merkulyeva, N.S.; Veshchitskii, A.S.; Kalinina, D.S.; Korzhevskii, D.E.; et al. Increased Dopamine Transmission and Adult Neurogenesis in Trace Amine-Associated Receptor 5 (TAAR5) Knockout Mice. *Neuropharmacology* **2021**, *182*, 108373. [CrossRef] [PubMed]
111. Efimova, E.V.; Kuvarzin, S.R.; Mor, M.S.; Katolikova, N.V.; Shemiakova, T.S.; Razenkova, V.; Ptukha, M.; Kozlova, A.A.; Murtazina, R.Z.; Smirnova, D.; et al. Trace Amine-Associated Receptor 2 Is Expressed in the Limbic Brain Areas and Is Involved in Dopamine Regulation and Adult Neurogenesis. *Front. Behav. Neurosci.* **2022**, *16*, 847410. [CrossRef]
112. Vaganova, A.N.; Murtazina, R.Z.; Shemyakova, T.S.; Prjibelski, A.D.; Katolikova, N.V.; Gainetdinov, R.R. Pattern of TAAR5 Expression in the Human Brain Based on Transcriptome Datasets Analysis. *Int. J. Mol. Sci.* **2021**, *22*, 8802. [CrossRef]
113. Maggi, S.; Bon, C.; Gustincich, S.; Tucci, V.; Gainetdinov, R.R.; Espinoza, S. Improved Cognitive Performances in Trace Amine-Associated Receptor 5 (TAAR5) Knock-out Mice. *Behav. Sci.* **2022**, *12*, 14708. [CrossRef]
114. Katolikova, N.V.; Vaganova, A.N.; Shafranskaya, D.D.; Efimova, E.V.; Malashicheva, A.B.; Gainetdinov, R.R. Expression Pattern of Trace Amine-Associated Receptors during Differentiation of Human Pluripotent Stem Cells to Dopaminergic Neurons. *Int. J. Mol. Sci.* **2023**, *24*, 15313. [CrossRef]
115. Cain, D.P. The Role of the Olfactory Bulb in Limbic Mechanisms. *Psychol. Bull.* **1974**, *81*, 654–671. [CrossRef]
116. Rolls, E.T. Limbic Systems for Emotion and for Memory, but No Single Limbic System. *Cortex* **2015**, *62*, 119–157. [CrossRef] [PubMed]
117. Morales-Medina, J.C.; Iannitti, T.; Freeman, A.; Caldwell, H.K. The Olfactory Bulbectomized Rat as a Model of Depression: The Hippocampal Pathway. *Behav. Brain Res.* **2017**, *317*, 562–575. [CrossRef] [PubMed]
118. Croy, I.; Hummel, T. Olfaction as a Marker for Depression. *J. Neurol.* **2017**, *264*, 631–638. [CrossRef] [PubMed]
119. Belov, D.R.; Efimova, E.V.; Fesenko, Z.S.; Antonova, K.A.; Kolodyazhny, S.F.; Lakstygal, A.M.; Gainetdinov, R.R. Putative Trace-Amine Associated Receptor 5 (TAAR5) Agonist α-NETA Increases Electrocorticogram Gamma-Rhythm in Freely Moving Rats. *Cell. Mol. Neurobiol.* **2020**, *40*, 203–213. [CrossRef] [PubMed]

120. Nicoli, A.; Weber, V.; Bon, C.; Steuer, A.; Gustincich, S.; Gainetdinov, R.R.; Lang, R.; Espinoza, S.; Di Pizio, A. Structure-Based Discovery of Mouse Trace Amine-Associated Receptor 5 Antagonists. *J. Chem. Inf. Model.* **2023**, *63*, 6667–6680. [CrossRef]
121. Efimova, E.V.; Katolikova, N.V.; Kanov, E.V.; Gainetdinov, R.R. Trace Amine-Associated Receptors at the Cross-Road between Innate Olfaction of Amines, Emotions, and Adult Neurogenesis. *Neural Regen. Res.* **2022**, *17*, 1257–1258. [CrossRef]

biomedicines MDPI

Article

Untangling Depression in Schizophrenia: The Role of Disorganized and Obsessive-Compulsive Symptoms and the Duration of Untreated Psychosis

Georgi Panov [1,2,*], Silvana Dyulgerova [1], Presyana Panova [3] and Sonia Stefanova [2]

1 Psychiatric Clinic, University Hospital for Active Treatment "Prof. Dr. Stoyan Kirkovich", Trakia University, 6000 Stara Zagora, Bulgaria
2 Medical Faculty, University "Prof. Dr. Asen Zlatarov", 8000 Burgas, Bulgaria
3 Medical Faculty, Trakia University, 6000 Stara Zagora, Bulgaria
* Correspondence: gpanov@dir.bg or drpanov2018@gmail.com

Abstract: Background: Schizophrenia is a complex disorder characterized by positive symptoms (e.g., hallucinations), negative symptoms (e.g., social withdrawal), and disorganized symptoms (e.g., thought disorder). Alongside these, cognitive and depressive symptoms often emerge, with depressive symptoms sometimes dominating the clinical picture. Understanding the factors that influence the development of depressive symptoms in schizophrenia could clarify the dynamics between depressive and psychotic symptoms and guide clinical interventions. **Methods:** A total of 105 patients with schizophrenia (66 women, 39 men) were assessed using several clinical scales: PANSS, BPRS, DOCS, DES, HAM-D, and the Luria-Nebraska Neuropsychological Battery for cognitive evaluation. Statistical analyses, including correlation and regression, were conducted using SPSS to determine the significance of associations. **Results:** Disorganized and obsessive-compulsive symptoms were identified as primary factors associated with depressive symptoms in patients with schizophrenia. Conversely, a longer duration of untreated psychosis was linked to a lower severity of depressive symptoms, suggesting that early intervention may alter the depressive symptom trajectory. **Conclusions:** Here, we suggest a complex interaction between psychotic and depressive symptoms, possibly indicating a biological antagonism. The association of depressive symptoms with disorganized and obsessive-compulsive features may reflect an adaptive psychological response, attempting to stabilize amidst the disintegration of schizophrenia. These insights support a more integrated approach to treatment, addressing both psychotic and depressive symptoms to improve patient outcomes.

Keywords: schizophrenia; psychosis; positive; negative; disorganized symptoms; obsessive-compulsive symptoms; duration of untreated psychosis; depressive symptoms; depression; biological antagonism

1. Introduction

Schizophrenia is a complex nosological entity that results from the interaction of genetic and epigenetic factors [1–4]. Genetic predisposition is easily detectable in the analysis of family history. This encumbrance in an etiological aspect cannot be accepted too categorically due to the influence of the impact of learned patterns of behavior, as well as the lack of stable parental role models. These factors can also be considered epigenetic impacts [5]. Analysis of the interaction of epigenetic influence and genetic polymorphism shows a relationship with both the development of the schizophrenia process and the effect of antipsychotic therapy [6]. The clinical picture of schizophrenic disorders is diverse, but positive, negative, and cognitive symptoms have been analyzed as the main storyline. In patients with schizophrenia, many other symptoms are also superimposed, such as anxiety, affective, and obsessive-compulsive disorders, as well as disorders in the perception of time and the perception of personal space [7,8]. All these deviations in mental status are also associated with changes in both metabolism and immunological markers [9,10]. All this multiplicity, both in the etiological and clinical aspects, poses the question of searching for a complex approach and therapeutic behavior that is consistent with the main and priority aspects in the clinical presentation [11–13].

Depressive symptoms and psychotic symptoms have many similarities and differences. These similarities and differences can be observed at the structural, functional, neurotransmitter, and metabolic levels. In both conditions, the analysis of structural disorders shows that we have a loss of gray brain matter in different parts of the brain, with a corresponding predilection for changes in them. In depression, changes are more pronounced in the hippocampus, prefrontal cortex [14], and the amygdala and white brain matter [15]. In schizophrenia, they are associated with gray matter loss and cortical thickness reduction [16], as well as hippocampal and temporal lobe changes [17]. Functional changes in depression are associated with hyperactivity in the default mode network (DMN) [18] and hypoactivity in the executive control network (ECN), as well as hyperactivation of the amygdala and anterior cingulate cortex (ACC) [19]. In psychosis, DMN hypoactivity and dysfunction [20] and dysregulation in the salience network (SN) [21] altered thalamocortical connectivity and dopamine system dysfunction [22]. Differences in the neurotransmitter system are also observed in both conditions. In depression, there are major changes in serotonin and norepinephrine [23], as well as in the glutamate and hypothalamic-pituitary-adrenocortical (HPA) axis [24]. In schizophrenia, the main neurotransmitter changes are found in dopamine and glutamate [25,26], as well as in the dysfunction of NMDA receptor activity [27]. Differences can be found in a purely metabolic aspect, related to the metabolism of kynurenic acid. Schizophrenia shows a KYNA elevation that interferes with receptor activity crucial to cognitive function and psychosis [28] while depression often shows a neurotoxic shift, increasing quinolinic acid [29]. These changes also warrant the search for therapeutic strategies to influence kynurenic acid metabolism [30–32].

Depressive symptoms are frequent and characteristic symptoms observed in patients with schizophrenia. On the one hand, they can be observed as clinically established symptoms in the post-psychotic period, reaching up to 50% in patients with first episodes and up to 25% in those with subsequent episodes. The presence of these episodes is associated, according to some authors, with a poor prognosis [33,34]. The opinion of other authors takes an opposite position, associating affective symptoms with a favorable course of schizophrenia [35–37], especially in those with high values on the depression scale [38] and in those with high values on the mania scale [39]. The importance of depressive symptoms in the development of the schizophrenic process has led to their special classification in ICD 10 and ICD 11 as post-schizophrenic depression [40,41]. These divergent data indicate that depressive symptoms themselves are most likely to have a diverse genesis, which in turn is associated with a different prognosis. On the other hand, apart from being a clinically evident phenomenon, depressive symptomatology can be observed as a subclinical persistent finding in the clinical picture of patients, not always demonstrably presented and mixed with the main symptomatology. A study conducted with the aim of analyzing depressive symptoms in patients with schizophrenia showed that they are moderately pronounced and persistent over time in patients with resistance to treatment and are relatively mild in those in remission [42]. These data give us reason to conclude that smoldering depressive symptoms are associated with resistance to the schizophrenic process, while the appearance of pronounced depressive and manic symptoms is associated with a good prognosis.

In the analysis of the factors related to the presence of depressive symptoms, the author team established a relationship between the negative subscale of the PANSS and the scale of general psychopathology with sociodemographic factors such as loneliness, isolation, and lack of support [43,44]. On the other hand, whether there is a connection with sociodemographic factors as a cause of depressive symptoms or whether sociodemographic factors are a consequence of the development of the schizophrenic process with the gradient loss of social connectivity associated with its progression is a question that can be discussed.

In this case, it is difficult to give an exact answer, as an analogy can be made with the question: "Which came first - the chicken or the egg?"″

There are multivariate analyses that present a different clinical value of depressive symptoms in patients with schizophrenia. This lack of consistency in research gave us reasons to look for and establish the relationship between depressive symptoms and other factors and symptoms in patients with schizophrenia.

In the analysis of the factors related to depressive symptoms, we considered it appropriate not to include the sociodemographic data. Due to the fact that they also appear as a result of the persistence of the main symptoms of the schizophrenia process, depressive complaints, in themselves and as the development of social maladaptation, appear to be directly deducible from the schizophrenic process.

2. Materials and Methods

We conducted a study of 105 patients with schizophrenia, of whom 66 were women and 39 were men. The examination and evaluation of the patients was carried out in the Psychiatric Clinic of the University General Hospital for Active Treatment —Stara Zagora. Patients were admitted for observation and treatment after consecutive psychotic episodes. The initial examination of the patients was performed in an outpatient setting, and after giving informed consent, they were admitted for treatment and assessment of the condition. Patients were recruited and followed for the period from 2017 to 2022.

All patients undertook the Hamilton depression and anxiety scales, the dissociation scale, the obsessive-compulsive symptom analysis scale (DOCS), and a memory assessment, using the Luria test [45–49].

The initial analysis and follow-up were performed in an inpatient setting, and later, the observation and follow-up of their condition were performed in an outpatient setting.

Patient inclusion criteria:

1. A series of psychotic episodes;
2. Evaluation of symptoms according to the PANSS and BPRS scales [50,51]
3. Prospective observation for at least 12 weeks;
4. Administration of at least two trials of antipsychotic drugs at a dose equivalent to or greater than 600 mg chlorpromazine equivalents to achieve remission and assess resistance.

Exclusion criteria:

1. Mental retardation;
2. Abuse of psychoactive substances;
3. Presence of organic brain damage;
4. Accompanying progressive neurological or severe somatic diseases;
5. Marked personality change (according to the DSM 5 and ICD 10 and ICD 11 diagnostic tools) [40,41,52,53];
6. First psychotic episode.

Statistical Analyses

For the purpose of the research, the capabilities of the statistical package SPSS version 26 were used. The methods used were tailored to the specifics and objectives of the research. Correlation analysis and regression analysis were used. Regression analysis was conducted, with the dependent variables being depressive complaints assessed with the Hamilton scale. Independent variables were age, disease onset, duration of untreated symptoms, duration of schizophrenia process, body mass index, PANSS positive, negative, and disorganized symptoms, dissociation scale, and obsessive-compulsive symptom scale. An assessment of the co-linearity index was also made to measure the significance and reliability of the obtained results. We have also used analysis of variance (ANOVA) as a statistical formula used to compare variances across the means (or average) of different variables. A correlation analysis was also conducted to find a relationship between the analyzed variables. On the other hand, correlation analysis and its results are a prerequisite for the choice of method when conducting regression analysis.

The same group of patients was studied in order to investigate other clinical indicators such as obsessive-compulsive, dissociative, and cognitive symptoms, lateralization of brain processes, the effect of the administration of the first antipsychotic drug, and the role of gender in patients with schizophrenia [42,54–60]. All patients gave written informed consent before being admitted to the clinical facilities and undergoing diagnostic tests and therapy.

The study was conducted in accordance with the Declaration of Helsinki and was approved by the Ethics Committee of the University Hospital "Prof. Dr. Stoyan Kirkovich" Stara Zagora, protocol code TR3-02-242/30 December 2021.

3. Results

3.1. Descriptive Statistics of the Sample

Out of a total of 105 patients with schizophrenia, 66 were female and 39 were male. The mean age of patients was 37.13 years (Table 1). The minimum age was 21 years and the maximum was 62 years.

Table 1. Some of the main characteristics of the group of patients.

Age (years)	37.13
Age of onset of SZ (years)	25.51
Duration of untreated period/months/	14.78
Duration of SZ (years)	11.77
BMI	26.9562
Height (cm)	168.55
Sex (M/F)	39/66

In males, we found that the average level of depression was 11.44, and the median was the same as in females, which was 12, with a standard deviation of 4.179.

We found a slightly higher level of depressive symptoms in females, but without statistical dependence on the level of depressive scores between the sexes.

3.2. Correlations Between Clinical Scales

We conducted a correlation analysis in order to assess the strength of the relationship between the scales we analyzed: the depression scale, the PANSS negative, positive, and disorganized scales, the dissociation scale, and the OCS scale, as well as short-term memory fixation (Tables 2–4).

This analysis reveals that depressive symptoms are modestly associated with longer illness duration, suggesting that the chronicity of schizophrenia may contribute to increased depressive symptoms over time. However, onset age and duration of untreated symptoms do not appear to have direct impacts on depression levels. These findings point to a potentially cumulative effect of long-term schizophrenia on depressive experiences, which could suggest treatment approaches that address the emotional impact of prolonged illness.

The analysis of data in Table 3 reveals that depressive symptoms are moderately associated with overall psychiatric severity (PANSS and BPRS), particularly with disorganized symptoms. The findings suggest that disorganization, along with positive symptoms, may play a more significant role in the experience of depressive symptoms in schizophrenia than negative symptoms do. These insights highlight the importance of addressing both mood and cognitive disorganization in managing depressive symptoms within this population.

The analysis reveals that depressive symptoms are strongly associated with anxiety and obsessive-compulsive symptoms. In contrast, there is little to no significant relationship between depressive symptoms and dissociation or fixation. The strong link between anxiety and depression highlights the importance of addressing both conditions in clinical settings, as they often exacerbate each other. The associations found between dissociation and obsessive-compulsive symptoms suggest that these constructs may warrant further exploration, particularly in their relationship with depressive experiences. Also striking is the negative correlation between depressive symptoms and short-term memory reflected by fixation in this analysis. Overall, we can say that these findings emphasize the interconnected nature of various psychiatric symptoms and the need for comprehensive assessment and treatment strategies.

Table 2. Degree of statistical significance between the depression scale and the onset of the illness, duration of the illness, and duration of untreated symptoms in patients with schizophrenia.

		Onset of the Illness	Duration of Untreated Symptoms	Duration of Sch	Hamilton D
Onset of the illness	Pearson Correlation	1	−0.350 **	−0.313 **	−0.039
	Sig. (2-tailed)		0.000	0.001	0.694
Duration of the untreated symptoms	Pearson Correlation	−0.350 **	1	0.148	−0.104
	Sig. (2-tailed)	0.000		0.133	0.292
Duration of the illness	Pearson Correlation	−0.313 **	0.148	1	0.196 *
	Sig. (2-tailed)	00.001	0.133		0.046
Hamilton D scale	Pearson Correlation	−0.039	−0.104	0.196 *	1
	Sig. (2-tailed)	0.694	0.292	0.046	

* $p < 0.05$, ** $p < 0.01$.

Table 3. Correlation between the Hamilton scale, the PANSS scale and its subscales, and the BPRS scale.

		Hamilton D	PANSS	PANSS Positive Subscale	PANSS Negative Subscale	PANSS Disorganized Subscale	BPRS
Hamilton D	Pearson Correlation	1	0.275 **	0.240 *	0.156	0.295 **	0.383 **
	Sig. (2-tailed)		0.005	0.014	0.113	0.002	0.000
PANSS	Pearson Correlation	0.275 **	1	0.835 **	0.806 **	0.954 **	0.911 **
	Sig. (2-tailed)	0.005		0.000	0.000	0.000	0.000
PANSS positive subscale	Pearson Correlation	0.240 *	0.835 **	1	0.493 **	0.738 **	0.785 **
	Sig. (2-tailed)	0.014	0.000		0.000	0.000	0.000
PANSS negative subscale	Pearson Correlation	0.156	0.806 **	0.493 **	1	0.730 **	0.719 **
	Sig. (2-tailed)	0.113	0.000	0.000		0.000	0.000
PANSS disorganized subscale	Pearson Correlation	0.295 **	0.954 **	0.738 **	0.730 **	1	0.888 **
	Sig. (2-tailed)	0.002	0.000	0.000	0.000		0.000
BPRS	Pearson Correlation	0.383 **	0.911 **	0.785 **	0.719 **	0.888 **	1
	Sig. (2-tailed)	0.000	0.000	0.000	0.000	0.000	

* $p < 0.05$, ** $p < 0.01$.

Table 4. Correlation between Hamilton depression rating scale and dissociation scale, fixation scale, Hamilton anxiety rating scale, and obsessive-compulsive symptoms rating scale.

		Hamilton D Scale	Dissociation Scale	Fixation Scale	Hamilton A Scale	OCS Scale
Hamilton D	Pearson Correlation	1	0.133	−0.139	0.719 **	0.256 **
	Sig. (2-tailed)		0.175	0.158	0.000	0.009
Dissociation scale	Pearson Correlation	0.133	1	−0.467 **	0.209 *	0.335 **
	Sig. (2-tailed)	0.175		0.000	0.032	0.000
Fixation	Pearson Correlation	−0.139	−0.467 **	1	−0.270 **	−0.121
	Sig. (2-tailed)	0.158	0.000		0.005	0.218
Hamilton anxiety scale	Pearson Correlation	0.719 **	0.209 *	−0.270 **	1	0.208 *
	Sig. (2-tailed)	0.000	0.032	0.005		0.033
OCS scale	Pearson Correlation	0.256 **	0.335 **	−0.121	0.208 *	1
	Sig. (2-tailed)	0.009	0.000	0.218	0.033	

* $p < 0.05$, ** $p < 0.01$.

In order to establish the most important factors influencing the appearance of depressive symptoms in patients with schizophrenia, we conducted a regression analysis. Regression analysis was conducted, with the dependent variables being depressive symptoms. Independent variables were age, age of onset, duration of untreated symptoms, duration of schizophrenia process, body mass index (BMI), PANSS positive, negative, and disorganized symptoms, dissociation scale, and obsessive-compulsive symptom scale. The results are presented in Tables 5 and 6.

Table 5. Results of the regression analysis. The factors with a statistically significant influence on the occurrence of depressive symptoms and their coefficients are presented.

	R2	β	t	p (sig)
Step 1 PANSS disorganized	0.295	0.148	3.136	0.002
Step 2 Duration of untreated symptoms	0.351	0.174	3.611	0.044
Step 3 OCS scale	0.409	0.150	3.098	0.022

Regression analysis identified three main predictors and models.

These predictors are:

1. PANSS Disorganized Symptoms: The strong positive impact of disorganized symptoms on depression highlights the significant role of cognitive and perceptual disorganization in contributing to depressive symptoms. This may reflect the distress and impairment that disorganized thinking and behavior impose, potentially fostering feelings of depressive complaints.
2. Duration of Untreated Symptoms: The negative relationship here suggests that individuals who experienced shorter periods of untreated psychosis report higher depressive symptoms. This finding could imply that early intervention mitigates long-term depressive symptoms, or that those who seek help sooner may be more likely to experience depression due to increased insight of their symptoms.

3. Obsessive-Compulsive Symptoms (OCS): The positive correlation between OCS scores and depressive symptoms implies that the presence of obsessive-compulsive symptoms may aggravate depressive symptoms, possibly due to the distress and mental strain associated with them.

Table 6. Statistical significance of established models when conducting regression analysis.

Model		Unstandardized Coefficients		Standardized Coefficients	t	Sig.
		B	Std. Error	Beta		
1	(Constant)	7.126	1.568		4.544	0.000
	PANSS disorganized	0.148	0.047	0.295	3.136	0.002
2	(Constant)	7.576	1.560		4.855	0.000
	PANSS disorganized	0.174	0.048	0.347	3.611	0.000
	Duration of untreated psychosis	−0.086	0.042	−0.196	−2.040	0.044
3	(Constant)	6.513	1.594		4.085	0.000
	PANS disorganized	0.150	0.048	0.299	3.098	0.003
	Duration of untreated psychosis	−0.098	0.042	−0.223	−2.351	0.021
	OCS scale	0.111	0.048	0.220	2.329	0.022

4. Discussion

Our study showed that gender distribution is not a factor related to the appearance of depressive symptoms in patients with schizophrenia. In the main population, there is evidence that there is a clear distinction between the sexes, with depressive symptoms being more characteristic of females. This is also directly deducible from the differences between the sexes, related to biological, psychological, and social factors, which are a prerequisite for the prevalence of depressive symptoms in persons of the female gender [61]. This is not the case in patients with schizophrenia. One study examines gender differences in the onset and progression of schizophrenia, including the expression of depressive symptoms, and suggests that typical gender differences in depression may not apply to individuals with schizophrenia [62]. Our results support this study by showing that schizophrenia patients did not differ in terms of the expression of depressive complaints. Other articles have also discussed how schizophrenia may diminish the usual gender differences seen in mood disorders, with a focus on the expression of depressive symptoms [63–65]. Other studies have attempted to analyze the reasons for the lack of differences in the occurrence of depressive symptoms in patients with schizophrenia. They examine and develop the concept of blunted gender differences in schizophrenia [66].

Another transcultural study also shows that there is a reduction of gender differences as a consequence of the influence of the schizophrenic process [67]. We also registered these blurred boundaries of gender differences in schizophrenia when conducting an assessment of the distribution of gender roles in patients with schizophrenia [57]. Our data also support the idea of blunted gender differences. The results of these studies give some authors reason to consider the idea of a strictly individual view and approach to these patients, not one based only on gender differences [68,69].

We find a directly proportional relationship between the expression of disorganized symptoms in schizophrenia and depressive symptoms. This dependence can be considered in the context that disorganized symptoms, unlike positive and negative symptoms, are directly related to functional impairment, which in turn leads to depressive complaints [70]. Negative symptoms are not perceived as ego-dystonic in the sense of suffering, and thus they do not lead to depressive complaints, although an overlap between depressive and negative symptoms may be observed outwardly, further impairing social functioning [71]. This close relationship between disorganized and depressive symptoms, as was shown in our previous study between disorganized and obsessive-compulsive symptoms [54], gives us reason to consider the idea of symptom formation as a consequence of the development of a process of "disintegration" in patients with schizophrenia. We can view depressive, positive, and obsessive-compulsive symptoms as defense mechanisms against the "disintegration" underlying the schizophrenic process [72–74].

This study also gives us an explanation of why we find obsessive-compulsive symptoms as a factor that is, to a large extent, a determinant of the appearance of depressive symptoms. Obsessive-compulsive symptoms themselves lead to severe stress and can further trigger the onset of depressive symptoms. Obsessive-compulsive symptoms in schizophrenia can also be seen as an adaptive phenomenon, a reaction against the chaos of disorganized symptoms [75].

We find the greatest association of depressive symptoms with disorganized and obsessive-compulsive symptoms. Another study of ours, which analyzed obsessive-compulsive symptoms in patients with schizophrenia, showed that they were also highly associated with the presence of disorganized symptoms [54]. Is it precisely the disorganized symptoms, symptoms without organization, that do not seek their secondary organization as psychotic, obsessive-compulsive, and depressive symptoms? Other studies also find a link between disorganized and depressive symptoms [76–81]. When conducting a correlation analysis, we found a high correlation dependence of depressive complaints, both with the individual subscales of the PANSS and with the BPRS scale. We found a higher correlation significance of depressive symptoms with disorganized symptoms and with the BPRS scale. The explanation of this observation can be found in the research that conducted a comparison between the PANSS and BPRS scales. The PANSS scale is much more specific than the BPRS. The BPRS scale reflects more the main psychopathology, which is also related to an overlap with some depressive and disorganized symptoms, which is the reason for their higher correlation coefficient [82–84].

Our study found that the duration of untreated symptoms was inversely related to the development of depressive symptoms. We find that the longer the duration of untreated psychosis, the lower the likelihood of developing depressive complaints. How should we analyze this observation?

In the context that psychosis is the primary and main disease, depressive symptomatology appears as an additional symptom in the course of the evolution of the disease or, on the other hand, as a side effect and as a symptom as a result of therapy. These relationships can be considered in the context of the relationship between dopamine blockade and depression, cognitive impairment associated with dopamine blockade, fatigue, sedation, motor side effects, etc. [78,85,86] . This is also the classic approach to looking at these relationships, and for this reason, in the F20 rubric of ICD 10 and 11, we have a sub-section on post-schizophrenic depression. Our data on the inverse correlation between depressive symptoms and duration of untreated psychosis prompts us to discuss another hypothesis. Since depressive symptomatology appears, on the one hand, as one of the main prodromal symptoms in schizophrenia, on the other hand, it represents a symptom that we can follow in the course of the schizophrenic process. From this point of view, the interrelationships between depressive and psychotic symptoms give us reason to ask the questionCan we not take a mirror look at these processes?

Depression is the primary disorder in which, in some cases, psychotic symptomatology is superimposed, which is clinically significant, expressed, and meets the diagnostic criteria of the main classification systems and, as such, requires antipsychotic therapy. In support of this observation comes the fact that often-expressed depression has psychotic symptoms that require antipsychotic therapy in parallel with the use of antidepressants [87–91].

On the other hand, the use of antidepressants has an effect on patients with schizophrenic disorder, even in the absence of clinically expressed depressive symptoms [92–95].

We can also judge the proximity of the two states by their prognosis. Both schizophrenia and psychotic depression have a similar prognosis, despite the presence of certain differences [96–99], which, again, gives us reason to question what is the primary underlying disorder. On the other hand, perhaps we should just accept that the question is largely rhetorical and that the two states are interwoven as one common entity.

These clinical observations give us reason to look at the biochemical disturbances in order to find similarities between them. In both conditions, a biochemical imbalance is established. In both conditions, there is a dopamine imbalance, disorders of serotonin, glutamate transmission, GABA mediation, an increased level of inflammatory factors, and a generally increased inflammatory background, associated with a change in cortisol secretion [100–103].

If we look at DMN changes in depression and psychosis, we find that they are opposite. While, in depression, we have hyperactivity [18], in schizophrenia, we have altered activity related to the loss of connectivity or altered activity to hypoactivity [20]. This process is most likely also related to the disorganization in the sense of "I", which provokes the creation of clinical symptoms such as positive or depressive or OCD [104]. How can we explain, from this perspective based on DMN dysfunction, the inverse relationship between the duration of untreated psychosis and depressive symptoms? The prolonged state of dysfunction of this neuronal network over time is related to strengthening the loss of connectivity at the functional and neuronal level, where it becomes even more difficult to react with "hyperfunction" of the same system and transition to depression.

In patients with resistant schizophrenia, depressive symptoms are registered in the range of moderately expressed [42]. These results can be commented on in light of our observation that schizophrenic disorder, which is essentially a form of disorganization of the psyche, finds its clinical expression in the construction of disorganized symptoms as a clinical phenomenon. The organism is not able to reach a new form of mental allostasis, regardless of whether it is a psychotic or depressive episode, and remains in an unbalanced state with persistent disorganized symptoms, which also show the highest degree of resistance in individual studies [105–107].

Limitation: The limitation of our study is related, on the one hand, to the number of observed patients. In order to answer fundamental questions related to the perception and analysis of the clinical dynamics of larger nosological categories, observation of a large number of patients with a long follow-up period is necessary, which we are currently unable to provide. The observation of these patients continues, which gives us the opportunity to follow the pathoplasticity of the described phenomenology, which we hope to be able to present in the future.

Another limitation of our study is that it is purely clinical, as we did not have the opportunity to analyze the functional connections in individual neuronal networks, metabolic disorders, and individual registered inflammatory markers characterizing these processes.

5. Conclusions

We found that the presence of disorganized and obsessive-compulsive symptoms is associated with the appearance of depressive symptoms in patients with schizophrenia. Additionally, an inverse relationship between the duration of untreated psychosis and the onset of depressive symptoms suggests that early intervention may impact the development of depressive features. These findings offer valuable insights for clinical practice, potentially enabling the prediction of individual symptom dynamics throughout the course of the schizophrenic process. Moreover, these observations prompt a reconsideration of the relationship between depression and psychosis as conditions that often exhibit convergent aspects in therapy. Rather than viewing them as separate entities, our results align with the concept of a single underlying pathology—a unified disease process that may express itself through varying symptom profiles over time. This perspective encourages a holistic approach to treatment, addressing core vulnerabilities that underpin both psychotic and depressive symptoms in a continuum of mental health disorders.

Author Contributions: Conceptualization, data collection, and analysis are by G.P.; data collection and analysis are by S.D.; writing, editing, and graphics are by P.P.; analysis and editing are by S.S. All authors listed have made a substantial, direct, and intellectual contribution to the work. All authors have read and agreed to the published version of the manuscript.

Funding: This research received no external funding.

Institutional Review Board Statement: The study was conducted following the Declaration of Helsinki and approved by the Ethical Committee of University Hospital "Prof. Dr. Stoyan Kirkovich" Stara Zagora, protocol code TR3-02-242/30 December 2021.

Informed Consent Statement: Informed consent was obtained from all subjects involved in the study.

Data Availability Statement: The raw data supporting the conclusions of this article will be made available by the authors upon reasonable request.

Conflicts of Interest: The authors declare no conflicts of interest.

References

1. O'sullivan, P.F.; Kendler, K.S.; Neale, M.C. Schizophrenia as a Complex Trait: Evidence from a Meta-Analysis of Twin Studies. *Arch. Gen. Psychiatry* **2003**, *60*, 1187–1192. [CrossRef] [PubMed]
2. Owen, M.J.; Sawa, A.; Mortensen, P.B. Schizophrenia. *Lancet* **2016**, *388*, 86–97. [CrossRef] [PubMed]
3. Akbarian, S.; Nestler, E.J. Epigenetic Mechanisms in Psychiatry. *Neuron* **2016**, *89*, 683–686. [CrossRef]
4. Jouroukhin, Y.; McFarland, R.; Ayhan, Y.; Pletnikov, M.V. Modeling gene-environment interaction in schizophrenia. In *Modeling the Psychopathological Dimensions of Schizophrenia: From Molecules to Behavior*; Pletnikov, M.V., Waddington, J., Eds.; Elsevier Academic Press: Amsterdam, The Netherlands, 2016; pp. 345–360. [CrossRef]
5. Mill, J.; Tang, T.; Kaminsky, Z.; Khare, T.; Yazdanpanah, S.; Bouchard, L.; Jia, P.; Assadzadeh, A.; Flanagan, J.; Schumacher, A.; et al. Epigenomic Profiling Reveals DNA-Methylation Changes Associated with Major Psychosis. *Am. J. Hum. Genet.* **2008**, *82*, 696–711. [CrossRef]
6. Föcking, M.; Doyle, B.; Munawar, N.; Dillon, E.T.; Cotter, D.; Cagney, G. Epigenetic Factors in Schizophrenia: Mechanisms and Experimental Approaches. *Mol. Neuropsychiatry* **2019**, *5*, 6–12. [CrossRef] [PubMed] [PubMed Central]
7. Amadeo, M.B.; Esposito, D.; Escelsior, A.; Claudio Claudio Campus; Inuggi, A.; Da Silva, B.P.; Serafini, G.; Amore, M.; Gori, M. Time in schizophrenia: A link between psychopathology, psychophysics and technology. *Transl. Psychiatry* **2022**, *12*, 331. [CrossRef]
8. Tanaka, M.; Vécsei, L. Editorial of special issue crosstalk between depression, anxiety, and dementia: Comorbidity in behavioral neurology and neuropsychiatry. *Biomedicine* **2021**, *9*, 517. [CrossRef]
9. Tanaka, M.; Tóth, F.; Polyák, H.; Szabó, Á.; Mándi, Y.; Vécsei, L. Immune influencers in action: Metabolites and enzymes of the tryptophan-kynurenine metabolic pathway. *Biomedicine* **2021**, *9*, 734. [CrossRef] [PubMed]
10. Correia, B.S.B.; Nani, J.V.; Waladares Ricardo, R.; Stanisic, D.; Costa, T.B.B.C.; Hayashi, M.A.F.; Tasic, L. Effects of psychostimulants and antipsychotics on serum lipids in an animal model for schizophrenia. *Biomedicines* **2021**, *9*, 235. [CrossRef]
11. Robertson, G.S.; Hori, S.E.; Powell, K.J. Schizophrenia: An integrative approach to modelling a complex disorder. *J. Psychiatry Neurosci.* **2006**, *31*, 157–167.
12. Tanaka, M.; Szabó, Á.; Vécsei, L. Integrating armchair, bench, and bedside research for behavioral neurology and neuropsychiatry: Editorial. *Biomedicine* **2022**, *10*, 2999. [CrossRef] [PubMed]
13. Tanaka, M.; Vécsei, L. Editorial of special issue 'dissecting neurological and neuropsychiatric diseases: Neurodegeneration and neuroprotection'. *Int. J. Mol. Sci.* **2022**, *23*, 6991. [CrossRef] [PubMed]
14. Schmaal, L.; Hibar, D.P.; Sämann, P.G.; Hall, G.B.; Baune, B.T.; Jahanshad, N.; Cheung, J.W.; van Erp, T.G.M.; Bos, D.; Ikram, M.A.; et al. Cortical abnormalities in adults and adolescents with major depression based on brain scans from 20 cohorts worldwide in the ENIGMA Major Depressive Disorder Working Group. *Mol. Psychiatry* **2017**, *22*, 900–909. [CrossRef] [PubMed] [PubMed Central]
15. Murphy, M.L.; Frodl, T. Meta-analysis of diffusion tensor imaging studies shows altered fractional anisotropy occurring in distinct brain areas in association with depression. *Biol. Mood Anxiety Disord.* **2011**, *1*, 3. [CrossRef] [PubMed] [PubMed Central]
16. van Erp, T.G.; Hibar, D.P.; Rasmussen, J.M.; Glahn, D.C.; Pearlson, G.D.; Andreassen, O.A.; Agartz, I.; Westlye, L.T.; Haukvik, U.K.; Dale, A.M.; et al. Subcortical brain volume abnormalities in 2028 individuals with schizophrenia and 2540 healthy controls via the ENIGMA consortium. *Mol Psychiatry* **2016**, *21*, 547–553; Erratum in *Mol. Psychiatry* **2016**, *21*, 585. [CrossRef] [PubMed] [PubMed Central]
17. Adriano, F.; Caltagirone, C.; Spalletta, G. Hippocampal Volume Reduction in First-Episode and Chronic Schizophrenia: A Review and Meta-Analysis. *Neuroscientist* **2012**, *18*, 180–200. [CrossRef]
18. Sheline, Y.I.; Price, J.L.; Yan, Z.; Mintun, M.A. Resting-State Functional MRI in Depression Unmasks Increased Connectivity in the Default Mode Network. *Proc. Natl. Acad. Sci. USA* **2010**, *107*, 11020–11025. [CrossRef]

19. Disner, S.G.; Beevers, C.G.; Haigh, E.A.; Beck, A.T. Neural mechanisms of the cognitive model of depression. *Nat. Rev. Neurosci.* **2011**, *12*, 467–477. [CrossRef] [PubMed]
20. Whitfield-Gabrieli, S.; Ford, J.M. Default mode network activity and connectivity in psychopathology. *Annu. Rev. Clin. Psychol.* **2012**, *8*, 49–76. [CrossRef] [PubMed]
21. Palaniyappan, L.; Simmonite, M.; White, T.P.; Liddle, E.B.; Liddle, P.F. Neural primacy of the salience processing system in schizophrenia. *Neuron* **2013**, *79*, 814–828. [CrossRef] [PubMed] [PubMed Central]
22. Woodward, N.D.; Heckers, S. Mapping Thalamocortical Functional Connectivity in Chronic and Early Stages of Psychotic Disorders. *Biol. Psychiatry* **2016**, *79*, 1016–1025. [CrossRef] [PubMed] [PubMed Central]
23. Krishnan, V.; Nestler, E.J. The molecular neurobiology of depression. *Nature* **2008**, *455*, 894–902. [CrossRef] [PubMed] [PubMed Central]
24. Ritter, C.; Buchmann, A.; Müller, S.T.; Volleberg, M.; Haynes, M.; Ghisleni, C.; Noeske, R.; Tuura, R.; Hasler, G. Evaluation of Prefrontal γ-Aminobutyric Acid and Glutamate Levels in Individuals with Major Depressive Disorder Using Proton Magnetic Resonance Spectroscopy. *JAMA Psychiatry* **2022**, *79*, 1209–1216. [CrossRef] [PubMed] [PubMed Central]
25. Perez, S.M.; Elam, H.B.; Lodge, D.J. Increased Presynaptic Dopamine Synthesis Capacity Is Associated with Aberrant Dopamine Neuron Activity in the Methylazoxymethanol Acetate Rodent Model Used to Study Schizophrenia-Related Pathologies. *Schizophr. Bull. Open* **2022**, *3*, sgac067. [CrossRef] [PubMed] [PubMed Central]
26. Panov, G.; Panova, P. Neurobiochemical Disturbances in Psychosis and their Implications for Therapeutic Intervention. *Curr. Top. Med. Chem.* **2024**, *24*, 1784–1798. [CrossRef] [PubMed]
27. Coyle, J.T. Glutamate and schizophrenia: Beyond the dopamine hypothesis. *Cell Mol. Neurobiol.* **2006**, *26*, 365–384. [CrossRef] [PubMed]
28. Erhardt, S.; Schwieler, L.; Imbeault, S.; Engberg, G. The kynurenine pathway in schizophrenia and bipolar disorder. *Neuropharmacology* **2017**, *112 Pt B*, 297–306. [CrossRef] [PubMed]
29. Wichers, M.C.; Koek, G.H.; Robaeys, G.; Verkerk, R.; Scharpé, S.; Maes, M. IDO and interferon-alpha-induced depressive symptoms: A shift in hypothesis from tryptophan depletion to neurotoxicity. *Mol. Psychiatry* **2005**, *10*, 538–544. [CrossRef] [PubMed]
30. Martos, D.; Tuka, B.; Tanaka, M.; Vécsei, L.; Telegdy, G. Memory Enhancement with Kynurenic Acid and Its Mechanisms in Neurotransmission. *Biomedicines* **2022**, *10*, 849. [CrossRef] [PubMed] [PubMed Central]
31. Tanaka, M.; Bohár, Z.; Martos, D.; Telegdy, G.; Vécsei, L. Antidepressant-like effects of kynurenic acid in a modified forced swim test. *Pharmacol. Rep.* **2020**, *72*, 449–455. [CrossRef] [PubMed]
32. Martos, D.; Lőrinczi, B.; Szatmári, I.; Vécsei, L.; Tanaka, M. The Impact of C-3 Side Chain Modifications on Kynurenic Acid: A Behavioral Analysis of Its Analogs in the Motor Domain. *Int. J. Mol. Sci.* **2024**, *25*, 3394. [CrossRef] [PubMed]
33. Upthegrove, R.; Birchwood, M.; Ross, K.; Brunett, K.; McCollum, R.; Jones, L. The evolution of depression and suicidality in first episode psychosis. *Acta Psychiatr. Scand.* **2010**, *122*, 211–218. [CrossRef] [PubMed]
34. Cardoso, C.S.; Caiaffa, W.T.; Bandeira, M.; Siqueira, A.L.; Silva, J.T.; Fonseca, J.O. Depression in schizophrenia: Prevalence and relationship to quality of life. *Cad. Saude Publica.* **2007**, *23*, 2035–2048. [CrossRef]
35. van Os, J.; Fahy, T.A.; Jones, P.; Harvey, I.; Sham, P.; Lewis, S.; Bebbington, P.; Toone, B.; Williams, M.; Murray, R. Psychopathological syndromes in the functional psychoses: Associations with course and outcome. *Psychol. Med.* **1996**, *26*, 161–176. [CrossRef] [PubMed]
36. Salvatore, P.; Khalsa, H.M.; Hennen, J.; Tohen, M.; Yurgelun-Todd, D.; Casolari, F.; Depanfilis, C.; Maggini, C.; Baldessarini, R.J. Psychopathology factors in first-episode affective and non-affective psychotic disorders. *J. Psychiatr. Res.* **2007**, *41*, 724–736. [CrossRef] [PubMed]
37. Jonsson, H.; Nyman, A.K. Predicting long-term outcome in schizophrenia. *Acta Psychiatr. Scand.* **1991**, *83*, 342–346. [CrossRef] [PubMed]
38. McIntosh, A.M.; Forrester, A.; Lawrie, S.M.; Byrne, M.; Harper, A.; Kestelman, J.N.; Best, J.J.; Johnstone, E.C.; Owens, D.G. A factor model of the functional psychoses and the relationship of factors to clinical variables and brain morphology. *Psychol. Med.* **2001**, *31*, 159–171. [CrossRef]
39. Allardyce, J.; McCreadie, R.G.; Morrison, G.; van Os, J. Do symptoms dimensions or categorical diagnoses best discriminate between known risk factors for psychosis? *Soc. Psychiatry Psychiatr. Epidemiol.* **2007**, *42*, 429–437. [CrossRef]
40. World Health Organization. *ICD-10: International Statistical Classification of Diseases and Related Health Problems: Tenth Revision*, 2nd ed.; World Health Organization: Geneva, Switzerland, 2004. Available online: https://iris.who.int/handle/10665/42980 (accessed on 24 September 2024).
41. World Health Organization. *ICD-11: International Classification of Diseases*, 11th ed.; World Health Organization: Geneva, Switzerland, 2022. Available online: https://icd.who.int/ (accessed on 24 September 2024).
42. Panov, G. Analysis of Depressive Symptoms in Treatment-Resistant Schizophrenia. *J. Psychiatr. Res.* **2022**, *150*, 100–110.
43. Golubović, B.; Golubović, Š. The Impact of Socio-Demographic Factors on Depressive Symptoms in Schizophrenia. *Psychiatr. Danub.* **2020**, *32* (Suppl. S2), 220–225.
44. Golubović, B.; Gajić, Z.; Ivetić, O.; Milatović, J.; Vuleković, P.; Đilvesi, Đ.; Golubović, S.; Vrban, F.; Subašić, A.; Rasulić, L. Factors associated with depression in patients with schizophrenia. *Acta Clin. Croat.* **2020**, *59*, 605–614. [CrossRef] [PubMed] [PubMed Central]

45. Van IJzendoorn, M.H.; Schuengel, C. The measurement of dissociation in normal and clinical populations: Meta-analytic validation of the Dissociative Experiences Scale (DES). *Clin. Psychol. Rev.* **1996**, *16*, 365–382. [CrossRef]
46. Hamilton, M. A rating scale for depression. *J. Neurol. Neurosurg. Psychiatry* **1960**, *23*, 56–62. [CrossRef] [PubMed]
47. Hamilton, M. The assessment of anxiety states by rating. *Br. J. Med. Psychol.* **1959**, *32*, 50–55. [CrossRef]
48. Abramowitz, J.S.; Deacon, B.J.; Olatunji, B.O.; Wheaton, M.G.; Berman, N.C.; Losardo, D.; Timpano, K.R.; McGrath, P.B.; Riemann, B.C.; Adams, T.; et al. Assessment of obsessive-compulsive symptom dimensions: Development and evaluation of the Dimensional Obsessive-Compulsive Scale. *Psychol. Assess.* **2010**, *22*, 180–198. [CrossRef] [PubMed]
49. Golden, C.J.; Hammeke, T.A. *The Luria-Nebraska Neuropsychological Battery: Theory and Clinical Applications*; Grune & Stratton: New York, NY, USA, 1984.
50. Overall, J.E.; Gorham, D.R. The Brief Psychiatric Rating Scale. *Psychol. Rep.* **1962**, *10*, 799–812. [CrossRef]
51. Kay, S.R.; Fiszbein, A.; Opler, L.A. The positive and negative syndrome scale (PANSS) for schizophrenia. *Schizophr. Bull.* **1987**, *13*, 261–276. [CrossRef]
52. Andrean, N.C.; Carpenter, W.T.; Kane, J.M., Jr.; Lasser, R.A.; Marder, S.R.; Weinberger, D.R. Remission in schizophrenia: Proposed criteria and rationale for consensus. *Am. J. Psychiatry* **2005**, *162*, 441–449. [CrossRef]
53. *Diagnostic and Statistical Manual of Mental Disorders: DSM-IV*; American Psychiatric Association: Washington, DC, USA, 2013.
54. Panov, G.; Panova, P. Obsessive-compulsive symptoms in patient with schizophrenia: The influence of disorganized symptoms, duration of schizophrenia, and drug resistance. *Front. Psychiatry.* **2023**, *14*, 1120974. [CrossRef]
55. Panov, G. Dissociative Model in Patients with Resistant Schizophrenia. *Front. Psychiatry* **2022**, *13*, 845493. [CrossRef]
56. Panov, G. Comparative Analysis of Lateral Preferences in Patients with Resistant Schizophrenia. *Front. Psychiatry* **2022**, *13*, 868285. [CrossRef] [PubMed]
57. Panov, G. Gender-associated role in patients with schizophrenia. Is there a connection with the resistance? *Front. Psychiatry* **2022**, *13*, 995455. [CrossRef] [PubMed]
58. Panov, G.P. Early Markers in Resistant Schizophrenia: Effect of the First Antipsychotic Drug. *Diagnostics* **2022**, *12*, 803. [CrossRef] [PubMed]
59. Panov, G.; Djulgerova, S.; Panova, P. The effect of education level and sex differences on resistance to treatment in patients with schizophrenia. *Bulg. Med.* **2022**, *12*, 22–29.
60. Panov, G.; Djulgerova, S.; Panova, P. Comparative anthropometric criteria in patients with resistant schizophrenia. *Bulg. Med.* **2022**, *12*, 30–39.
61. Kuehner, C. Why is depression more common among women than among men? *Lancet Psychiatry* **2017**, *4*, 146–158. [CrossRef]
62. Hafner, H.; van der Heiden, W.; Behrens, S.; Gattaz, W.F.; Hambrecht, M.; Loffler, W.; Maurer, K. Causes and consequences of the gender difference in age at onset of schizophrenia. *Schizophr. Bull.* **1999**, *24*, 99–113. [CrossRef]
63. Goldstein, J.M.; Tsuang, M.T.; Faraone, S.V. Gender and schizophrenia: Implications for understanding the heterogeneity of the illness. *Psychiatr. Clin. N. Am.* **1989**, *12*, 205–221. [CrossRef]
64. Cotton, S.M.; Lambert, M.; Schimmelmann, B.G.; Filia, K.M.; Rayner, V.; Hides, L.; McGorry, P.D. Gender differences in premorbid, entry, treatment, and outcome characteristics in a treated epidemiologicl sample of 661 patients with first-episode psychosis. *Schizophr. Res.* **2009**, *114*, 17–24. [CrossRef]
65. Leung, A.; Chue, P.; Xiang, Y.T. Gender differences in schizophrenia: A review of the literature. *J. Psychiatry Neurosci.* **2010**, *35*, 322–330.
66. Seeman, M.V. Psychopathology in women and men: Focus on female hormones. *Am. J. Psychiatry* **1997**, *154*, 1641–1647. [CrossRef] [PubMed]
67. Hambrecht, M.; Maurer, K.; Häfner, H.; Sartorius, N. Gender differences in schizophrenia in three cultures: Results of the WHO ten-country study. *Acta Psychiatr. Scand.* **1992**, *86*, 287–292.
68. Perlick, D.A.; Rosenheck, R.A.; Kaczynski, R.; Swartz, M.S.; Cañive, J.M.; Lieberman, J.A. Components and correlates of family burden in schizophrenia. *Psychiatr. Serv.* **2006**, *57*, 1117–1125. [CrossRef] [PubMed]
69. Conus, P.; Berk, M.; McGorry, P.D. Psychological treatment of comorbid depression and substance use disorder. *J. Clin. Psychiatry* **2014**, *75*, 134–141.
70. Addington, J.; Addington, D. Neurocognitive and social functioning in schizophrenia: A 2.5 year follow-up study. *Schizophr. Res.* **2000**, *44*, 47–56. [CrossRef]
71. Ventura, J.; Nuechterlein, K.H.; Subotnik, K.L.; Green, M.F.; Gitlin, M.J. Symptom dimensions in recent-onset schizophrenia: Associations with social functioning. *Schizophr. Res.* **2000**, *45*, 107–119.
72. Lysaker, P.H.; Lysaker, J.T. Schizophrenia and alterations in self-experience: A comparison of 6 perspectives. *Schizophr. Bull.* **2010**, *36*, 331–340. [CrossRef] [PubMed]
73. Sass, L.A.; Parnas, J. Schizophrenia, consciousness, and the self. *Schizophr. Bull.* **2003**, *29*, 427–444. [CrossRef]
74. van der Meer, L.; de Vos, A.E.; Stiekema, A.P.; Pijnenborg, G.H.; van Tol, M.J.; Nolen, W.A.; Aleman, A. Insight in schizophrenia: Involvement of self-reflection networks? *Schizophr. Bull.* **2013**, *39*, 1288–1295. [CrossRef]
75. Poyurovsky, M.; Koran, L.M. Obsessive-compulsive disorder in schizophrenia. *CNS Drugs* **2005**, *19*, 997–1008. [CrossRef]
76. Geddes, J.; Mercer, G.; Frith, C.D.; Macmillan, F.; Owens, D.G.C.; Johnstone, E.C. Prediction of outcome following a first episode schizophrenia; a follow-up study of Northwick Park first episode study subjects. *Br. J. Psychiatry* **1994**, *165*, 664–668. [CrossRef] [PubMed]

77. Buckley, P.F.; Miller, B.J.; Lehrer, D.S.; Castle, D.J. Schizophrenia and comorbid conditions. *Schizophr. Bull.* **2009**, *35*, 383–402. [CrossRef]
78. Siris, S.G. Depression in schizophrenia: Perspective in the era of atypical antipsychotic agents. *Am. J. Psychiatry* **2000**, *157*, 1379–1389. [CrossRef] [PubMed]
79. Rector, N.A.; Beck, A.T. Cognitive behavioral therapy for schizophrenia: An empirical review. *J. Nerv. Ment. Dis.* **2001**, *189*, 278–287. [CrossRef] [PubMed]
80. Upthegrove, R.; Marwaha, S.; Birchwood, M. Depression and schizophrenia: Cause, consequence, or trans-diagnostic issue? *Schizophr. Bull.* **2017**, *43*, 240–244. [CrossRef]
81. Addington, D.; Addington, J.; Maticka-Tyndale, E. Cognitive functioning and positive and negative symptoms in schizophrenia. *Schizophr. Res.* **1993**, *9*, 179–185. [CrossRef]
82. Leucht, S.; Kane, J.M.; Kissling, W.; Hamann, J.; Etschel, E.; Engel, R. Clinical implications of Brief Psychiatric Rating Scale scores. *Br. J. Psychiatry* **2005**, *187*, 366–371. [CrossRef] [PubMed]
83. Leucht, S.; Engel, R.R.; Kane, J.M. Measuring schizophrenia—What difference does the choice of the scale make? *Schizophr. Res.* **2008**, *100*, 251–258.
84. Emsley, R.; Rabinowitz, J.; Medori, R. PANSS factors predictive of response to risperidone in schizophrenia: Evidence from a large, long-term, randomized trial. *Schizophr. Res.* **2007**, *92*, 65–73.
85. Meltzer, H.Y. Treatment of schizophrenia with atypical antipsychotic drugs: Influence on cognition, depression, and negative symptoms. *Am. J. Manag. Care* **2001**, *7* (Suppl. S11), S253–S257.
86. Schennach, R.; Obermeier, M.; Seemüller, F.; Jäger, M.; Schmauss, M.; Laux, G.; Riedel, M. Change of subjective well-being under antipsychotic treatment in schizophrenia. *Eur. Psychiatry* **2012**, *27*, 247–256.
87. Kane, J.M.; Kishimoto, T.; Correll, C.U. Non-adherence to medication in patients with psychotic disorders: Epidemiology, contributing factors and management strategies. *World Psychiatry* **2013**, *12*, 216–226. [CrossRef] [PubMed]
88. Leucht, S.; Cipriani, A.; Spineli, L.; Mavridis, D.; Örey, D.; Richter, F.; Samara, M.; Barbui, C.; Engel, R.R.; Geddes, J.R.; et al. Comparative efficacy and tolerability of 15 antipsychotic drugs in schizophrenia: A multiple-treatments meta-analysis. *Lancet* **2013**, *382*, 951–962. [CrossRef] [PubMed]
89. Correll, C.U.; Rubio, J.M.; Kane, J.M. What is the risk-benefit ratio of long-term antipsychotic treatment in people with schizophrenia? *World Psychiatry* **2018**, *17*, 149–160. [CrossRef]
90. Miyamoto, S.; Duncan, G.E.; Marx, C.E.; Lieberman, J.A. Treatments for schizophrenia: A critical review of pharmacology and mechanisms of action of antipsychotic drugs. *Mol. Psychiatry* **2005**, *10*, 79–104. [CrossRef] [PubMed]
91. Lieberman, J.A.; Stroup, T.S.; McEvoy, J.P.; Swartz, M.S.; Rosenheck, R.A.; Perkins, D.O.; Keefe, R.S.E.; Davis, S.M.; Davis, C.E.; Lebowitz, B.D.; et al. Effectiveness of antipsychotic drugs in patients with chronic schizophrenia. *N. Engl. J. Med.* **2005**, *353*, 1209–1223. [CrossRef]
92. Gallagher, P.; Jones, L.; O'Connor, R.; Cowen, P.J. A pilot study of antidepressant efficacy in patients with schizophrenia and depressive symptoms: Mirtazapine combined with risperidone. *J. Psychopharmacol.* **2006**, *20*, 683–688.
93. Zisook, S.; Kasckow, J.W. Intriguing role of antidepressants in schizophrenia treatment. *J. Clin. Psychiatry* **2009**, *70*, 514–522.
94. Wijkstra, J.; Lijmer, J.; Burger, H.; Geddes, J.; Nolen, W.A. Pharmacological treatment for major depressive disorder and depressive symptoms in schizophrenia: A systematic review and meta-analysis. *Br. J. Psychiatry* **2013**, *204*, 255–259.
95. Schennach, R.; Meyer, S.; Seemüller, F.; Jäger, M.; Schmauss, M.; Laux, G.; Riedel, M. Antidepressant treatment in schizophrenic patients with predominantly negative symptoms. *Pharmacopsychiatry* **2015**, *48*, 141–149.
96. Rothschild, A.J. Challenges in the treatment of major depressive disorder with psychotic features. *Schizophr. Bull.* **2013**, *39*, 787–796. [CrossRef] [PubMed]
97. Meyers, B.S.; Flint, A.J. The epidemiology of psychotic depression: Age, race, gender, and risk for chronicity. *Am. J. Geriatr. Psychiatry* **1991**, *7*, 5–13.
98. Coryell, W.; Leon, A.C.; Turvey, C.; Akiskal, H.S.; Mueller, T.; Endicott, J. The significance of psychotic features in unipolar major depression: A report from the National Institute of Mental Health collaborative depression study. *J. Clin. Psychiatry* **2001**, *62*, 521–527.
99. Tew, J.D.; Mulsant, B.H. Current approaches to the treatment of major depression with psychotic features. *J. Clin. Psychiatry* **2007**, *68* (Suppl. S3), 12–17.
100. Meyer-Lindenberg, A. From maps to mechanisms through neuroimaging of schizophrenia. *Nature* **2010**, *468*, 194–202. [CrossRef]
101. Howes, O.D.; Kapur, S. The dopamine hypothesis of schizophrenia: Version III—The final common pathway. *Schizophr. Bull.* **2009**, *35*, 549–562. [CrossRef]
102. Sanacora, G.; Banasr, M. From pathophysiology to novel antidepressant drugs: Glial contributions to the pathology and treatment of mood disorders. *Biol. Psychiatry* **2013**, *73*, 1172–1179. [CrossRef]
103. Gibbons, A.; Dean, B. The role of glutamate in schizophrenia and the likely impact of glutamatergic dysfunction on the development of the disorder. *Biochem. Cell Biol.* **2016**, *94*, 92–97.
104. Zhou, Y.; Liang, M.; Jiang, T.; Tian, L.; Liu, Y.; Liu, Z.; Liu, H.; Kuang, F. Functional dysconnectivity of the dorsolateral prefrontal cortex in first-episode schizophrenia using resting-state fMRI. *Neurosci Lett.* **2007**, *417*, 297–302. [CrossRef] [PubMed]
105. Metsanen, M.; Wahlberg, K.E.; Hakko, H.; Saarento, O.; Tienari, P. Thought disorder index: A longitudinal study of severity levels and schizophrenia factors. *J. Psychiatr. Res.* **2006**, *40*, 258–266. [CrossRef]

106. Reed, R.A.; Harrow, M.; Herbener, E.S.; Martin, E.M. Executive function in schizophrenia: Is it linked to psychosis and poor life functioning? *J. Nerv. Ment. Dis.* **2002**, *190*, 725–732. [CrossRef] [PubMed]
107. Shenton, M.E.; Kikinis, R.; Jolesz, F.A.; Pollak, S.D.; LeMay, M.; Wible, C.G.; Hokama, H.; Martin, J.; Metcalf, D.; Coleman, M.; et al. Abnormalities of the left temporal lobe and thought disorder in schizophrenia. A quantitative magnetic resonance imaging study. *N. Engl. J. Med.* **1992**, *327*, 604–612. [CrossRef] [PubMed]

biomedicines

MDPI

Article

Resveratrol and Its Metabolite as Potential Allosteric Regulators of Monoamine Oxidase A Activity in the Brain and Liver Under Chronic Predator Stress

Jurica Novak [1,*], Olga B. Tseilikman [2], Vladislav A. Shatilov [2], Maxim S. Zhukov [2], Vadim A. Shevyrin [3], Zuhra R. Khismatullina [4], Albina M. Fedorova [4], Georgiy N. Patrikyan [2], Timur L. Khaibullin [2] and Vadim E. Tseilikman [2,5,6,*]

[1] Centre for Informatics and Computing, Ruđer Bošković Institute, Bijenička Cesta 54, 10000 Zagreb, Croatia
[2] Faculty of Fundamental Medicine, Chelyabinsk State University, 454001 Chelyabinsk, Russia
[3] Chemical Technology Institute, Ural Federal University Named after the First President of Russia B. N. Yeltsin, 620062 Yekaterinburg, Russia
[4] Institute of Nature and Man, Ufa University of Science and Technology, 450076 Ufa, Russia
[5] Scientific and Educational Center 'Biomedical Technologies', School of Medical Biology, South Ural State University, 454080 Chelyabinsk, Russia
[6] Zelman Faculty of Medicine and Psychology, Novosibirsk State University, 630090 Novosibirsk, Russia
* Correspondence: jnovak@irb.hr (J.N.); vadimed@yandex.ru (V.E.T.)

Abstract: Background: Resveratrol has been shown to modulate stress-related anxiety by reducing brain monoamine oxidase A (MAO-A) activity. However, the molecular mechanism underlying this neurochemical effect remains unknown. In this study, we employed in silico approaches to investigate the binding affinity of resveratrol and its predominant blood metabolite, resveratrol glucuronide, to specific sites on MAO-A. **Methods**: For the in silico analysis, we employed molecular docking and molecular dynamics simulations. Within the liver–brain axis, we investigated the role of hepatic MAO-A in the development of anxiety. The activity of whole-brain MAO-A was compared with its activity in specific brain regions, including the amygdala, hippocampus, and prefrontal cortex. **Results**: Our findings suggest the presence of an allosteric site on the enzyme that accommodates these compounds. Furthermore, in vivo experiments demonstrated that high-dose resveratrol suppresses MAO activity not only in the brain but also in the liver of stress-exposed rats. The in vivo results are interpreted in the context of an allosteric site on MAO-A in both the brain and liver, which may mediate the interaction with resveratrol and its metabolite. **Conclusions**: The primary outcomes of the study include the identification of the role of hepatic MAO-A in the development of anxiety-like behavior, as well as the determination of resveratrol dose ranges at which it functions as an allosteric modulator of MAO-A activity.

Keywords: resveratrol; monoamine oxidase; serotonin; *trans*-resveratrol-3-*O*-glucuronide; allostery

1. Introduction

Resveratrol (*trans*-3,4′,5-trihydroxystilbene) (Figure 1) is a naturally occurring phenolic compound belonging to the stilbene family, predominantly found in various plant sources, including grape skins, berries, cocoa, and nuts [1–3]. Its levels in plants often increase in response to various environmental stressors, such as ultraviolet radiation, ozone exposure, and pathogen attacks [4,5]. Resveratrol (RES) has been recognized as one of the most promising chemopreventive agents against cancer. In addition, it exhibits antidiabetic, antiviral, cardioprotective, anti-inflammatory, and neuroprotective properties. Notably, its neuroprotective effects are largely attributed to its ability to enhance neuroplasticity [6–8].

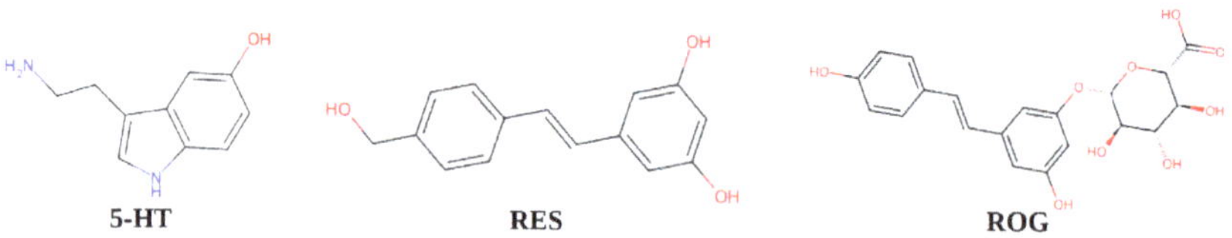

5-HT **RES** **ROG**

Figure 1. Two-dimensional structures of serotonin (5-HT), resveratrol (RES), and *trans*-resveratrol-3-*O*-glucuronide (ROG).

Due to its neuroprotective and antioxidant properties, RES has demonstrated therapeutic potential in neurodegenerative disorders as well as in the correction of stress-related behavioral disorders [9,10]. Recent studies from our group have established the efficacy of RES in alleviating anxiety disorders induced by chronic predator stress, an experimental model of post-traumatic stress disorder (PTSD) [11,12]. These findings identified monoamine oxidases (MAOs) in the brain as key molecular targets of RES. Our results further revealed that stress-induced anxiety correlates with increased MAO-A activity, whereas RES administration effectively reduced MAO-A activity in parallel with behavioral improvements. Importantly, the anxiolytic effects of RES exceeded those of selective serotonin reuptake inhibitors (SSRIs), which are currently considered the first-line pharmacological treatment for PTSD. Notably, RES shares a common target with SSRIs—the serotonin transporter (SERT)—which is responsible for serotonin reuptake.

Despite its remarkable therapeutic potential, the clinical application of RES remains challenging due to its rapid metabolism and poor bioavailability [13,14]. Pharmacokinetic studies indicate significant losses of RES during absorption, with only a small fraction of the compound being absorbed through the intestinal epithelium without undergoing metabolism. Experiments on an isolated rat intestinal model have shown that 96.5% $\pm$ 4.6% of the absorbed RES was detected as its glucuronide conjugate, highlighting its susceptibility to glucuronidation during transport across the jejunal epithelium [13].

Interestingly, *trans*-resveratrol-3-*O*-glucuronide (ROG) itself exhibits biological activity, including well-documented anticancer properties [15–17]. In our studies, a correlation was observed between the levels of ROG in the blood of stressed animals and anxiety-related behavioral parameters in the elevated plus maze test, a widely used model for assessing anxiety in chronic predator stress [18]. However, the precise mechanisms underlying the behavioral effects of ROG under chronic stress conditions remain unknown.

Traditionally, the relationship between brain MAO-A and the regulation of behavioral activity has been the primary focus of research, with particular emphasis on the enzyme's ability to metabolize monoamine neurotransmitters. However, the potential contribution of hepatic MAO-A to behavioral regulation has been largely overlooked. In the liver, MAO-A is involved in the oxidative deamination of trace amines of intestinal origin that reach the liver via the portal circulation. To date, the therapeutic effects of resveratrol on anxiety disorders have not been associated with its modulation of MAO-A activity in peripheral organs. Furthermore, paradoxical findings—such as resveratrol's ability to reduce MAO-A activity despite an upregulation of its gene expression—remain insufficiently addressed.

Given that MAO-A has been identified as a key target of RES, we conducted an in silico comparative analysis to evaluate the binding interactions of RES and ROG with MAO-A. The computational results were further correlated with the experimental findings on RES and ROG levels in stressed animals and their impact on MAO-A activity.

2. Materials and Methods

2.1. Animals

Experiments were conducted on male Wistar rats, weighing 210–230 g and three months of age at the onset of the study. The use of males was justified by the fact that applying the same experimental protocol to females would require additional time to synchronize the estrous cycle. In this study, male Wistar rats were housed in individually ventilated cages, with each enclosure accommodating three to four animals. The rodents had unrestricted access to tap water and a nutritionally balanced diet (Beaphar Care Plus Rat Food, Raalte, The Netherlands). Environmental conditions within the vivarium were carefully regulated, maintaining a temperature range of 22–25 °C and a relative humidity of 55%. The light–dark cycle was set to 12:12 h, with illumination commencing at 07:00 and concluding at 19:00.

2.2. Chronic Predator Stress Paradigm

In this study, a chronic predator stress (PS) paradigm was employed. While cat urine has been conventionally used as a predator odor source in post-traumatic stress disorder (PTSD) research, its efficacy in eliciting an immediate anxiety response following prolonged stress exposure has been limited. Prior research demonstrated that prolonged exposure to cat odor led to a diminished sensitivity to this stimulus in stressed rats by the conclusion of the PS paradigm. Furthermore, time-dependent sensitization—recognized as a key feature of PTSD—only became evident two weeks after the exposure period. To provoke an immediate behavioral response characterized by acute stress-induced anxiety, cat urine was replaced with fox urine, which exhibits a stronger anxiogenic effect.

2.3. Fox Urine Collection and Application

Urine was obtained from sexually mature males of domesticated silver-black foxes (*Vulpes vulpes*). Collection took place during the autumn season from multiple individuals, after which the samples were aliquoted and stored at −18 °C for a maximum duration of one month. Prior to use, the urine was thawed immediately. To deliver the stressor, 100 μL of urine was deposited onto a cotton pad and placed within a plastic Petri dish covered by a nylon mesh to allow the release of volatile compounds. The Petri dish was positioned inside the animals' home cages for a duration of 10 min each day across a 10-day period, starting on the fifth day of the experiment.

2.4. Timeline of Predator Stress Exposure, Resveratrol Treatment, and Plasma Resveratrol Concentration Assessment

To evaluate the effects of RES treatment on anxiety-like behavior and monoamine oxidase A (MAO-A) activity in the brain and liver, rats were subjected to a 10-day predator stress (PS) paradigm. The animals were assigned to the following experimental groups:

1. Control (n = 7): Rats received vehicle treatment for 10 consecutive days without exposure to predator stress.
2. PS (n = 7): Rats were subjected to chronic predator stress.
3. RES + PS 20 mg/kg (n = 7): Rats were administered resveratrol (20 mg/kg) via intraperitoneal injection one hour prior to each predator stress exposure.
4. RES + PS 50 mg/kg (n = 7): Rats were administered resveratrol (50 mg/kg) via intraperitoneal injection one hour prior to each predator stress exposure.
5. RES + PS 100 mg/kg (n = 7): Rats were administered resveratrol (100 mg/kg) via intraperitoneal injection one hour prior to each predator stress exposure.

The rationale for administering RES one hour prior to the onset of stressor exposure was based on the brief duration of a single stressor session. It was essential for RES to be present in the system at the time of stressor exposure. The PS-exposed animals were divided into two groups: one received daily intraperitoneal injections of RES at doses of 20, 50, or 100 mg/kg ("PS + RES" group), while the other received vehicle only ("PS" group). Control animals were also administered vehicle injections.

Trans-resveratrol was obtained from Sigma Aldrich Ltd. (St. Louis, MO, USA). Daily intraperitoneal injections of RES were administered over the first 10 days of the experiment. Fresh solutions were prepared on a weekly basis and stored at room temperature until use. RES was dissolved in 99% DMSO to achieve a final injection volume of 1 mL/kg of body weight, corresponding to a dosage of 20, 50, and 100 mg/kg [18].

Plasma concentrations of RES and its primary metabolite, ROG, were quantified in the "PS + RES" group. Correlations were examined between RES and ROG levels and various behavioral parameters, as well as MAO-A activity in the brain and liver.

2.5. Behavioral Testing

Anxiety-like behavior was assessed using the elevated plus maze (EPM) test, employing a standard apparatus (model TS0502-R3, OpenScience, Russia; http://www.openscience.ru/index.php?page=ts&item=002 (accessed on 9 May 2025)). The EPM consisted of two open and two closed arms (arm length: 0.5 m; arm width: 0.14 m) elevated 0.55 m above the floor, with the height of the closed arm walls measuring 0.3 m and the side rails of the open arms measuring 0.01 m [19]. At the beginning of each trial, animals were placed in the central platform facing an open arm. An entry into an arm was recorded when all four paws of the rat were within the arm. Behavioral tracking and analysis were performed using the 3D animal tracking system "EthoStudio" (http://ethostudio.com/new/en/about/ (accessed on 9 May 2025)). The test was performed over a 10-min period. The rationale for selecting the behavioral tests was based on their established suitability for assessing anxiety levels and fear responses. To minimize potential bias, control and experimental groups were assessed concurrently under blinded conditions.

Key metrics for behavioral assessment included:

- Frequency of entries into the open and closed arms of the EPM;
- Duration of time spent within the open and closed arms.

Following the completion of each testing session, the surface of the EPM or the open field arena was thoroughly wiped with gauze soaked in ethanol to eliminate any residual traces left by the previous animal.

2.6. Blood and Tissue Collection and Storage

The rats were sacrificed by an overdose of diethyl ether, decapitated, and blood was collected for further analysis. During necropsy, samples of blood and liver tissue were collected from the rats. The blood was processed by centrifugation to isolate plasma, which was then transferred into Eppendorf tubes and stored at −70 °C. Liver tissue was preserved in two forms: one part was fixed in 10% buffered formalin for histopathological examination, while the remaining tissue was rapidly frozen in liquid nitrogen and stored at −70 °C for subsequent biochemical analysis.

Brain and liver tissues were rapidly frozen in liquid nitrogen and stored at −70 °C for biochemical investigations. The hippocampus, prefrontal cortex, and amygdala were dissected from freshly excised brains cooled on ice, based on anatomical landmarks defined in the Paxinos and Watson atlas [20]. These brain regions were immediately frozen in liquid nitrogen and stored at −70 °C for neurochemical analysis, which was conducted within seven days of tissue collection.

2.7. Quantification of RES and RES-O-Glucuronide in Rat Plasma

The concentrations of RES and its metabolite, ROG, in rat plasma were determined using high-performance liquid chromatography (HPLC) with a diode array ultraviolet (UV) detector (Agilent 1260 Infinity II, Agilent Technologies, Santa Clara, CA, USA). The separation process utilized a gradient elution approach on a Poroshell 120 EC-C_{18} reversed-phase column (3.0 mm × 100 mm × 2.7 μm; Agilent Technologies, 695975-302), coupled with a 5 mm guard column for system protection. The mobile phase comprised two eluents: solvent A (aqueous 0.1% *v*/*v* acetic acid) and solvent B (methanol containing 0.1% *v*/*v* acetic acid). A linear gradient elevated solvent B concentration from 15% to 100% over 14.3 min, and maintained at 100% for an additional 1.7 min. Operational parameters included a 0.7 mL/min flow rate and column thermostatting at 30 °C. Analyses employed 5 μL injections with ultraviolet detection configured at 304 nm.

Calibration standards were generated through spiking 50 μL of a methanol-dissolved RES working solution (Sigma-Aldrich, St. Louis, MO, USA, 98% purity) into 150 μL portions of blank plasma. This procedure yielded plasma calibration standards spanning 0.05–20.0 μg/mL RES concentrations. For sample processing, 200 μL of either plasma or prepared standards were aliquoted into 2.0 mL centrifugation vials. Each vial received 50 μL of pterostilbene internal standard solution (Sigma-Aldrich, St. Louis, MO, USA, 97% purity) at 20 μg/mL. Following 15 s vortex agitation, 0.8 mL of acetonitrile was introduced, and the mixture was vortex-mixed again for an additional 15 s. Samples were processed by centrifugation at 10,000 rpm for 15 min using a Thermo ST16R unit (Thermo Scientific, Waltham, MA, USA). Supernatants were harvested, transferred to fresh tubes, and dried under nitrogen gas at 45 °C via an NDK200 concentrator (Hangzhou MIU Instruments Co., Hangzhou, China). Dried residues were resolubilized in 0.2 mL of methanol:water (1:1 *v*/*v*), transferred to autosampler vials, and subjected to analysis.

Quantification of RES plasma levels utilized a calibration curve derived from the relationship between analyte-to-internal standard peak area ratios and corresponding analyte concentrations. ROG concentrations were calculated using the RES calibration framework, presuming equivalent detector responses between the two analytes. Identification of RES and pterostilbene chromatographic peaks was verified through retention time alignment and UV spectral matching (200–400 nm range) against reference standards.

ROG characterization was performed using an Agilent 6545 Q-TOF LC-MS system (Agilent Technologies, Santa Clara, CA, USA) with negative-ion electrospray ionization. Chromatographic parameters remained consistent with previously outlined separation conditions. Mass analysis detected a deprotonated molecular ion $[M-H]^-$ at m/z 403.1036 (Δ = 0.42 ppm). Under collision-induced dissociation parameters, the MS/MS spectrum displayed elimination of a glucuronic acid moiety (176 Da), generating a fragment ion at m/z 227.0712 (Δ = 0.74 ppm), corresponding to deprotonated resveratrol $[M-H]^-$.

2.8. Monoamine Oxidase Activity Measurement

MAO-A enzymatic activity was quantified in purified brain and liver mitochondrial preparations. Mitochondrial isolation from tissue homogenates followed established protocols from Satav and Katyare [21]. Evaluation of MAO-A activity in both brain and liver tissues was conducted using methodologies adapted from Tipton et al. [22].

For MAO-A assessment, cerebral tissue homogenates were incubated with 100 μL of 0.5 μM L-deprenyl (a MAO-B-specific inhibitor) for 60 min at 37 °C prior to analysis. The reaction was initiated by introduction of 5-hydroxytryptamine creatinine sulfate (4 mM) as the MAO-A-specific substrate. Spectrophotometric quantification at 278 nm determined enzymatic activity, expressed as nanomoles of serotonin catabolized (via MAO-A pathway) per milligram protein per minute.

A graphical overview of the experimental design, including group allocation (control and treatment groups) and the sequence of behavioral and biochemical assessments, is presented in Figure 2.

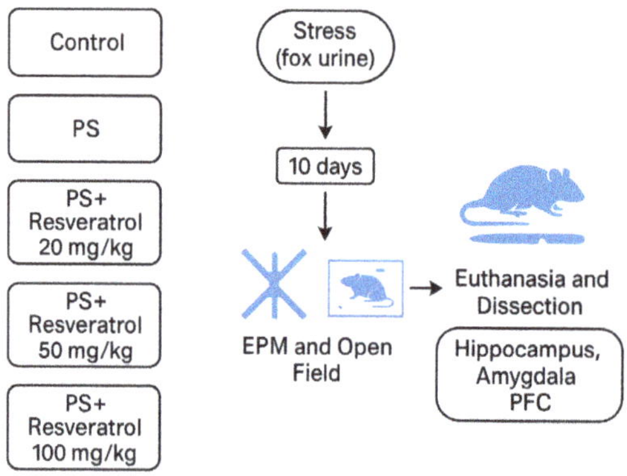

Figure 2. Graphical representation of the experimental workflow.

2.9. Statistical Analysis

Data were analyzed using SPSS 24.0 (SPSS Inc., Chicago, IL, USA), STATISTICA 10.0 (StatSoft Inc., Tulsa, OK, USA), and MS Excel 2010 (Microsoft Inc., Redmond, WA, USA) software. Quantitative data are expressed as the mean ± standard deviation (SD). Comparisons among groups were performed using the Kruskal–Wallis test, followed by Dunn's post hoc tests for pairwise comparisons. Spearman's rank correlation coefficient was used to assess the relationships between variables.

The effect size was estimated based on preliminary data obtained in previous studies conducted in our laboratory, in accordance with established recommendations and relevant literature from comparable research [23].

2.10. Molecular Docking Protocol

The high-resolution three-dimensional (3D) structure of monoamine oxidase A (MAO-A) was retrieved from the RCSB Protein Data Bank [24]. For molecular docking studies, the crystal structure of MAO-A (PDB ID: 2Z5X) [25] was selected. In this structure, the active site of MAO-A is occupied by the co-crystallized ligand HRM (7-methoxy-1-methyl-9*H*-*β*-carboline). Only the A chain of the MAO-A protein was retained for docking, while all water molecules and small ligands, except for the bound prosthetic group flavin adenine dinucleotide (FAD), were removed. Protein preparation was performed using Chimera 1.14 [26], which included the assignment of Gasteiger charges to each atom and the merging of all non-polar hydrogen atoms. Atom types were assigned according to the AutoDock force field, and the processed receptor structures were saved in `pdbqt` format for subsequent docking simulations.

The 3D structures of resveratrol (RES), *trans*-resveratrol-3-*O*-glucuronide (ROG), and serotonin (5-HT) were retrieved from the PubChem database [27]. Ligand preparation was carried out using the Python script mk_prepare_ligand.py version 0.6.1, developed by the Forli lab at the Center for Computational Structural Biology (CCSB) [28]. This script was employed to assign Gasteiger charges, define atom types according to the AutoDock force field, and generate the required `pdbqt` files for molecular docking simulations.

The center of the docking grid for MAO-A was defined at coordinates (40.6, 26.9, −14.5) Å, while the grid box dimensions were set to $75 \times 60 \times 55$ Å^3 to encompass the entire binding site and allow sufficient conformational flexibility for ligand binding.

Molecular docking simulations were conducted using AutoDock Vina version 1.2.5 [29], with an exhaustiveness parameter of 600 and a total of 100 docking modes per ligand to ensure a thorough exploration of binding conformations. Docked conformations were retained only if their binding affinity was within 4 kcal mol^{-1} of the highest-ranked pose, ensuring the selection of energetically favorable binding modes.

To assess different binding scenarios, docking simulations were performed for three sets of multiple ligands (5-HT, RES, ROG; 5-HT, RES; 5-HT, ROG) and a single-ligand (5-HT) system. Following docking, all generated poses were visually inspected, and the conformations with the lowest binding energy were selected for subsequent structural and energetic analyses.

2.11. Molecular Dynamics Protocol

The molecular dynamics (MD) simulations were conducted using the Amber 22 package [30].

Prior to the simulations, the protonation states of protein side chains were determined using the PDB2PQR web server [31], ensuring accurate assignment based on physiological pH conditions. Ligand parameterization was performed with the Antechamber module of Amber 22 [32], employing the General Amber Force Field 2 (GAFF2) [33] for atom type assignment. Partial atomic charges were derived using the restrained electrostatic potential (REsP) fitting method, a widely used approach that optimally reproduces the electrostatic potential around molecules. The protein was parametrized using the Amber ff19SB force field [34], which provides improved accuracy for protein–ligand interactions. To reduce computational complexity, the hydrophobic *N*-terminal helix (Val498–Leu524), which anchors MAO-A to the mitochondrial membrane was removed.

The protein–ligand complexes were solvated in an octahedral water box, maintaining a minimum distance of 12 Å between the solute and the box boundary. The OPC water model was employed due to its superior compatibility with the ff19SB force field [35]. The systems were neutralized by adding three Na^+ counterions and subsequently adjusted to a physiological salt concentration (0.15 M NaCl) following the protocol by Machado and Pantano [36].

Four independent MD simulations were performed for the following systems: MAO-A complexed with 5-HT, RES, and ROG (MAO-A:5-HT:RES:ROG), MAO-A with 5-HT and RES (MAO-A:5-HT:RES), MAO-A with 5-HT and ROG (MAO-A:5-HT:ROG), and MAO-A bound to 5-HT alone (MAO-A:5-HT).

Each system underwent energy minimization using periodic boundary conditions, with harmonic restraints (k = 10.0 kcal mol^{-1} Å^{-2}) applied to the protein, FAD, and ligands. A total of 10,000 minimization steps were performed, consisting of 4000 steps using the steepest descent algorithm, followed by 6000 steps using the conjugate gradient method.

Following minimization, the systems were gradually heated from 0 K to 310 K over 500 ps without positional restraints, ensuring a smooth transition to physiological temperature. The heating phase was followed by a 500 ps equilibration phase to allow stabilization of temperature and pressure.

A 300 ns production MD simulation was performed for each system under constant pressure (1 atm) and temperature (310 K), maintained using a Langevin thermostat with a collision frequency of 1 ps^{-1}. The time step for numerical integration was set to 2 fs. Bond lengths involving hydrogen atoms were constrained using the SHAKE algorithm [37], allowing for a stable 2 fs time step. Non-bonded interactions were computed using an 11 Å cutoff, while long-range electrostatic interactions were handled using the Particle Mesh Ewald (PME) method [38]. Periodic boundary conditions were applied in all directions.

To enhance statistical reliability, all simulations were conducted in triplicate, yielding a cumulative simulation time of 900 ns. MD simulations were executed on the Supek supercomputer at the University Computing Center (SRCE), University of Zagreb, Croatia.

2.12. Free Energy of Binding Calculation

The binding free energy (ΔG_{bind}) between the protein and 5-HT was calculated using the molecular mechanics/generalized Born surface area (MM/GBSA) method, implemented via the MMPBSA.py script from the AmberTools package [39]. The calculation followed a single-trajectory approach with the following formula:

$$\Delta G_{bind} = \Delta H - T\Delta S \quad (1)$$

$$\Delta E_{MM} = \Delta E_{inter} + \Delta E_{ele} + \Delta E_{vdW} \quad (2)$$

$$\Delta G_{sol} = \Delta G_{GB} + \Delta G_{SA} \quad (3)$$

In these formulas, ΔE_{MM} represents the change in molecular mechanics energy, which includes bond, angle, and dihedral contributions (ΔE_{inter}), along with electrostatic (ΔE_{ele}) and van der Waals (ΔE_{vdW}) energies. The solvation free energy change, ΔG_{sol}, is composed of two parts: the polar (ΔG_{GB}, electrostatic solvation energy) and the non-polar (ΔG_{SA}, non-electrostatic solvation energy) components. Finally, $T\Delta S$ accounts for the entropic contribution to binding.

During the production phase, the trajectory was divided into six segments, each spanning 50 ns. From each segment, 100 snapshots were extracted at regular intervals to ensure comprehensive sampling of conformational space. Binding free energy (ΔG_{bind}) calculations were performed for each snapshot, and the final ΔG_{bind} value was reported as the mean ± standard deviation across all six segments for the three independent replicates.

Additionally, the MM/PBSA binding free energy was decomposed on a per-residue basis to evaluate the contribution of individual residues to the overall binding free energy. This decomposition enabled the identification of specific interactions and energetic contributions. Due to the high computational cost associated with calculating the entropy term, it was omitted from the analysis.

3. Results

3.1. In Vivo

3.1.1. Levels of Resveratrol and Resveratrol Glucuronide in the Plasma of Stressed Animals Treated with Resveratrol at Doses of 20, 50, and 100 mg/kg

The concentrations of resveratrol and its metabolite, resveratrol glucuronide, are shown in (Table 1). At the investigated doses of RES, the concentration of its metabolite predominates, accounting for more than 95% of the total content of these stilbenoids.

Table 1. Levels of resveratrol (RES) and resveratrol glucuronide (ROG) in plasma of rats (M ± m) [1].

Group	RES (mkg/mL)	ROG (mkg/mL)
PS + RES 100 mg/kg	0.73 ± 0.14 (3.5%)	19.67 ± 2.2 (96.5%)
PS + RES 50 mg/kg	0.49 ± 0.11 (3.3%)	14.21 ± 1.14 (96.7%)
PS + RES 20 mg/kg	0.26 ± 0.07 (3.1%)	8.11 ± 2.3 (96.1%)

[1] The percentage content of RES and ROG relative to their total content is given in parentheses.

3.1.2. Effects of Resveratrol on Anxiety-like Behavior and MAO-A Activity in Stressed Rats

Behavioral outcomes in PS-exposed animals treated with RES at doses of 20 mg/kg, 50 mg/kg, and 100 mg/kg are summarized in Table 2 and Figure 3. Chronic PS induced anxiety-like behavior, as evidenced by increased freezing behavior, prolonged time spent in the closed arms, and reduced exploration of the open arms in the elevated plus maze. Additionally, chronic PS reduced the time spent in the center of the open field (OF) arena ($F_{4,30}$ = 9.45; p = 0.0001), while increasing the frequency of freezing behavior ($F_{4,30}$ = 14.13; p = 0.0001) and anxiety-induced defecation ($F_{4,30}$ = 21.86; p = 0.0001).

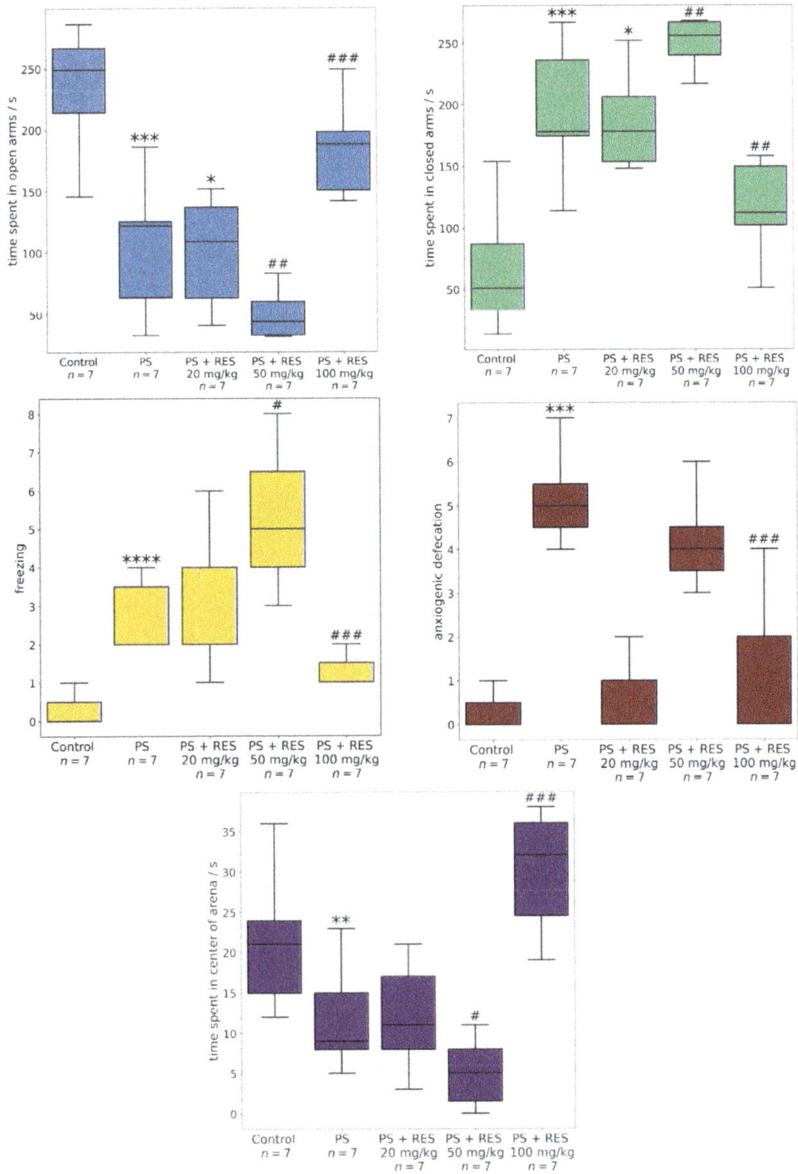

Figure 3. Effect of resveratrol treatment at doses of 20, 50, and 100 mg/kg on behavioral outcomes in rats subjected to predator stress. Behavioral performance was assessed using the elevated plus maze and open field tests to evaluate anxiety-like responses. * = effect between groups PS and control; # = effect between groups PS and PS + RES; * $p < 0.01$; ** $p < 0.05$; *** $p < 0.001$; **** $p < 0.0001$; # $p < 0.05$; ## $p < 0.01$; ### $p < 0.001$.

Table 2. Effect of resveratrol treatment at doses of 20, 50, and 100 mg/kg on the behavior of rats subjected to PS.

Group	Entries in the Open Arms	Entries in the Closed Arms
Control (*n* = 7)	3.1 ± 0.21	2.45 ± 0.62
PS (*n* = 7)	1.3 ± 0.09	2.11 ± 0.41
PS + RES 20 mg/kg (*n* = 7)	1.9 ± 0.9	1.73 ± 0.97
PS + RES 50 mg/kg (*n* = 7)	1.45 ± 0.21	1.6 ± 0.34
PS + RES 100 mg/kg (*n* = 7)	2.73 ± 0.48	1.93 ± 0.61

RES administration at 20 mg/kg did not significantly affect the number of entries into the light and dark arms or the time spent in the open and closed arms. Resveratrol at this dose did not exert a significant effect on the behavioral parameters in the OF test. However, treatment with 50 mg/kg RES exacerbated the anxiogenic effects of chronic stress, further decreasing time spent in the open arms and increasing time in the closed arms compared to both the control and PS groups. Furthermore, resveratrol at this dose exacerbated anxiety disorders and the expression of fear, as evidenced by the OF test. In the PS + RES 50 mg/kg group, compared to the PS group, there was a reduced time spent in the center of the arena and increased levels of anxiety-induced defecation and freezing behavior. In contrast, 100 mg/kg RES alleviated stress-induced anxiety-like behavior, restoring time spent in the open and closed arms to control levels.

Figure 4 illustrates the effects of different RES doses on MAO-A activity in the brain and liver. In stressed animals, a significant increase in MAO-A activity was observed in the brain. RES treatment at 20 mg/kg failed to prevent stress-induced elevation of MAO-A activity. Notably, administration of 50 mg/kg RES resulted in a twofold increase in brain MAO-A activity compared to control levels ($F_{2,36} = 4.21$; $p = 0.022$). In contrast, 100 mg/kg RES completely mitigated the stress-induced rise in brain MAO-A activity.

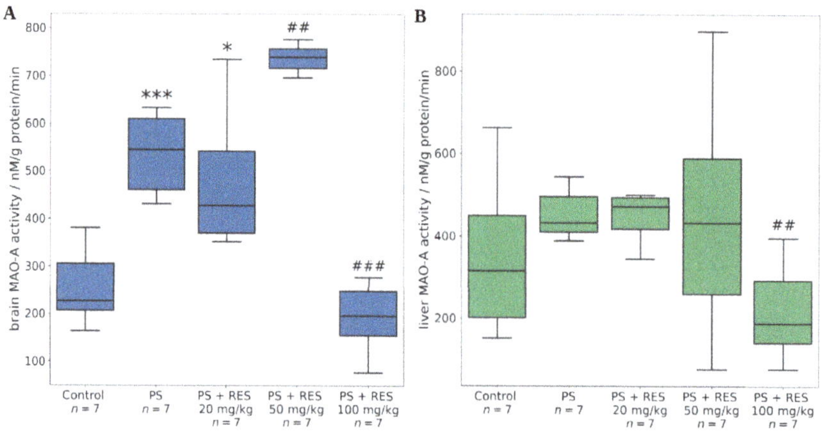

Figure 4. Effect of predator stress (PS) and resveratrol (RES) at doses of 20, 50, and 100 mg/kg on MAO-A activity in the brain (**A**) and liver (**B**). * = effect between groups PS and control; # = effect between groups PS and PS + RES; * $p < 0.01$; *** $p < 0.001$; ## $p < 0.01$; ### $p < 0.001$.

Unlike the brain, the liver of stressed animals did not exhibit increased MAO-A activity. However, administration of 100 mg/kg RES led to a twofold reduction in hepatic MAO-A activity. Lower doses of RES (20 mg/kg and 50 mg/kg) did not produce significant changes in hepatic MAO-A activity.

Figure 5 illustrates changes in MAO-A activity in the amygdala, hippocampus, and prefrontal cortex. It was found that PS was associated with increased MAO-A activity in both the hippocampus and amygdala. Resveratrol at a dose of 100 mg/kg reduced MAO-A activity, whereas resveratrol at a dose of 50 mg/kg enhanced MAO-A activity in all brain regions examined. Resveratrol at a dose of 20 mg/kg had no effect on MAO-A activity in these brain regions.

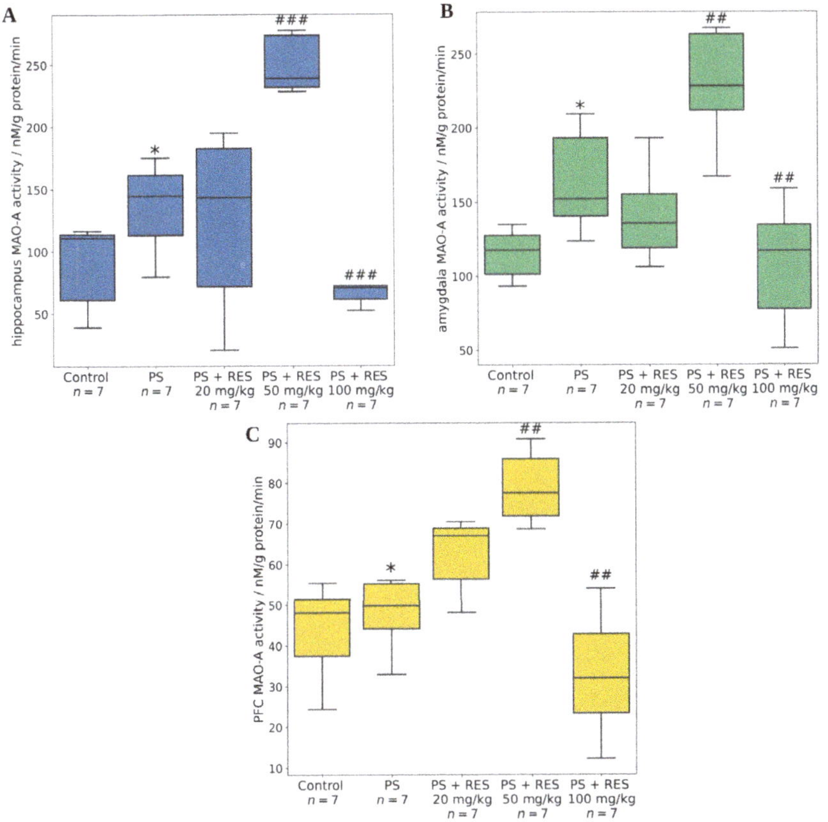

Figure 5. Effect of predator stress (PS) and resveratrol (RES) at doses of 20, 50, and 100 mg/kg on MAO-A activity in the hippocampus (**A**), amygdala (**B**), and prefrontal cortex (PFC, (**C**)). * = effect between groups PS and control; # = effect between groups PS and PS + RES; * $p < 0.05$; ## $p < 0.05$; ### $p < 0.001$.

3.2. *In Silico*

Molecular docking revealed that 5-HT binds to the active site of the MAO-A enzyme in all simulated complexes, located in close proximity to the prosthetic group FAD Figure S1. In the MAO-A:5-HT:ROG complex, the ligand ROG adopts a position almost parallel to α-helix H3 and is situated near helix H24 (for nomenclature see Figure S2) at the C-terminal region of the enzyme. A similar binding position is observed for the ligand RES in the MAO-A:5-HT:RES complex, where it also binds at the same site between H3 and H24. In contrast, in the complex with three ligands (MAO-A:5-HT:RES:ROG), RES binds to the surface of the enzyme near residue Asp36, while ROG remains bound within the same pocket as in the two-ligand complex. The position of 5-HT is highly conserved across all complexes, with only minor differences in the relative orientation of its NH_2 group. These docked geometries were subsequently used as input structures for molecular dynamics (MD) simulations.

To investigate the influence of RES and its derivative, ROG, on the binding of 5-HT to MAO-A, we performed four sets of molecular dynamics (MD) simulations. These included the MAO-A complex with serotonin alone (MAO-A:5-HT), as well as systems where serotonin was co-bound with resveratrol (MAO-A:5-HT:RES), its derivative (MAO-A:5-HT:ROG), or both compounds simultaneously (MAO-A:5-HT:RES:ROG).

Each system was subjected to 300 ns of MD simulations, conducted in triplicate, to ensure statistical robustness. Our primary objective was to assess how the presence of RES and/or ROG modulates the stability and binding interactions of 5-HT within the MAO-A active site. To this end, we analyzed the structural dynamics, binding free energies, and key intermolecular interactions in each complex, providing insights into potential allosteric effects or competition among the ligands.

To assess the structural stability of the MAO-A:ligand complexes, we monitored the root mean square deviation (RMSD) of the protein backbone over 300 ns for all four systems (Figure 6). The RMSD profiles indicate that all complexes reached equilibrium within the first 50 ns, after which they exhibited stable fluctuations. The MAO-A:5-HT complex displayed the lowest RMSD values, suggesting minimal conformational rearrangements upon serotonin binding. The addition of RES resulted in slightly increased RMSD values, indicating moderate structural adaptation. The presence of ROG, either alone or in combination with RES, led to higher RMSD fluctuations, particularly in one replicate of the MAO-A:5-HT:ROG complex, where RMSD exhibited a sudden increase after 50 ns and fluctuated around 4 Å. This suggests that ROG binding induces greater conformational flexibility in MAO-A, potentially altering its binding pocket dynamics. Notably, the MAO-A:5-HT:RES:ROG complex exhibited a relatively stable RMSD profile compared to MAO-A:5-HT:ROG, implying that RES may mitigate the structural perturbations introduced by ROG.

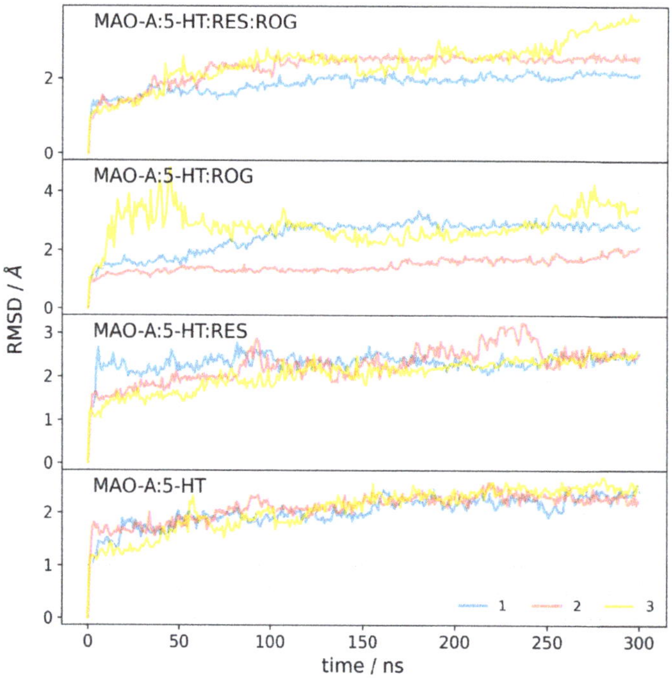

Figure 6. Root mean square deviation (RMSD) profiles of MAO-A complexes over 300 ns molecular dynamics simulations in triplicate.

The structural compactness and overall stability of the MAO-A complexes were assessed through the analysis of the radius of gyration (R_g, Figure S3) and solvent-accessible surface area (SASA) over the 300 ns MD simulations, performed in triplicate. R_g values remained relatively stable throughout the simulations, indicating that no major conformational changes or unfolding events occurred in the protein-ligand complex during the simulation. The low standard deviations further support the consistency of the protein's compact structure across the different runs (Table 3). SASA refers to the surface area of a biomolecule that is accessible to a solvent (water in our case). It is a crucial metric in understanding the exposure of residues or ligands to the solvent environment and is often used in MD simulations to monitor structural changes over time. The mean SASA values show that the protein's surface exposure to the solvent also remained relatively unchanged. The small variations in SASA suggest that no large-scale structural changes took place, which is in agreement with the R_g data.

Table 3. Average values and standard deviations of RMSD (in Å), radius of gyration (R_g) (in Å), solvent-accessible surface area (SASA) (in Å^2), root-mean-square fluctuation (RMSF) (in Å) and number of hydrogen bonds for the MAO-A:ligand complexes, calculated from 300 ns molecular dynamics trajectories performed in triplicate.

	RMSD	R_g	SASA	RMSF	H-bond
MAO-A:5-HT:RES:ROG	2.21 ± 0.51	23.2 ± 0.1	22150 ± 446	1.30 ± 0.84	1.32 ± 1.01
MAO-A:5-HT:ROG	2.27 ± 0.75	23.2 ± 0.2	22150 ± 446	1.31 ± 0.94	1.81 ± 1.11
MAO-A:5-HT:RES	2.21 ± 0.29	23.3 ± 0.1	21962 ± 517	1.25 ± 0.81	1.39 ± 1.08
MAO-A:5-HT	2.07 ± 0.34	23.2 ± 0.1	21842 ± 521	1.31 ± 0.78	1.90 ± 1.30

The root mean square fluctuation (RMSF) analysis was conducted to investigate residue-level flexibility in MAO-A across all four complexes Figure S4. The RMSF profiles demonstrate consistent trends across the replicates, underscoring the reproducibility of the simulations. As shown in the plots, residues located at the *N*- and *C*-terminal regions exhibit higher RMSF values, indicative of increased flexibility in these unstructured regions. In contrast, residues within the core structured regions of the protein, particularly those forming secondary structure elements such as α-helices and β-sheets, display lower RMSF values, signifying their relative rigidity. Prior to the simulation, a *N*-terminal helix (Val498–Leu524), which is typically embedded in the mitochondrial membrane, was removed to reduce the system size. This helix is known to play a role in stabilizing the protein's position in the membrane environment. Its removal may have led to increased flexibility and movement of the nearby unstructured regions, particularly the loop, resulting in a conformational shift and the corresponding jump in RMSD. However, these structural changes are located far from the active site and binding pocket, suggesting that they are unlikely to have a significant impact on the binding energy estimation or the stability of the ligand within the binding pocket. Interestingly, residues in proximity to the active site exhibit minimal fluctuations, suggesting that this region remains structurally stable during the simulations. This stability is critical for maintaining the enzymatic function of MAO-A and ensuring proper ligand binding.

Visual inspection of the simulation trajectories supports the RMSF analysis, revealing that the most significant structural changes occur at the *C*-terminus, which exhibits high flexibility across all complexes. In the MAO-A:5-HT:ROG complex, ROG is bound between α-helix H3 and the unstructured loop preceding helix H24 (Figure S2). This loop undergoes a conformational shift, moving away from the protein surface and contributing to increased RMSD and R_g values. Similarly, in the MAO-A:5-HT:RES complex, RES occupies the same binding pocket as ROG, and this loop also displays notable flexibility. In contrast, in the MAO-A:5-HT complex without ROG or RES, this loop remains the most flexible region, suggesting that its dynamic nature may be intrinsic to its structural role. Interestingly, in complexes without ROG or RES, the C-terminus becomes the most flexible region, as indicated by elevated RMSF values. Across all systems, residues spanning Val481 to Ser497 consistently show high flexibility, highlighting their dynamic behavior. These findings suggest that while ligand binding induces localized structural changes, particularly in loop regions near the binding pocket, the C-terminus may possess intrinsic flexibility independent of ligand presence. In addition to these measures, secondary structure conservation was analyzed using the DSSP algorithm [40], which assigns secondary structure elements based on hydrogen bond patterns and backbone geometries. The analysis (Figure S5) confirmed that the protein's secondary structure remained conserved across all triplicates, further supporting the conclusions drawn from the R_g and SASA data.

These results suggest that serotonin binding alone does not significantly perturb MAO-A stability, whereas the presence of ROG induces structural fluctuations, potentially affecting ligand binding and enzymatic function.

The analysis of hydrogen bonds between 5-HT and MAO-A reveals a moderate interaction strength throughout the MD simulations. The MAO-A:5-HT complex maintains a mean of 1.9 hydrogen bonds during interactions, higher than complexes with allosteric ligands (1.3–1.8). The free energy decomposition analysis (Table 4) identified FAD (flavin adenine dinucleotide), aromatic residues (Phe208, Phe352, Tyr408), aliphatic residues (Ile180, Leu337), and polar residues (Gln215, Asn181) as the primary contributors to ligand binding in MAO-A. The flavin cofactor (FAD) exhibited the strongest contribution, attributed to electrostatic interactions critical for substrate oxidation. Aromatic residues (Phe208, Phe352, Tyr408) dominated via π–π stacking and hydrophobic packing, stabilizing the ligand within the hydrophobic core of the binding pocket. Aliphatic residues (Ile180, Leu337) enhanced binding through van der Waals interactions, optimizing shape complementarity. This synergy between hydrophobic stabilization and localized polar interactions underscores MAO-A's reliance on aromatic-rich motifs for substrate recognition, with FAD's electrostatic role aligning with its catalytic function in neurotransmitter metabolism.

Table 4. Contributions (in kcal mol^{-1}) of the most crucial amino acid residues for the binding of 5-HT to MAO-A.

MAO-A:5-HT:RES:ROG		MAO-A:5-HT:ROG		MAO-A:5-HT:RES		MAO-A:5-HT	
FAD	−1.67	Gln215	−1.74	FAD	−1.73	FAD	−1.52
Phe208	−1.09	FAD	−1.19	Gln215	−1.44	Tyr408	−1.05
Phe352	−0.92	Phe208	−1.08	Phe208	−0.91	Ile180	−1.02
Ile180	−0.89	Asn181	−1.06	Phe352	−0.89	Phe208	−1.01
Gln215	−0.88	Ile180	−0.74	Leu337	−0.79	Gln215	−0.99

The MM/GBSA binding free energy analysis for the MAO-A:5-HT complex (Table 5), both in the presence and absence of resveratrol and its metabolite *trans*-resveratrol-3-*O*-glucuronide, revealed key energetic contributions governing ligand binding. The total binding free energy (ΔG_{bind}) for the MAO-A:5-HT complex was calculated as -17.9 ± 2.6 kcal mol^{-1}, with van der Waals interactions (ΔE_{vdW}) being the dominant stabilizing factor (-24.7 ± 1.8 kcal mol^{-1}), followed by electrostatic interactions (ΔE_{ele}, -20.7 ± 7.4 kcal mol^{-1}). The solvation free energy ($\Delta G_{GB} + \Delta G_{SA}$) contributed unfavorably, particularly the polar desolvation energy (ΔG_{GB}), which counteracted favorable electrostatic contributions. The presence of RES and ROG slightly modulated these interactions, with minor variations in binding energy, suggesting that their inclusion does not drastically alter the fundamental binding mode of 5-HT. However, the slight decrease in ΔG_{bind} upon adding ROG (-15.5 ± 2.3 kcal mol^{-1}) suggests a minor destabilization effect.

Table 5. Energy analysis for binding of 5-HT to MAO-A as obtained by MM/GBSA method. All units are kcal mol^{-1}.

	MAO-A:5-HT:RES:ROG	MAO-A:5-HT:ROG	MAO-A:5-HT:RES	MAO-A:5-HT
ΔE_{vdW}	-24.9 ± 2.0	-24.3 ± 1.8	-24.1 ± 2.0	-24.7 ± 1.8
ΔE_{ele}	-17.6 ± 3.3	-18.4 ± 3.7	-18.0 ± 4.3	-20.7 ± 7.4
ΔG_{GB}	29.3 ± 2.9	30.7 ± 3.2	29.1 ± 3.2	31.0 ± 6.0
ΔG_{SA}	-3.5 ± 0.2	-3.6 ± 0.3	-3.5 ± 0.2	-3.5 ± 0.2
ΔG_{bind}	-16.7 ± 2.9	-15.5 ± 2.3	-16.6 ± 2.6	-17.9 ± 2.6

These findings align well with the binding free energy decomposition analysis, which identified key residues contributing to ligand stabilization. The dominance of van der Waals interactions is consistent with the significant roles of hydrophobic residues such as Phe208, Phe352, Ile180, Leu337, and Tyr408, which facilitate ligand binding via π–π stacking and nonpolar stabilization. Meanwhile, the electrostatic contributions reflect the involvement of polar residues such as Gln215 and Asn181. The unfavorable desolvation energy further emphasizes the importance of the hydrophobic environment within the binding pocket, which protects 5-HT from solvent exposure. The relatively stable binding energy across conditions suggests that the core interactions between 5-HT and MAO-A remain largely conserved, reinforcing the critical role of identified residues in defining ligand affinity. These insights provide a detailed energetic framework for understanding serotonin binding and could guide future modifications aimed at optimizing interactions within the MAO-A active site.

4. Discussion

This article is part of a comprehensive study demonstrating the therapeutic effects of RES. In earlier works, we have shown the protective effects of RES in experimental PTSD and under conditions of chronic stress, which serve as a trigger in this PTSD model. Overall, it has been established that RES reduces anxiety-like behavior by modulating the regulation of key enzymes such as 11β-hydroxysteroid dehydrogenase type 1 (11β-HSD-1) and monoamine oxidase. Thus, RES exerts anti-anxiogenic effects by modulating the metabolism of glucocorticoids and monoamines in both the brain and liver [18].

Furthermore, under conditions of predator stress and PTSD, the therapeutic effects of RES were manifested in hepatoprotective activity, evidenced by a reduction in necrotic liver damage and inflammation in the organ. It was also found that chronic exposure to predator stress led to a significant increase in serotonin levels and upregulation of the expression of the SERT and 5-HT$_{3A}$ receptors. SSRIs were unable to prevent anxiety or reduce serotonin levels, partly due to suppressed SERT expression. RES reduced the regulation of SERT and 5-HT$_{3A}$ expression to a lesser extent than SSRIs, but effectively decreased anxiety and restored serotonin levels, likely through upregulation of MAO-A expression. Furthermore, this study compared the therapeutic effects of RES with those of SSRIs. It was found that none of the four analyzed drugs were able to effectively influence behavioral disorders under stress conditions. Therefore, the therapeutic effect of RES was superior to that of the other drugs. However, in these studies, a bidirectional effect of RES at a dose of 100 mg/kg on gene expression and MAO-A activity was identified [12].

Despite the observed increase in MAO-A gene expression, administration of RES in stressed animals resulted in a paradoxical reduction in MAO-A activity, which correlated with an attenuation of stress-induced anxiety-like behavior. Under conditions of increased MAO-A production, a substantial enhancement of the enzyme's activity is likely. Consistent with this hypothesis, our previous studies demonstrated that RES upregulates MAO-A gene expression while downregulating serotonin transporter (SERT) gene expression in the hippocampus of chronically stressed animals [12,41]. Through increased MAO-A expression and activity, RES may exert pro-anxiogenic effects, particularly given that serotonin is a primary substrate of MAO-A. Notably, in our experimental model, MAO-A activity was measured based on the oxidative deamination of serotonin, and a reduction in serotonin levels is well-documented to contribute to stress-related anxiety and depressive disorders [42].

Therefore, in the present study, we intentionally narrowed the focus to a comparison of in silico predictions with in vivo findings regarding the modulation of MAO-A activity. Anxiety-related behaviors were evaluated using a range of behavioral paradigms, including the elevated plus maze and the open field test. Predatory stress was associated with a marked decrease in the time spent in the open arms of the EPM and the center of the OF arena. Additionally, a significant increase in spontaneous freezing behavior—a validated index of fear response—was observed in the OF test.

RES exerted a dose-dependent effect on behavioral markers of anxiety and fear. At a dose of 100 mg/kg, RES demonstrated robust anxiolytic properties and concurrently reduced fear-related responses. In contrast, at a dose of 50 mg/kg, RES elicited pro-anxiogenic effects in both the EPM and OF paradigms. Administration of resveratrol at 20 mg/kg had no statistically significant impact on behavioral activity.

The in vivo findings further demonstrated that RES modulates MAO-A activity in a dose-dependent manner across several tissues and brain regions, including the liver, whole brain, amygdala, hippocampus, and prefrontal cortex. The amygdala is a central brain structure involved in the generation of anxiety-related behaviors, and its activity is regulated through its neuronal interactions with the prefrontal cortex and hippocampus.

It was found that PS significantly increased MAO-A activity in the amygdala and hippocampus, but not in the prefrontal cortex. Positive correlations were identified between MAO-A activity in the amygdala and the time spent in the closed arms of the EPM ($r = 0.72$; $p < 0.05$), MAO-A activity in the hippocampus and the freezing response ($r = 0.69$; $p < 0.05$), and MAO-A activity in the liver and the level of anxiety-related defecation ($r = 0.79$; $p < 0.05$).

RES exerted dose-dependent corrective effects on MAO-A activity in the aforementioned brain regions. A significant reduction in MAO-A activity was observed in the amygdala, hippocampus, prefrontal cortex, and whole brain following administration of RES at 100 mg/kg. Conversely, MAO-A activity was increased at a dose of 50 mg/kg. No significant effect was observed with the 20 mg/kg dose in any of the brain regions examined.

In the present study, we extended our analysis by assessing hepatic MAO-A activity in addition to its enzymatic activity in the brain. A novel correlation was identified between hepatic MAO-A activity and the time spent in the dark arms of the elevated plus maze ($r = 0.85$, $p < 0.05$). Furthermore, a positive correlation was found between hepatic MAO-A activity and plasma concentrations of ROG ($r = 0.77$, $p < 0.05$).

Based on these findings, we propose that RES and its metabolites interact with an allosteric site on MAO-A, leading to enzyme inhibition. This hypothesis is supported by our in silico analyses, which provide further evidence for resveratrol-mediated allosteric modulation of MAO-A activity.

Statistical analysis using a *t*-test revealed that the calculated binding free energies (ΔG_{bind}) for the different complexes were not significantly different, indicating that the presence of resveratrol (RES) and its metabolite trans-resveratrol-3-O-glucuronide (ROG) does not substantially alter the thermodynamic stability of serotonin (5-HT) binding to MAO-A. However, experimentally observed reductions in MAO-A activity in the presence of RES and ROG suggest an additional regulatory mechanism not accounted for in the present study. Given that our analysis focused on binding free energy calculations, we explored the potential for allosteric modulation by RES and ROG rather than direct competitive inhibition. Nevertheless, we did not explicitly investigate the influence of these compounds as competitive inhibitors, leaving open the possibility that their impact on enzyme activity could arise from alternative mechanisms such as conformational changes or indirect effects on enzyme dynamics. Further studies integrating kinetic assays and enhanced sampling molecular dynamics simulations would be required to fully elucidate these effects.

Notably, in addition to RES, its glucuronide metabolite exhibits a distinct affinity for the allosteric site of MAO-A. Our previous studies demonstrated significant correlations between behavioral activity measures and plasma concentrations of ROG in stressed animals. Specifically, a negative correlation was observed between time spent in the open arms of the elevated plus maze and plasma levels of ROG.

The potential allosteric effects of RES/ROG identified in silico may represent integral components of the molecular and systemic mechanisms underlying the anxiolytic effects of RES. The molecular mechanisms of RES's action are primarily associated with its ability to function as a ligand for sirtuins—deacetylase enzymes. In various types of neuronal cultures, the protective effects of RES against mitochondrial dysfunction, oxidative stress, and apoptosis have been shown to be enhanced via upregulation of SIRT1 expression [43]. SIRT1, in turn, activates multiple molecular pathways and mediates a range of neuroprotective effects of RES treatment.

These neuroprotective effects are closely linked to the improvement of mitochondrial function. RES enhances mitochondrial efficiency through activation of the SIRT1/AMPK/PGC-1α signaling axis. Additionally, RES promotes neuroplasticity via the SIRT1/AMPK/CREB/BDNF pathway, thereby supporting synaptic plasticity and overall neurotransmission. By downregulating NF-κB, RES reduces the release of pro-inflammatory cytokines from glial cells, alleviating neuroinflammation and oxidative stress—processes that are critically involved in the pathophysiology of stress-related anxiety disorders. The restoration of neurotransmission under such conditions constitutes a key neuroprotective mechanism of RES.

The systemic mechanisms underlying the anxiolytic effects of RES have been comprehensively reviewed [44]. This analysis convincingly demonstrated that key components of the pathogenesis of stress-related anxiety disorders—including neuroinflammation, oxidative stress, mitochondrial dysfunction, impaired neuroplasticity, dysregulated neuronal circuitry and neurotransmitter levels, altered cerebral blood flow, dysfunction of the liver–hypothalamic–pituitary–adrenal (LHPA) axis, and disturbances in the gut–brain and liver–brain axes—are amenable to modulation by RES [44].

The therapeutic actions of RES are primarily based on its capacity to counteract neuroinflammation, oxidative stress, and mitochondrial dysfunction. As a potent antioxidant, RES may exert its protective effects via direct scavenging of reactive oxygen species. Oxidative stress is a major contributor to mitochondrial dysfunction, and it is noteworthy that MAO-A is localized on the outer mitochondrial membrane. This spatial proximity allows for the direct mitochondrial penetration of RES and its potential interaction with allosteric sites on MAO-A.

RES has also been shown to enhance synaptic structure and function by increasing dendritic spine density and upregulating the expression of postsynaptic density protein 95 (PSD95) and brain-derived neurotrophic factor (BDNF), thereby mitigating paclitaxel-induced synaptic damage [45]. Beyond BDNF and glial-cell-line-derived neurotrophic factor (GDNF), RES activates signaling pathways such as ERK1/2 and CREB [46]. In vitro, the neuroprotective effects of RES are associated with increased levels of SIRT1, phosphorylated CREB (p-CREB), total CREB, and BDNF, as well as reduced expression of miR-134 [46]. Moreover, RES enhances the expression of synaptic plasticity-related proteins, including SynGAP, PSD95, synapsin-1, and synaptotagmin-1 in the hippocampus, in a SIRT1-dependent manner [45,47].

The ability of RES to improve synaptic plasticity is particularly relevant for addressing stress-related anxiety disorders, where synaptic stability is critical for efficient neurotransmitter function. Collectively, these neuroprotective properties contribute to the therapeutic potential of RES in alleviating anxiety symptoms through enhanced synaptic resilience and improved neurotransmission.

The localization of MAO-A on the outer mitochondrial membrane is a crucial factor influencing its activity, as the enzyme is highly sensitive to the state of its lipid microenvironment [22]. Previous in vivo and in vitro studies have demonstrated that oxidative stress-induced lipid peroxidation in mitochondrial membranes can lead to MAO-A inactivation [22]. Given resveratrol's lipophilic nature, it readily penetrates mitochondria and acts as a free radical scavenger, exerting potent antioxidant effects [48]. In this context, RES likely serves a protective role not only for MAO-A but also for other mitochondrial membrane proteins.

However, MAO-A is an oxidase that generates H_2O_2 as a byproduct, which, in the presence of Fe^{2+} and Cu^{2+} ions, can contribute to oxidative stress. RES may provide additional protection against the auto-oxidation of MAO-A [49]. This raises the possibility that the observed upregulation of MAO-A activity in response to RES is mediated through multiple mechanisms. One such mechanism could involve the SIRT1/NHLH2/MAO-A pathway, in which SIRT1-induced deacetylation of NHLH2 transcription factors leads to increased MAO-A expression and decreased 5-HT levels in neurons, potentially exacerbating anxiety-like behaviors [44,50].

It is plausible that the anxiogenic effects of RES at a dose of 50 mg/kg are mediated through this mechanism. Notably, at this dose, RES increased MAO-A activity in the amygdala, hippocampus, and prefrontal cortex, as well as in whole-brain homogenates, but not in the liver. Glucocorticoids are known to enhance MAO-A gene expression in multiple brain regions [51]. Therefore, RES at 50 mg/kg may potentiate both the SIRT1/NHLH2/MAO-A signaling axis and glucocorticoid synthesis [52]. In turn, elevated glucocorticoid levels further upregulate MAO-A expression.

Importantly, administration of RES at 50 mg/kg also increased spontaneous freezing behavior in the OF test, a response indicative of heightened fear. Such fear responses are known to be potentiated by glucocorticoid dysregulation [53].

In contrast, at a dose of 100 mg/kg, the putative allosteric effects of RES may be engaged, as reflected by the generalized suppression of MAO-A enzymatic activity across all investigated brain regions and the liver.

Mechanistically, the association between brain MAO-A activity/expression and anxiety-related behaviors is well established due to its role in neurotransmitter metabolism. However, the involvement of hepatic MAO-A in anxiety regulation is less apparent. Nevertheless, it is important to highlight the ability of hepatic MAO-A to catalyze the oxidative deamination of monoamines of intestinal origin, which are produced through the decarboxylation of amino acids by the gut microbiota [54]. Thus, it can be hypothesized that hepatic MAO-A plays a key role in regulating the gut–liver–brain axis by modulating the levels of trace amines such as tyramine, tryptamine, phenylethylamine, and others. These amines enter the liver via the portal vein, where they are partially metabolized by hepatic MAO-A before reaching the systemic circulation and subsequently crossing the blood–brain barrier (Figure 7). In the brain, trace amines interact with their specific receptor system-trace amine-associated receptors (TAAR), which comprise nine known subtypes.

Notably, TAAR1 colocalizes with dopamine D2 receptors, and its activation has been implicated in anti-addictive, antipsychotic, anxiolytic, and antidepressant effects [55]. Moreover, recent studies have demonstrated that TAAR1 agonists can ameliorate experimental PTSD [56].

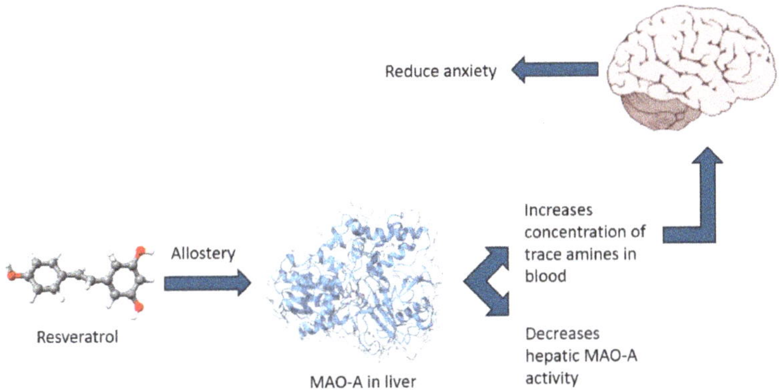

Figure 7. Proposed mechanism of hepatic MAO-A contribution to reduced anxiety.

Given the strong positive correlation between hepatic MAO-A activity and anxiety-related behaviors (r = 0.85, $p < 0.05$), we propose the existence of a distinct mechanism underlying anxiety development during chronic stress. Hepatic MAO-A, through oxidative deamination, may reduce the availability of trace amines necessary for brain function under chronic stress conditions. Simultaneously, brain MAO-A dysregulates neurotransmitter metabolism, further exacerbating anxiety-like behaviors.

The anxiolytic effects of RES appear to be mediated not only through inhibition of brain MAO-A but also via suppression of hepatic MAO-A activity. Interestingly, RES significantly inhibited both hepatic and brain MAO-A activity only at the highest dose (100 mg/kg), whereas no statistically significant differences were observed between stressed (PS) and resveratrol-treated (PS + RES) groups at lower doses. In silico analyses provide valuable insights into this phenomenon, suggesting that the allosteric binding sites of MAO-A may exhibit sensitivity to high concentrations of RES. This hypothesis may also extend to ROG.

Based on the comparison of in vivo data with in silico findings, a hypothesis emerged suggesting that the differences in cellular conditions (such as pH and ion composition) between the liver and brain, or the varying concentrations of RES and its metabolite, ROG, in these tissues, could explain the observed differences in their sensitivity to resveratrol and its metabolite. This is supported by the distinct correlation patterns observed: RES was correlated exclusively with brain MAO-A, while ROG was associated only with hepatic MAO-A. Future studies will further investigate this hypothesis and explore the broader biological effects of resveratrol glucuronide.

Currently, most research focuses on the protective effects of RES, while its metabolites remain relatively understudied. Nevertheless, emerging evidence highlights the therapeutic potential of ROG. Notably, preconditioning neuronal cultures with low concentrations (0.01–10 nM) of ROG protected neurons from serum withdrawal-induced apoptosis via cAMP-mediated signaling pathways [57]. It is plausible that the neuroprotective effects of ROG underlie its ability to mitigate stress-related behavioral alterations. Furthermore, the systemic effects of RES and its metabolite may be integrated within the gut–liver–brain axis, emphasizing the need for further research in this area.

The therapeutic mechanisms of RES presented herein have been characterized primarily in male subjects. Whether resveratrol elicits comparable effects in females remains an open question. This issue is of particular importance given that post-traumatic stress disorder (PTSD) and anxiety disorders often present with greater severity in females compared to males. Moreover, estrogens are known to regulate MAO-A activity [58], suggesting potential sex-specific differences in the neurobiological response to RES.

5. Conclusions

In this study, we provided an in silico rationale for the potential binding of resveratrol and its metabolite, resveratrol glucuronide, to the allosteric site of MAO-A. In experimental studies conducted on a chronic predator stress model, we demonstrated that the anti-anxiogenic effects of resveratrol are associated with the inhibition of not only the brain but also the liver isoform of MAO-A activity. Thus, we uncovered new insights into the involvement of the liver–brain axis. Further research will explore the relationship between liver MAO activity levels and the concentrations of trace amines in the blood, liver, and brain. Additionally, in silico investigations will be conducted to determine the binding sites of resveratrol and resveratrol glucuronide on MAO-B. This is particularly important in the context of MAO-B's role in trace amine metabolism.

Supplementary Materials: The following supporting information can be downloaded at: https://www.mdpi.com/article/10.3390/biomedicines13051196/s1, Figure S1: Geometries of docked complexes. MAO-A:5-HT:RES:ROG (A), MAO-A:5-HT:ROG (B), MAO-A:5-HT:RES (C), MAO-A:5-HT (D); Figure S2: Secondary structure of the MAO-A protein (pdb ID: 2Z5X). Figure is generated using PDBsum web server [59]; Figure S3: Radius of gyration (R_g) profiles of MAO-A complexes over 300 ns molecular dynamics simulations in triplicate; Figure S4: Root mean square fluctuation (RMSF) profiles of MAO-A complexes over 300 ns molecular dynamics simulations in triplicate; Figure S5: Changes in the secondary structure of the MAO-A:ligand complexes during molecular dynamics simulations in triplicates. MAO-A:5-HT:RES:ROG (A), MAO-A:5-HT:ROG (B), MAO-A:5-HT:RES (C), MAO-A:5-HT (D).

Author Contributions: Conceptualization, J.N., V.E.T.; methodology, J.N., V.E.T.; investigation, J.N., V.A.S. (Vladislav A. Shatilov), V.A.S. (Vadim A. Shevyrin), M.S.Z., G.N.P., T.L.K., A.M.F., Z.R.K.; writing—original draft J.N., O.B.T., V.E.T.; writing—editing, J.N., V.E.T.; visualization, J.N. All authors have read and agreed to the published version of the manuscript.

Funding: This work was supported by the Russian Scientific Foundation, regional grant, Chelyabinsk Region (#23-15-20040).

Institutional Review Board Statement: The study was conducted according to the guidelines of the Declaration of Helsinki and approved by the Ethical Committee for Animal Experiments of South Ural State University, Chelyabinsk, Russia (project #0425-2018-0011 of 17 May 2018, protocol number 36/645).

Informed Consent Statement: Not applicable.

Data Availability Statement: The Amber trajectories of MAO-A:ligand complexes are openly available in the FULIR repository at https://urn.nsk.hr/urn:nbn:hr:241:401110 (accessed on 26 March 2025).

Acknowledgments: J.N. acknowledges the support of the Croatian Science Foundation (grant IP-2022-4658), and the University of Zagreb, University Computing Center – SRCE, for granting access to the Supek supercomputer. During the preparation of this work, the authors used ChatGPT 3.5 in order to improve the grammar, readability, and language throughout the manuscript. It was not employed to generate original research content or to conduct data analysis. After using this service, the authors reviewed and edited the content as needed and take full responsibility for the content of the publication.

Conflicts of Interest: The authors declare no conflicts of interest.

References

1. Soleas, G.J.; Diamandis, E.P.; Goldberg, D.M. Resveratrol: A molecule whose time has come? And gone? *Clin. Biochem.* **1997**, *30*, 91–113. [CrossRef] [PubMed]
2. Soleas, G.J.; Diamandis, E.P.; Goldberg, D.M. Wine as a biological fluid: History, production, and role in disease prevention. *J. Clin. Lab. Anal.* **1997**, *11*, 287–313. [CrossRef]
3. Sovak, M. Grape Extract, Resveratrol, and Its Analogs: A Review. *J. Med. Food* **2001**, *4*, 93–105. [CrossRef]
4. Tang, K.; Zhan, J.C.; Yang, H.R.; Huang, W.D. Changes of resveratrol and antioxidant enzymes during UV-induced plant defense response in peanut seedlings. *J. Plant Physiol.* **2010**, *167*, 95–102. [CrossRef]
5. Duan, D.; Fischer, S.; Merz, P.; Bogs, J.; Riemann, M.; Nick, P. An ancestral allele of grapevine transcription factorMYB14promotes plant defence. *J. Exp. Bot.* **2016**, *67*, 1795–1804. [CrossRef]
6. Lin, J.K.; Tsai, S.H. Chemoprevention of cancer and cardiovascular disease by resveratrol. *Proc. Natl. Sci. Counc. Repub. China B* **1999**, *23*, 99–106.
7. Harikumar, K.B.; Aggarwal, B.B. Resveratrol: A multitargeted agent for age-associated chronic diseases. *Cell Cycle* **2008**, *7*, 1020–1035. [CrossRef]
8. Howes, M.J.R.; Simmonds, M.S. The role of phytochemicals as micronutrients in health and disease. *Curr. Opin. Clin. Nutr. Metab. Care* **2014**, *17*, 558–566. [CrossRef]
9. Grosso, C.; Santos, M.; Barroso, M.F. From Plants to Psycho-Neurology: Unravelling the Therapeutic Benefits of Bioactive Compounds in Brain Disorders. *Antioxidants* **2023**, *12*, 1603. [CrossRef]
10. Bhandari, U.R.; Danish, S.M.; Ahmad, S.; Ikram, M.; Nadaf, A.; Hasan, N.; Kesharwani, P.; Ahmad, F.J. New opportunities for antioxidants in amelioration of neurodegenerative diseases. *Mech. Ageing Dev.* **2024**, *221*, 111961. [CrossRef]
11. Tseilikman, V.E.; Shatilov, V.A.; Zhukov, M.S.; Buksha, I.A.; Epitashvily, A.E.; Lipatov, I.A.; Aristov, M.R.; Koshelev, A.G.; Karpenko, M.N.; Traktirov, D.S.; et al. Limited Cheese Intake Paradigm Replaces Patterns of Behavioral Disorders in Experimental PTSD: Focus on Resveratrol Supplementation. *Int. J. Mol. Sci.* **2023**, *24*, 14343. [CrossRef] [PubMed]
12. Tseilikman, V.E.; Tseilikman, O.B.; Karpenko, M.N.; Traktirov, D.S.; Obukhova, D.A.; Shatilov, V.A.; Zhukov, M.S.; Manuilov, G.V.; Yegorov, O.N.; Aristov, M.R.; et al. Unraveling the Serotonergic Mechanism of Stress-Related Anxiety: Focus on Co-Treatment with Resveratrol and Selective Serotonin Reuptake Inhibitors. *Biomedicines* **2024**, *12*, 2455. [CrossRef] [PubMed]
13. Kuhnle, G.; Spencer, J.P.; Chowrimootoo, G.; Schroeter, H.; Debnam, E.S.; Srai, S.S.; Rice-Evans, C.; Hahn, U. Resveratrol Is Absorbed in the Small Intestine as Resveratrol Glucuronide. *Biochem. Biophys. Res. Commun.* **2000**, *272*, 212–217. [CrossRef] [PubMed]
14. Gambini, J.; Inglés, M.; Olaso, G.; Lopez-Grueso, R.; Bonet-Costa, V.; Gimeno-Mallench, L.; Mas-Bargues, C.; Abdelaziz, K.M.; Gomez-Cabrera, M.C.; Vina, J.; et al. Properties of Resveratrol:In VitroandIn VivoStudies about Metabolism, Bioavailability, and Biological Effects in Animal Models and Humans. *Oxidative Med. Cell. Longev.* **2015**, *2015*, 837042. [CrossRef]
15. Calamini, B.; Ratia, K.; Malkowski, M.; Cuendet, M.; Pezzuto, J.; Santarsiero, B.; Mesecar, A. Pleiotropic mechanisms facilitated by resveratrol and its metabolites. *Biochem. J.* **2010**, *429*, 273–282. [CrossRef]
16. Polycarpou, E.; Meira, L.B.; Carrington, S.; Tyrrell, E.; Modjtahedi, H.; Carew, M.A. Resveratrol 3-*O*-D-glucuronide and resveratrol 4′-*O*-D-glucuronide inhibit colon cancer cell growth: Evidence for a role of A3 adenosine receptors, cyclin D1 depletion, and G1 cell cycle arrest. *Mol. Nutr. Food Res.* **2013**, *57*, 1708–1717. [CrossRef]
17. Xie, Q.; Yang, Y.; Wang, Z.; Chen, F.; Zhang, A.; Liu, C. Resveratrol-4-O-D-(2′-galloyl)-glucopyranoside Isolated from Polygonum cuspidatum Exhibits Anti-Hepatocellular Carcinoma Viability by Inducing Apoptosis via the JNK and ERK Pathway. *Molecules* **2014**, *19*, 1592–1602. [CrossRef]
18. Tseilikman, V.E.; Tseilikman, O.B.; Shevyrin, V.A.; Yegorov, O.N.; Epitashvili, A.A.; Aristov, M.R.; Karpenko, M.N.; Lipatov, I.A.; Pashkov, A.A.; Shamshurin, M.V.; et al. Unraveling the Liver–Brain Axis: Resveratrol's Modulation of Key Enzymes in Stress-Related Anxiety. *Biomedicines* **2024**, *12*, 2063. [CrossRef]
19. Ullmann, E.; Perry, S.W.; Licinio, J.; Wong, M.L.; Dremencov, E.; Zavjalov, E.L.; Shevelev, O.B.; Khotskin, N.V.; Koncevaya, G.V.; Khotshkina, A.S.; et al. From Allostatic Load to Allostatic State—An Endogenous Sympathetic Strategy to Deal with Chronic Anxiety and Stress? *Front. Behav. Neurosci.* **2019**, *13*. [CrossRef]
20. Paxinos, G.; Watson, C. *The Rat Brain in Stereotaxic Coordinates*; Elsevier Science: Amsterdam, The Netherlands, 2013.
21. Satav, J.G.; Katyare, S.S. Effect of experimental thyrotoxicosis on oxidative phosphorylation in rat liver, kidney and brain mitochondria. *Mol. Cell. Endocrinol.* **1982**, *28*, 173–189. [CrossRef]
22. Tipton, K.F.; Davey, G.; Motherway, M. Monoamine Oxidase Assays. *Curr. Protoc. Pharmacol.* **2000**, *9*, 3.6.1–3.6.42. [CrossRef] [PubMed]
23. Zhang, X.; Hartmann, P. How to calculate sample size in animal and human studies. *Front. Med.* **2023**, *10*, 1215927. [CrossRef] [PubMed]
24. Berman, H.M. The Protein Data Bank. *Nucleic Acids Res.* **2000**, *28*, 235–242. [CrossRef] [PubMed]

25. Son, S.Y.; Ma, J.; Kondou, Y.; Yoshimura, M.; Yamashita, E.; Tsukihara, T. Structure of human monoamine oxidase A at 2.2-Å resolution: The control of opening the entry for substrates/inhibitors. *Proc. Natl. Acad. Sci. USA* **2008**, *105*, 5739–5744. [CrossRef]
26. Pettersen, E.F.; Goddard, T.D.; Huang, C.C.; Couch, G.S.; Greenblatt, D.M.; Meng, E.C.; Ferrin, T.E. UCSF Chimera—A visualization system for exploratory research and analysis. *J. Comput. Chem.* **2004**, *25*, 1605–1612. [CrossRef]
27. Kim, S.; Chen, J.; Cheng, T.; Gindulyte, A.; He, J.; He, S.; Li, Q.; Shoemaker, B.A.; Thiessen, P.A.; Yu, B.; et al. PubChem 2023 update. *Nucleic Acids Res.* **2022**, *51*, D1373–D1380. [CrossRef]
28. Forli Lab. Meeko: A Python Library for Preparing Molecules for AutoDock-GPU and AutoDock Vina. 2024. Available online: https://github.com/forlilab/Meeko (accessed on 30 September 2024).
29. Morris, G.M.; Huey, R.; Lindstrom, W.; Sanner, M.F.; Belew, R.K.; Goodsell, D.S.; Olson, A.J. AutoDock4 and AutoDockTools4: Automated docking with selective receptor flexibility. *J. Comput. Chem.* **2009**, *30*, 2785–2791. [CrossRef]
30. Case, D.A.; Aktulga, H.M.; Belfon, K.; Ben-Shalom, I.; Berryman, J.; Brozell, S.; Cerutti, D.S.; Cheatham, T.E., III; Cisneros, G.A.; Cruzeiro, V.; et al. Amber 2022. 2022. Available online: https://ambermd.org (accessed on 9 May 2025).
31. Dolinsky, T.J.; Czodrowski, P.; Li, H.; Nielsen, J.E.; Jensen, J.H.; Klebe, G.; Baker, N.A. PDB2PQR: Expanding and upgrading automated preparation of biomolecular structures for molecular simulations. *Nucleic Acids Res.* **2007**, *35*, W522–W525. [CrossRef]
32. Case, D.A.; Aktulga, H.M.; Belfon, K.; Cerutti, D.S.; Cisneros, G.A.; Cruzeiro, V.W.D.; Forouzesh, N.; Giese, T.J.; Götz, A.W.; Gohlke, H.; et al. AmberTools. *J. Chem. Inf. Model.* **2023**, *63*, 6183–6191. [CrossRef]
33. Wang, J.; Wolf, R.M.; Caldwell, J.W.; Kollman, P.A.; Case, D.A. Development and testing of a general amber force field. *J. Comput. Chem.* **2004**, *25*, 1157–1174. [CrossRef]
34. Tian, C.; Kasavajhala, K.; Belfon, K.A.A.; Raguette, L.; Huang, H.; Migues, A.N.; Bickel, J.; Wang, Y.; Pincay, J.; Wu, Q.; et al. ff19SB: Amino-Acid-Specific Protein Backbone Parameters Trained against Quantum Mechanics Energy Surfaces in Solution. *J. Chem. Theory Comput.* **2019**, *16*, 528–552. [CrossRef] [PubMed]
35. Izadi, S.; Anandakrishnan, R.; Onufriev, A.V. Building Water Models: A Different Approach. *J. Phys. Chem. Lett.* **2014**, *5*, 3863–3871. [CrossRef] [PubMed]
36. Machado, M.R.; Pantano, S. Split the Charge Difference in Two! A Rule of Thumb for Adding Proper Amounts of Ions in MD Simulations. *J. Chem. Theory Comput.* **2020**, *16*, 1367–1372. [CrossRef] [PubMed]
37. Andersen, H.C. Rattle: A "velocity" version of the shake algorithm for molecular dynamics calculations. *J. Comput. Phys.* **1983**, *52*, 24–34. [CrossRef]
38. Darden, T.; York, D.; Pedersen, L. Particle mesh Ewald: An Nlog(N) method for Ewald sums in large systems. *J. Chem. Phys.* **1993**, *98*, 10089–10092. [CrossRef]
39. Miller, B.R.; McGee, T.D.; Swails, J.M.; Homeyer, N.; Gohlke, H.; Roitberg, A.E. MMPBSA.py: An Efficient Program for End-State Free Energy Calculations. *J. Chem. Theory Comput.* **2012**, *8*, 3314–3321. [CrossRef]
40. Kabsch, W.; Sander, C. Dictionary of protein secondary structure: Pattern recognition of hydrogen-bonded and geometrical features. *Biopolymers* **1983**, *22*, 2577–2637. [CrossRef]
41. Shih, J.H.; Ma, K.H.; Chen, C.F.F.; Cheng, C.Y.; Pao, L.H.; Weng, S.J.; Huang, Y.S.; Shiue, C.Y.; Yeh, M.K.; Li, I.H. Evaluation of brain SERT occupancy by resveratrol against MDMA-induced neurobiological and behavioral changes in rats: A 4-[18F]-ADAM/small-animal PET study. *Eur. Neuropsychopharmacol.* **2016**, *26*, 92–104. [CrossRef]
42. Tseilikman, V.; Lapshin, M.; Klebanov, I.; Chrousos, G.; Vasilieva, M.; Pashkov, A.; Fedotova, J.; Tseilikman, D.; Shatilov, V.; Manukhina, E.; et al. The Link between Activities of Hepatic 11beta-Hydroxysteroid Dehydrogenase-1 and Monoamine Oxidase-A in the Brain Following Repeated Predator Stress: Focus on Heightened Anxiety. *Int. J. Mol. Sci.* **2022**, *23*, 4881. [CrossRef]
43. Rasouri, S.; Lagouge, M.; Auwerx, J. SIRT1/PGC-1: Un axe neuroprotecteur? *Med. Sci.* **2007**, *23*, 840–844. [CrossRef]
44. Tseilikman, V.E.; Tseilikman, O.B.; Yegorov, O.N.; Brichagina, A.A.; Karpenko, M.N.; Tseilikman, D.V.; Shatilov, V.A.; Zhukov, M.S.; Novak, J. Resveratrol: A Multifaceted Guardian against Anxiety and Stress Disorders—An Overview of Experimental Evidence. *Nutrients* **2024**, *16*, 2856. [CrossRef] [PubMed]
45. Zhang, F.; Wang, Y.Y.; Liu, H.; Lu, Y.F.; Wu, Q.; Liu, J.; Shi, J.S. Resveratrol Produces Neurotrophic Effects on Cultured Dopaminergic Neurons through Prompting Astroglial BDNF and GDNF Release. *Evid.-Based Complement. Altern. Med.* **2012**, *2012*, 1–7. [CrossRef] [PubMed]
46. Kulkarni, S.S.; Cantó, C. The molecular targets of resveratrol. *Biochim. Biophys. Acta–Mol. Basis Dis.* **2015**, *1852*, 1114–1123. [CrossRef]
47. Hsieh, C.P.; Chang, W.T.; Chen, L.; Chen, H.H.; Chan, M.H. Differential inhibitory effects of resveratrol on excitotoxicity and synaptic plasticity: Involvement of NMDA receptor subtypes. *Nutr. Neurosci.* **2019**, *24*, 443–458. [CrossRef]
48. Ungvari, Z.; Labinskyy, N.; Mukhopadhyay, P.; Pinto, J.T.; Bagi, Z.; Ballabh, P.; Zhang, C.; Pacher, P.; Csiszar, A. Resveratrol attenuates mitochondrial oxidative stress in coronary arterial endothelial cells. *Am. J. Physiol.-Heart Circ. Physiol.* **2009**, *297*, H1876–H1881. [CrossRef]

49. Dean, R.T.; Thomas, S.M.; Garner, A. Free-radical-mediated fragmentation of monoamine oxidase in the mitochondrial membrane Roles for lipid radicals. *Biochem. J.* **1986**, *240*, 489–494. [CrossRef] [PubMed]
50. Li, W.; Guo, B.; Tao, K.; Li, F.; Liu, Z.; Yao, H.; Feng, D.; Liu, X. Inhibition of SIRT1 in hippocampal CA1 ameliorates PTSD-like behaviors in mice by protections of neuronal plasticity and serotonin homeostasis via NHLH2/MAO-A pathway. *Biochem. Biophys. Res. Commun.* **2019**, *518*, 344–350. [CrossRef]
51. Higuchi, Y.; Soga, T.; Parhar, I.S. Potential Roles of microRNAs in the Regulation of Monoamine Oxidase A in the Brain. *Front. Mol. Neurosci.* **2018**, *11*, 339. [CrossRef]
52. Li, D.; Dammer, E.B.; Sewer, M.B. Resveratrol Stimulates Cortisol Biosynthesis by Activating SIRT-Dependent Deacetylation of P450scc. *Endocrinology* **2012**, *153*, 3258–3268. [CrossRef]
53. Battaglia, S.; Fazio, C.D.; Borgomaneri, S.; Avenanti, A. Cortisol Imbalance and Fear Learning in PTSD: Therapeutic Approaches to Control Abnormal Fear Responses. *Curr. Neuropharmacol.* **2025**, *23*, 835–846. [CrossRef]
54. Bugda Gwilt, K.; González, D.P.; Olliffe, N.; Oller, H.; Hoffing, R.; Puzan, M.; El Aidy, S.; Miller, G.M. Actions of Trace Amines in the Brain-Gut-Microbiome Axis via Trace Amine-Associated Receptor-1 (TAAR1). *Cell. Mol. Neurobiol.* **2019**, *40*, 191–201. [CrossRef] [PubMed]
55. Harmeier, A.; Obermueller, S.; Meyer, C.A.; Revel, F.G.; Buchy, D.; Chaboz, S.; Dernick, G.; Wettstein, J.G.; Iglesias, A.; Rolink, A.; et al. Trace amine-associated receptor 1 activation silences GSK3β signaling of TAAR1 and D2R heteromers. *Eur. Neuropsychopharmacol.* **2015**, *25*, 2049–2061. [CrossRef]
56. Peng, L.; Zhang, J.; Feng, J.; Ge, J.; Zou, Y.; Chen, Y.; Xu, L.; Zeng, Y.; Li, J.X.; Liu, J. Activation of trace amine-associated receptor 1 ameliorates PTSD-like symptoms. *Biochem. Pharmacol.* **2024**, *228*, 116236. [CrossRef]
57. Gopalakrishna, R.; Aguilar, J.; Oh, A.; Lee, E.; Hou, L.; Lee, T.; Xu, E.; Nguyen, J.; Mack, W.J. Resveratrol and its metabolites elicit neuroprotection via high-affinity binding to the laminin receptor at low nanomolar concentrations. *FEBS Lett.* **2024**, *598*, 995–1007. [CrossRef]
58. Hernández-Hernández, O.T.; Martínez-Mota, L.; Herrera-Pérez, J.J.; Jiménez-Rubio, G. Role of Estradiol in the Expression of Genes Involved in Serotonin Neurotransmission: Implications for Female Depression. *Curr. Neuropharmacol.* **2019**, *17*, 459–471. [CrossRef]
59. Laskowski, R.A.; Jabłońska, J.; Pravda, L.; Vařeková, R.S.; Thornton, J.M. PDBsum: Structural summaries of PDB entries. *Protein Sci.* **2017**, *27*, 129–134. [CrossRef]

MDPI AG
Grosspeteranlage 5
4052 Basel
Switzerland
Tel.: +41 61 683 77 34

Biomedicines Editorial Office
E-mail: biomedicines@mdpi.com
www.mdpi.com/journal/biomedicines

www.ingramcontent.com/pod-product-compliance
Lightning Source LLC
Chambersburg PA
CBHW061615210926
51850CB00009B/2332
9783725848515